Therapeutic Management of Incontinence and Pelvic Pain

D1592383

Springer
London
Berlin
Heidelberg
New York
Barcelona
Hong Kong
Milan
Paris
Singapore
Tokyo

J. Laycock and J. Haslam (Eds)

Therapeutic Management of Incontinence and Pelvic Pain

Pelvic Organ Disorders

With 95 Figures

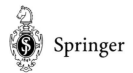 Springer

J. Laycock, OBE, PhD, FCSP
The Culgaith Clinic, Culgaith,
Penrith, Cumbria, UK

J. Haslam, MPhil, Grad Dip Phys, MCSP, SRP
Centre for Rehabilitation Science, University of Manchester,
Central Manchester Healthcare Trust, Manchester, UK

British Library Cataloguing in Publication Data
Therapeutic management of incontinence and pelvic pain:
    pelvic organ disorders
    1. Urinary incontinence 2. Fecal incontinence 3. Pelvic pain
    4. Urinary incontinence – Treatment 5. Fecal incontinence –
    Treatment 6. Pelvic pain – Treatment
    I. Laycock, J. II. Haslam, J.
    616.6′06
    ISBN 1852332247

Library of Congress Cataloging-in-Publication Data
Therapeutic management of incontinence and pelvic pain: pelvic organ disorders/J.
    Laycock and J. Haslam, eds.
        p.; cm.
    Includes bibliographical references and index.
    ISBN 1-85233-224-7 (alk. paper)
    1. Pelvis–Diseases–Treatment. 2. Pelvic pain–Treatment. 3. Urinary
    incontinence–Treatment. 4. Fecal incontinence–Treatment. I. Laycock, J. (Jo), 1941– II.
    Haslam, J. (Jeanette), 1949–
    [DNLM: 1. Pelvic Pain–therapy. 2. Urinary Incontinence–therapy. 3. Fecal
    Incontinence–therapy. 4. Pelvis–physiopathology. 5. Prolapse. WJ 146 T398 2002]
    RC946.T47 2002
    617.5′5–dc21
                                                                    2001049604

ISBN 1-85233-224-7 Springer-Verlag London Berlin Heidelberg
a member of BertelsmannSpringer Science+Business Media GmbH
www.springer.co.uk

Typeset by EXPO Holdings, Malaysia
Printed and bound at The Cromwell Press, Trowbridge, Wiltshire
28/3830-54 Printed on acid-free paper SPIN 11414841

To David and Bob
with all our love
and thanks for your support

Foreword

As medical knowledge advances we tend to compartmentalise our specialties into smaller units; but, hand in hand with this, there is a growing understanding between the different disciplines within the caring professions. Thus we are able to share our special skills to the benefit of patients. This book is an excellent example of the advantage of interdisciplinary communication and demonstrates a refreshing holistic approach to the problems of incontinence and pelvic pain. Written with physiotherapists in mind, the editors have invited contributions from many distinguished experts in their own field. These have been compiled into a comprehensive book, which will appeal to many healthcare professionals.

I have had great pleasure in reading this book. During the time that I have been involved with 'pelvic dysfunction' there have been many exciting advances. These are all included in a most readable sequence, some presented with a refreshing new twist. In particular, I would like to bring to your attention the section on 'pelvic pain'. Because of our lack of understanding it has been a problem that is too often ignored and here at last are some practical ideas for therapeutic management.

There is still much progress to be made in the field of incontinence and pelvic pain and as yet, no editors can be expected to produce a definitive work. However, I would like to recommend this book most strongly. It has a new approach to this topic, which is still a major problem for many people.

Angela Shepherd, MD, FRCOG, MCSP
Southmead Hospital, Bristol

Preface

In times past incontinence was a taboo subject, never to be mentioned in public, to family or friends. Going to a doctor with a complaint of either urinary or faecal incontinence usually resulted either in advice to use pads or being referred for surgery. Times have now changed, men and women demand ever more of the healthcare system, and research evidence has shown that incontinence can be well managed and in many cases cured by the use of appropriate therapies. Likewise, other pelvic floor disorders, leading to constipation, pelvic pain and prolapse can be treated by a variety of healthcare professionals, each bringing different skills to ameliorate their patients' symptoms. There is a growing body of research evidence and consensus on which to base clinical practice, and there are also several "alternative" therapies, which need scientific evaluation.

The purpose of this book is for many different specialists including doctors, nurses, physiotherapists and researchers within various fields of work to present their work with a critical review of the literature, and to identify and give recommendations for both practice and possible further research.

The book provides a clear, concise and practical clinical introduction to the assessment and conservative treatment of pelvic floor disorders in both men and women.

Section I looks at the prevalence, anatomy and aetiology of urinary incontinence, including the neurological patient and the elderly. Clear guidance is given regarding assessment and the investigations available. Section II contains chapters that look at specific therapeutic management strategies by exercise, biofeedback, vaginal cones and electrical stimulation. The importance of patient compliance to therapy is discussed and the use of plugs and devices considered, as are the appropriate types of surgery available. The male patient receives particular consideration as does bladder training, voiding problems and drugs acting on the lower urinary tract. Section III considers colorectal disorders, including an overview of the possible problems and the therapies available. Section IV is concerned with all aspects of pelvic pain and its therapeutic treatment and management, and section V looks at the various aspects of pelvic organ prolapse. Section VI considers osteopathy and the diversity of alternative therapies that are at present practised by clinicians with specialist knowledge and training: these include acupuncture, reflex therapy and homeopathy relating to pelvic disorders. The final section looks at the issues that need to concern health professionals including research trials, audit and infection control issues.

The book is written primarily for physiotherapists working in this specialist field. However, it is hoped that anyone working with patients suffering with incontinence or other pelvic disorders, such as nurse continence specialists, students of 'alternative' therapies, osteopaths, urologists, gynaecologists and general practitioners will increase their knowledge and all find something of use within its covers.

We are most grateful to Angela Shepherd for agreeing to write the foreword. Dr Shepherd initially qualified as a physiotherapist before medical training, becoming renowned internationally as a specialist urogynaecologist; she is the ideal person to give words of wisdom on the subject.

Jo Laycock and Jeanette Haslam

Contents

List of Contributors

Ray Addison
Consultant Nurse, The Lancaster Suite,
Mayday University Hospital, Croyden, Surrey,
UK

Phil Assassa
Consultant Urogynaecologist, Pinderfields
and Pontefract NHS Trust, Pontefract,
Yorkshire, UK
rpa2@le.ac.uk

Patricia King
Physical Therapist, Winchester, VA, USA

Lynda Barkess-Jones
Senior Infection Control Nurse Specialist,
Infection Control Department, Royal Albert
Edward Infirmary, Wigan, Lancashire, UK
Lynda.BarkessJones@wiganlhs-
tr.nwest.nhs.uk

Josephine D. Barlow
Chief Clinical Physiologist, Department of GI
Physiology, Hope Hospital, Salford, UK
jbarlow@fs1.ho.man.ac.uk

Chris Betts
Consultant Urological Surgeon, Department
of Urology, Hope Hospital, Salford, UK

Kelvin Boos
Consultant Obstetrician and Gynaecologist,
Royal Sussex County Hospital, Brighton, UK

Linda Cardozo
Professor of Urogynaecology. King's College
Hospital, London, UK
Lcardozo@compuserve.com

Pauline Chiarelli
Senior Lecturer, Discipline of Physiotherapy,
Faculty of Health , University of Newcastle,
NSW, Australia
pauline.chiarelli@newcastle.edu.au

Jane M Clayton
Research Fellow in Nursing, School of Health
and Social Care, Sheffield Hallam University,
Southbourne, Sheffield, UK
j.m.clayton@talk21.com

Mark Comerford
Director Kinetic Control, Southampton,
Hants, UK

John O.L. DeLancey
Norman F. Miller Professor of Gynecology,
Department of Obstetrics and Gynecology,
University of Michigan Medical Center,
L4100 Womens Hospital, Ann Arbor, MI, USA
DeLancey@umich.edu

Yves Dereix
Consultant Physiotherapist. Hawksworth
Physiotherapy & Sports Clinic, Ilkley,
Yorkshire, UK
HPSC@dereix.fsnet.co.uk

Nadia Ellis
Private Physiotherapy Practitioner. High
Wycombe, Buckinghamshire, UK
nadiaellis@freenet.co.uk

Carol A. Glowacki
Clinical Instructor. Department of
Gynecology, Stanford Hospitals, Stanford,
CA, USA
cglowacki@stanford.edu

Gerard Gorniak
DPT Program Director, University of St
Augustine for Health Sciences, St Augustine,
FL, USA
gcgornia@usa.edu

Elizabeth (Dee) Heaton Hartman
Specialist Physical Therapist in Womens
Health, Healthy Expectations, Naperville, IL,
USA
healthyexp@aol.com

Jeanette Haslam
Clinical Specialist Women's Health
(Physiotherapy), Centre for Rehabilitation
Science, University of Manchester, Central
Manchester Healthcare Trust, Manchester,
UK
ejhaslam@attglobal.net

Doreeen Isherwood
Chartered Physiotherapist specialising in
women's health, The Westminster
Physiotherapy Centre, London, UK
doreenisherwood@hotmail.com

Shahid Islam
Specialist Registrar in Urology, Department
of Urology, Hope Hospital, Salford, UK

Ruth C. Jones
Director RJ Manipulative Physiotherapy
Clinic and Kinetic Control, Ruth Jones
Physiotherapy, The Hampshire Tennis and
Health Club, Southampton, UK
ruth@ruthjonesphysio.co.uk

Vik Khullar
Senior Lecturer in Obstetrics and
Gynaecology, Subspecialist in
Urogynaecology, Faculty of Medicine, ICSM,
St. Mary's Hospital, London, UK
vik.khullar@ic.ac.uk

Stephanie Knight
Physiotherapist, Physiotherapy Department,
Bradford Royal Infirmary, Bradford, UK
sknightawright@pelican2.freeserve.co.uk

Davinder Kumar
Colorectal Surgeon. St Georges Hospital,
London, UK

Jo Laycock
Private Physiotherapy Practitioner. The
Culgaith Clinic, Culgaith, Penrith, UK
jolaycock@enterprise.net

Fiona Mensah
Medical statistician, Department of
Epidemiology and Public Health, University
of Leicester, Leicester, UK

Christine Norton
Nurse Consultant, St. Mark's Hospital,
Harrow, UK

Sarah I Perry
Honorary Visiting Fellow, Department of
Epidemiology and Public Health, University
of Leicester, Leicester, UK

Ursula M. Peschers
Oberaerztin. Ludwig-Maximilians-
Universitaet, Women's Hospital, Muenchen,
Germany
Ursula.Peschers@fk-i.med.uni-muenchen.de

Ruth R. Sapsford
Physiotherapist for Pelvic Floor Dysfunction,
Physiotherapy Department, Mater
Misericordiae Hospital, South Brisbane,
Queensland, Australia
rsapsford@ozemail.com.au

Beth Shelly
Director of Women's Health Services, Rock
Valley Physical Therapy, Moline, IL, USA
bethshelly@prodigy.net

Angela Shepherd
Urodynamics Unit, Southmead Hospital,
Bristol, UK
angela@pinecottage.freeserve.co.uk

Douglas G. Tincello
Senior Lecturer/Honorary Consultant in
Obstetrics and Gynaecology, University of
Leicester. Department of Obstetrics and
Gynaecology, Leicester General Hospital,
Leicester, UK

David B. Vodusek
Professor of Neurology, Medical Director,
Division of Neurology, University Medical
Centre, Ljubljana, Slovenia
david.vodusek@kclj.si

Adrian Wagg
Senior Lecturer in Geriatric Medicine,
Department of Geriatric Medicine,
University College Hospital, London, UK
a.wagg@ucl.ac.uk

Lewis Wall
Department of Obstetrics and Gynecology,
Cedars-Sinai Medical Center, Los Angeles,
CA
Lewis.Wall@cshs.org

Kathe Wallace
Physical Therapist, Physical Therapy
Resources, Seattle, WA, USA
kwallace@nwlink.com

Gail Wetzler
Physical Therapist, Physical Therapy Clinic,
Newport Beach, CA, USA

Jeni Worden
General Practitioner, Highcliffe Medical
Centre, Christchurch, Dorset, UK

List of Abbreviations

ADL	activities of daily living	MTP	myofascial trigger point
ASIS	anterior superior iliac spine	NMES	neuromuscular electrical stimulation
BPH	benign prostatic hypertrophy		
BC	bulbocavernosus	NSP	non-starch polysaccharides
CMG	Cystometrogram	OTC	over-the-counter
CVA	cerebrovascular accident	PET	Positron Emission Tomography
CISC	clean intermittent self catheterisation	PMUS	painful male urethral syndrome
		PFM	pelvic floor muscle
CRPS	complex regional pain syndrome	PFME	pelvic floor muscle exercises
CRDs	complex repetitive discharges	PMC	pontine micturition centre
CT	computed tomography	PMD	post-micturition dribble
CSS	constipation scoring system	PVR	post-void residual
DBs	decelerating bursts	RCT	randomised controlled trials
DHIC	detrusor hyperactivity with impaired contractility	ROM	range of motion
		RAIR	recto-anal inhibitory reflex
DSD	detrusor sphincter dyssynergia	RCP	Royal College of Physicians
EMG	electromyography	ROI	regions of interest
EAS	external anal sphincter	RU	residual urine
GMC	General Medical Council	ROC	ring of continence
HBM	health belief model	RCOG	Royal College of Obstetricians and Gynaecologists
HRT	hormone replacement therapy		
IAS	Internal Anal Sphincter	SMRC	sacral micturition reflex centre
ICS	International Continence Society	SI	sacroiliac
IPD	idiopathic Parkinsons' disease	SCFA	short-chain fatty acids
IVBD	intravaginal balloon device	SCI	spinal cord injury
IVU	intravenous urogram	SEMG	surface electromyography
LM	Lumbar Multifidus	TrA	transversus abdominis
LUT	lower urinary tract	TCM	Traditional Chinese Medicine
MRI	magnetic resonance imaging	TPPP	typical pelvic pain posture
MED	male erectile dysfunction	UPP	urethral pressure profilometry
MVC	maximum voluntary contraction	UTI	urinary tract infection
MS	multiple sclerosis	VCU	videocystourethrography
MSA	multiple system atrophy		

I Urinary Incontinence

1 Prevalence of Urinary Incontinence: A Review of the Literature

S.I. Perry

Epidemiological studies investigate the occurrence of disease in populations. The frequencies with which diseases occur are described in terms of their prevalence and incidence. Prevalence refers to the proportion of a defined population with a disease within a specified time period. Prevalence measures are useful for assessing the size of a problem or level of burden in a given population and potential service needs. Incidence refers to the rate at which new cases occur within a specified time. Such measures can indicate whether an epidemic is in progress (e.g. rise in new cases) or whether prevention programmes are working (e.g. fall in new cases).

Urinary incontinence is a symptom rather than a disease or condition. As such it is one of a number of symptoms which act as markers for different underlying conditions. The symptoms; urinary incontinence, urgency, frequency and nocturia can indicate conditions as wide ranging as genuine stress incontinence, detrusor instability, reflex incontinence and overflow incontinence. Prevalence studies of urinary incontinence measure the level of symptoms reported rather than the burden of a specific disease in a defined population at one point in time.

A number of reviews on the prevalence of urinary incontinence have been conducted.[1-6] They have found that prevalence estimates vary considerably in the literature. There are five main reasons for this:

1   differences in the definitions used – some authors refer to *any* leakage, some to particular *types* of leakage (e.g. stress or urge), some to leakage of a certain *severity* (e.g. monthly occurrence or large volumes) and others to leakage which is perceived to be a social or hygienic *problem*

2   differences in the prevalence measure used – some studies refer to *point* prevalence (i.e. current), others to *period* prevalence (i.e. last 12 months), others to *historical* prevalence (i.e. life history) and others do not reference the time period at all

3   differences in study design – some studies use postal questionnaires and others home interviews and studies may use self-reported, clinical and/or proxy information

4   differences in sampling procedures – surveys often use different sampling frames, have different exclusion criteria and do not always account for non-response bias;

5   the scarcity of well-validated measures (rarely tested for validity and reliability).

It is difficult, therefore, to make comparisons across studies. Despite this, patterns do emerge: the prevalence of urinary incontinence is more common in women than in men,[7] is more common in institutional settings than among people living independently at home,[4] and tends to be more severe in old age than in middle age.[8-10] The evidence suggests that approximately 14% of women and 5% of men report urinary incontinence on a regular basis (monthly or more often).[1-4] In nursing homes, however, this figure may be 30–60% of the population,[4,11-14] and almost half of those with urinary incontinence will also experience faecal incontinence.[11]

The prevalence of urinary incontinence in men increases with age. About 2% of middle-aged men report regular incontinence, compared to 9% of elderly men aged 75 years or over.[7] In women, however, it appears to peak at 45–55 years of age, then slumps between ages 55–70 and increases again in the elderly.[7,8,10] Peaks followed by declines suggest that some underlying disorders may recover naturally over time, or that adaptation occurs to some extent. These age–sex differences suggest that although men and women of different ages report urinary incontinence, they may have different underlying conditions. Thus, symptoms of stress incontinence are more common in younger than in older women, whereas urge and mixed incontinence predominate in older women.[8,9,10,15] Less is known about the prevalence of types of incontinence in men, but urge incontinence and post-micturition dribble appear to predominate and stress incontinence is relatively rare.[3,16,17]

Assessing the prevalence of need for treatment in the community is even more problematic. Distinctions have been made between definitions of need which are symptom-based, those which focus on problematic symptoms (i.e. symptoms which are perceived to be bothersome or socially disabling) and those based on perceived need for help (i.e. potential service demand) and current patterns of service utilisation. Prevalence estimates vary tremendously (see Table 1.1). Thus 40% of the population may report any incontinence, but only 2% may find their symptoms socially disabling. The evidence suggests that it is not practical to treat minor incontinence that has little impact on an individual's quality of life.[18] It may be more appropriate to encourage people with more severe symptoms that have an impact on quality of life to seek help.

Currently, only about a quarter of women with urinary incontinence seek professional help for their symptoms (see Table 1.2). Symptoms are often perceived to be trivial, or a normal part of the ageing process. People often develop their own ways of managing symptoms, they are not aware that symptoms are treatable and that services are available and they experience difficulties talking to professionals about these sorts of problems.

Most of the research in this area has concentrated on women.[15,23,26,29–33] Less is known about the prevalence of incontinence and levels of need among men.

Table 1.1. Prevalence of urinary incontinence and need in women

Definition	Prevalence estimates in women (%)
Any urinary incontinence[3]	Range: 12–53 Median: 40.5
Regular urinary incontinence: monthly or more often[3]	Range: 4.5–37 Median 14.0
Bothersome urinary incontinence[8,10,19–21]	Range: 5–25 Median: 8.5
Socially disabling urinary incontinence[10,20–24]	Range: 0.1–5 Median: 2.0

Table 1.2. The percentage of women with urinary incontinence seeking help from a health professional

Study	Age (years)	% who seek help[a]
Yarnell et al. (1981)[10]	18+	9
Lara and Nancy (1994)[25]	18+	26
Holst and Wilson (1988)[15]	18+	35
Harrison et al. (1994)[20]	20+	13
Seim et al. (1995)[26]	20+	20
Samuelsson et al. (1997)[19]	20–59	9
Brocklehurst (1993)[22]	30+	47
Rekers et al. (1992)[23]	35–79	28
Roberts (1998)[27]	50+	13
Lagro-Janssen et al. (1990)[21]	50–65	32
Bogren (1997)[28]	65	25

[a] Range: 9–47%; median 25%.

Despite research in this field, most prevalence estimates of urinary incontinence are crude and do not differentiate between symptoms; stress incontinence, urge incontinence, mixed incontinence, functional incontinence, unconscious incontinence, nocturnal enuresis, continuous dribbling, post-micturition dribble and severity; frequency or volume of leakage and level of disability experienced. This is unfortunate, because it is likely that these symptoms have different aetiologies, natural histories, impact on quality of life and potential service needs. For example, a number of studies have found that urge incontinence is perceived to be more problematic than stress incontinence.[10,34–37]

Prevalence studies have tended to concentrate on the symptoms of stress and urge incontinence, but the exploration of symptom groups (e.g. urge incontinence, urgency and frequency) may be more beneficial in terms of screening for underlying conditions (e.g. detrusor instability). Little is known about the prevalence of other incontinence symptoms (e.g. nocturnal enuresis, unconscious incontinence, continuous dribbling, post-micturition dribble and functional incontinence).

A self-reported questionnaire properly validated on a community population is required to enable more confident predictions of need for services in the community. Similarly, definitions of symptoms need to be standardised to enable cross-study and cross-cultural comparisons. Longitudinal studies on the natural history of urinary incontinence symptoms are also necessary in order to assess which symptoms are self-limiting and require a more watchful waiting approach and those which are enduring and necessitate conservative treatments or more invasive interventions.

To conclude, urinary incontinence is a common symptom in the community. However, the prevalence of urinary incontinence which requires treatment is probably much lower. Further studies should concentrate on determining the latter level of need in the community and target specific groups where need is likely to be the greatest, such as elderly people and those living in institutional settings.

References

1. Thom D (1998) Variations in estimates of urinary incontinence prevalence in the community: effects of differences in definition, population characteristics and study type. J Am Geriatr Soc 46: 473–80.
2. Hampel C, Wienhold D, Benken N, Eggersman C, Thuroff JW (1997) Prevalence and natural history of female incontinence. Eur Urol 32 (Suppl 2): 3–12.
3. Hampel C, Wienhold D, Benken N, Eggersman C, Thuroff JW (1997) Definition of overactive bladder and epidemiology of urinary incontinence. Urology 50 (Suppl 6A): 4–14.
4. Royal College of Physicians (1995) Incontinence: Causes, management and provision of services. Royal College of Physicians, London.
5. Sandvik H (1995) Female urinary incontinence. In: Studies of Epidemiology And Management In General Practice. University of Bergen, Norway.
6. Mohide EA (1986) The prevalence and scope of urinary incontinence. Clin Geriatr Med 2: 639–55.
7. Thomas TM, Plymat KR, Blannin J, Meade TW (1980) Prevalence of urinary incontinence. BMJ 281: 1243–5.
8. Sandvik H, Hunskaar S, Seim A et al. (1995) Validation of a severity index in female urinary incontinence and its implementation in an epidemiological survey. J Epidemiol Community Health 47: 497–9.
9. Sommer P, Bauer T (1990) Nielson et al. Voiding patterns and prevalence of incontinence in women. A questionnaire survey. Br J Urol 66: 12–15.
10. Yarnell JWG, Voyle GJ, Richards CJ, Stephenson TP (1981) The prevalence and severity of urinary incontinence in women. J Epidemiol Community Health 35: 71–4.
11. Peet S, Castledon CM, McGrother CW (1995) Prevalence of urinary and faecal incontinence in hospitals and residential and nursing homes for older people. BMJ 311: 1063–4.
12. Stott DJ, Dutton M, Williams BO, Macdonald J (1990) Functional capacity and mental status of elderly people in long-term care in west Glasgow. Health Bull 48: 17–24.
13. Capewell AE, Primrose WR, Macintyre C (1986) Nursing dependency in registered nursing homes and long-term care geriatric wards in Edinburgh. BMJ 292: 1719–21.
14. Clarke M, Hughes AO, Dodd KJ et al. (1979) The elderly in residential care: patterns of disability. Health Trends 11: 17–20.
15. Holst K, Wilson PD (1998) The prevalence of female urinary incontinence and reasons for not seeking treatment. NZ Med J 101: 756–8.
16. Schulman C, Claes H, Matthijs J (1997) Urinary ncontinence in Belgium: a population based epidemiological survey. Eur Urol 32: 315–20.
17. Jolleys JV, Donovan JL, Nanchahal K, Peters TJ, Abrams P (1994) Urinary symptoms in the community how bothersome are they? Br J Urol 74: 551–5.
18. Abrams P (1997) Lower urinary tract symptoms in women: who to investigate and how. Br J Urol 80 (Suppl)(1): 43–8.
19. Samuelsson E, Victor A, Tibblin GA (1997) A population study of urinary incontinence and nocturia among women aged 20-59 years. Acta Obstet Gynecol Scand 76: 74–80.
20. Harrison GL, Memel DS (1994) Urinary incontinence in women: its prevalence and its management in a health promotion clinic. Br J Gen Pr 44: 149–52.
21. Lagro-Janssen TLM, Smits AJA, Weel C Van (1990) Women with urinary incontinence: self-perceived worries and general practitioners' knowledge of the problem. Br J Gen Pr 40: 331–4.
22. Brocklehurst JC (1993) Urinary incontinence in the community–analysis of a MORI poll. BMJ 306: 832–4.
23. Rekers H, Drogendijk AC, Valkenburg H, Riphagen F (1992) Urinary incontinence in women from 35 to 79 years of age: prevalence and consequences. J Obstet Gynecol Reprod Biol 43: 229–34.
24. Lam GW, Foldspang A, Elving LB, Mommsen S (1992) Social context, social abstention and problem recognition correlated with adult female urinary incontinence. Dan Med Bull 39: 565–70.
25. Lara C, Nancy J (1994) Ethnic differences between Maori, Pacific Island and European New Zealand women in prevalence and attitudes to urinary incontinence. NZ Med J 107: 374–6.
26. Seim A, Sandvik H, Hermstad R, Hunskaar S (1995) Female urinary incontinence–consultation behaviour and patient experiences: an epidemiological survey in a Norwegian community. Fam Pr 12: 18–21.
27. Roberts RO, Jacobsen SJ, Rhodes T et al. (1998) Urinary incontinence in a community-based cohort: prevalence and healthcare seeking. J Am Geriatr Soc 46: 467–72.
28. Bogren MA, Hvarfwen E, Fridlund B (1997) Urinary incontinence among a 65 year old Swedish population: medical history and psychosocial consequences. Vard I Norden 17: 14–17.
29. Reymert J, Hunskarr S (1994) Why do only a minority of perimenopausal women with urinary incontinence consult a doctor? Scand J Prim Health Care 12: 180–3.
30. Burgio KL, Ives DG, Locher JL, Arena VC, Kuller LH (1994) Treatment seeking for urinary incontinence in older adults. J Am Geriatr Soc 42: 208–12.
31. Goldstein M, Hawthorne ME, Engeberg S, McDowell BJ, Burgio KL (1992) Urinary incontinence. Why people do not seek help. J Gerontol Nurs 18: 15–20.
32. Jolleys JV (1988) Reported prevalence of urinary incontinence in women in a general practice. BMJ 296: 1300–2.
33. McGrother C, Castleden CM, Duffin H, Clarke M (1987) A profile of disordered micturition in the elderly at home. Age Ageing 16: 105–11.
34. Lagro-Janssen ALM, Debruyne FMJ, Weel C Van (1992) Psychosocial aspects of female urinary incontinence in general practice. Br J Urol 70: 499–502.
35. Hunskar S, Vinsnes RN (1991) The quality of life in women with urinary incontinence as measured by the sickness impact profile. J Am Geriatr Soc 39: 378–82.
36. Wyman JF, Harkins SW, Taylor JR, Fantl A (1987) Psychosocial impact of urinary incontinence in women. Obstet Gynecol 70: 378.
37. Frazer MI, Sutherst JR, Holland EFN (1987) Visual analogue scores and urinary incontinence. BMJ 295: 582.

2 Anatomy

U.M. Peschers and J.O.L. DeLancey

The pelvic floor is a complex structure, having not only to allow the passage of urine or stool at appropriate times but also to preserve continence daily. It is necessary for sexual activity, conception and fertility and is also the birth passage at the time of vaginal delivery.

The following descriptions offer a brief overview of some clinically relevant aspects of pelvic floor structure that help us to understand the normal and abnormal behaviour of this system.

2.1 Female Pelvic Anatomy

2.1.1 Pelvic Viscera

The lower urinary tract can be divided into the bladder and urethra. At the junction of these two continuous yet discrete structures lies the vesical neck. The bladder consists of the detrusor muscle, which is covered by a serosa layer at its dome and lined by a submucosa and transitional epithelium. Two prominent bands on the dorsal aspect of the bladder that are derived from the outer longitudinal layer pass beside the urethra to form a loop on its anterior aspect, called the detrusor loop.[1] On the anterior aspect of this loop, some detrusor fibres leave the region of the vesical neck and attach to the pubic bones and pelvic walls; these are called the pubovesical muscles.

The trigone is a structure at the bladder neck whose visible apices are formed by the ureteric orifices and the internal urinary meatus. The urethra is a complex tubular viscus with its upper third clearly separate from the vagina and the lower two-thirds intimately connected to the lower anterior vaginal wall. Embedded within its substance are a number of elements that are important

Table 2.1. Topography of urethral and paraurethral structures

Approximate location	Region of the urethra	Paraurethral structures
0–20	Intramural urethra	Urethral lumen traverses the bladder wall
20–60	Midurethra	Sphincter urethrae muscle Pubovesical muscle Vaginolevator attachment
60–80	Perineal membrane	Compressor urethrae muscle Urethrovaginal sphincter muscle
80–100	Distal urethra	Bulbocavernosus muscle

to lower urinary tract dysfunction,[2] summarised in Table 2.1.

2.1.2 Striated Urogenital Sphincter

The outer layer of the urethra is formed by the muscle of the striated urogenital sphincter (Fig. 2.1). In its upper two-thirds, the sphincter fibres lie in a primarily circular orientation; distally, they leave the confines of the urethra and either encircle the vaginal wall as the urethrovaginal sphincter, or extend along the inferior pubic ramus above the perineal membrane (urogenital diaphragm) as the compressor urethrae.

The sphincter is composed largely of slow-twitch muscle fibres,[3] which are well suited to maintaining the constant tone as well as allowing voluntary increases in urethral constriction when increased closure pressure is needed. In the distal urethra, this striated muscle compresses the urethra from above, and proximally, it constricts the lumen. It has been suggested that it is responsible for approximately one-third of resting urethral closure pressure.[4]

a

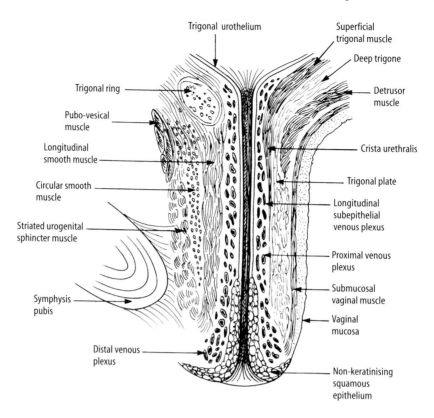

b

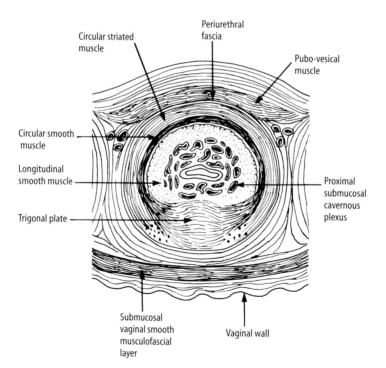

Figure 2.1 Sagittal section (**a**) and axial section (**b**) of a female urethra. [Strohbehn K, DeLancey JOL. The Anatomy of Stress Incontinence. Operative Techniques in Gynecologic Surgery 1997; 2: 5–16.]

2.1.3 Urethral Smooth Muscle

The smooth muscle of the urethra is contiguous with that of the trigone and detrusor. The fibres of the inner layer are directed longitudinally and are surrounded by a thinner circular layer. The smooth muscles lie inside the striated urogenital sphincter muscle, and are present throughout the upper four-fifths of the urethra. The configuration of the circular muscle suggests a role in constricting the lumen, and the longitudinal muscle may help shorten and funnel the urethra during voiding although its exact function is not known.

2.1.4 Submucosal Vasculature

Lying within the urethra is a well-developed vascular plexus which is more prominent than expected for the ordinary demands of so small an organ.[5] The flow of blood into the large venules can be controlled, assisting in forming a watertight closure of the mucosal surfaces.

2.1.5 Mucosa

The mucosal lining of the urethra is continuous with the transitional epithelium of the bladder and with the squamous epithelium of the vestibule below. The mucosa is hormonally sensitive and undergoes significant change depending on its state of stimulation.

2.1.6 Vesical Neck

The vesical neck is the area at the base of the bladder, where the urethral lumen passes through the thickened musculature of the bladder base. Therefore, it is sometimes considered as part of the bladder musculature, but also contains the urethral lumen studied during urethral pressure profilometry. It is a region where the detrusor musculature, including the detrusor loop, surrounds the trigonal ring and the urethral meatus. The vesical neck has come to be considered separately from the bladder and urethra because of its unique functional characteristics.

2.2 Vagina and Uterus

The distal third of the vagina is fused with the urethra anteriorly, to the perineal body posteriorly and the perineal membrane and levator ani muscles laterally, it is lined with stratefied non-keratininzing squamous epithelium. The support of the vagina varies at different levels. In the upper third of the vagina, it is suspended on its lateral wall to the pelvic sidewall by the paracolpium, an ill-defined body of connective tissue that also contains smooth muscle, elastic fibres, nerves and vessels. The cervix is directly connected to the vaginal wall. Posterior to the cervix, the vaginal wall is covered on its dorsal wall with the perineum of the cul-de-sac. As the vagina is directed posteriorly in a normal woman, the upper third of the vagina and the cul-de-sac are closed like a flap-valve by intraabdominal pressure by being compressed against the rectum and levator plate. The middle of the vagina is connected laterally to the pelvic walls by the pubocervical and rectovaginal fascias.

2.2.1 Rectum and Anal Sphincters

The rectum is located posteriorly in the pelvis and is composed of a mucosa, a submucosa, a circular and a longitudinal layer of smooth muscle and a serosa. The anterior wall of the rectum is located directly adjacent to the posterior vaginal wall.

The anal sphincters are a complex system for faecal continence, with the anal canal having a pressure level to secure a waterproof closure. The innermost layer is the mucocutaneous lining of the anal sphincter complex. The mucosa is surrounded by the internal anal sphincter muscle, a thickened prolongation of the circular smooth muscle layer of the bowel. The function of the internal anal sphincter has been discussed for decades, just as the detailed anatomy of the anal canal was a subject of debate. Currently the internal sphincter is thought to be responsible for 75% of resting pressure of the anal sphincter system.[6,7] The smooth muscle of the internal sphincter is well suited to its job of generating a constant tension over long periods of time. Between the internal and the external anal sphincter are the fused longitudinal fibres of the intestinal wall and levator ani muscles that continue into the superficial part of the external anal sphincter muscle. The external anal sphincter composition has been discussed for a long time, and several anatomic models have been proposed.[8–10] In our opinion, supported by studies of sectional anatomic specimens, the external sphincter is mainly composed of two parts: a deep part and a superficial part, separated by a connective tissue layer. The superficial part forms a round structure at the edge and below the caudal end of the internal sphincter. Both parts send connective tissue fibres to the tip of the coccyx. In the female the external anal sphincter is shorter anteriorly than posteriorly.[11]

The third part of the anal continence mechanism is the puborectalis muscle that forms a sling around the rectum. The puborectalis muscle and the deep part of the external sphincter muscle form the characteristic double bump in a sagittal image (Fig. 2.2).

The internal anal sphincter is responsible for the maintenance of resting pressure, but both the external anal sphincter and the puborectalis muscle actively contract and thereby increase anal pressure in situations of faecal urgency. It is well accepted that childbirth leads to neurogenic damage to the innervation of the external anal sphincter[12,13] and to disruption of the internal and external sphincters.[14] However, little is known about the impact of vaginal delivery on internal sphincter innervation and function. Resting anal sphincter tonus is associated with internal sphincter function and is known to be lower in women after vaginal birth complicated by a third-degree perineal tear compared to controls without rupture of the sphincters.[15]

2.3 Pelvic Floor Muscles

2.3.1 Levator Ani Muscle

The levator ani muscle provides the main muscular support for the pelvic organs and is of crucial importance for pelvic floor re-education. It can be divided into two parts: the pubovisceral muscle and the ileococcygeal muscle.[16] On its inferior and supe- rior surfaces the levator ani muscle is covered by connective tissue, which forms respectively the infe- rior and superior fascia of the levator ani fascia. The layer formed by the muscle and its fascial layers (superior and inferior) is referred to as the "pelvic diaphragm".

The pubovisceral muscle is a thick U-shaped muscle, which arises from the pubic bones on either side of the midline. It passes behind the rectum forming a sling-like arrangement and also attaches to the walls of the vagina, perineal body and anal sphincter complex (Fig. 2.2).

Laterally, the iliococcygeus arises from a fibrous band on the pelvic wall (arcus tendineus levator ani) and forms a relatively horizontal sheet that spans the opening within the pelvis and provides a shelf on which the organs may rest (Fig. 2.3).

The pubovisceral muscle has several components. Clinicians have often referred to the entire pubovis- ceral muscle by the term pubococcygeus. This term is somewhat misleading because it signifies a muscle that would connect two relatively immovable struc- tures (pubis and coccyx). Functionally it therefore cannot contribute to any lifting of the pelvic organs, but might contribute to pelvic support by isotonic contraction. The puborectalis portion of the pubo- visceral muscle passes beside the vagina, with some attachment to the lateral vaginal walls. The muscle then continues dorsally where some fibres insert into the rectum between the internal and external sphincter while others pass behind the anorectal junction. The vagina attaches to the medial portion of the pubovisceral muscle and the fibres between

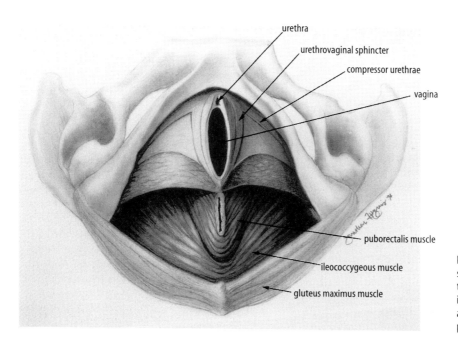

urethra
urethrovaginal sphincter
compressor urethrae
vagina
puborectalis muscle
ileococcygeous muscle
gluteus maximus muscle

Figure 2.2 Levator ani muscles seen from below. That portion of the pubovisceral muscle which inserts into the rectum and forms a "U" behind it is called the puborectalis.

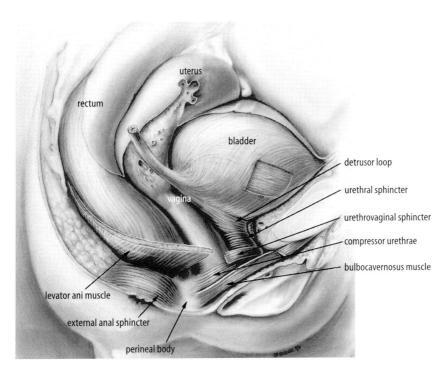

Figure 2.3 Lateral view of the pelvic organs and their relation to the pelvic floor.

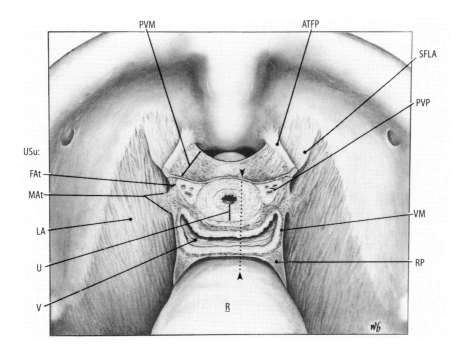

Figure 2.4 Drawing of the urethra (U), vagina (V) and levator ani muscles (LA) just below the vesical neck. The pubovesical muscles (PVM) can be seen anterior to the urethra and the periurethral vascular plexus (PVP) and attach to the arcus tendineus fasciae pelvis (ATFP). Urethral supports (USu) run underneath (dorsal to) the urethra and vessels. Some of its fibres (MAt) attach to the muscle of the levator ani (LA), while others (FAt) are derived from the vaginal wall and vaginal surface of the urethra (U) and attach to the superior fascia of the levator ani (SFLA). [DeLancey JOL. Pubovesical Ligament: A separate structure from urethral supports. Neurology and Urodynamics 1989; 8: 53–61.]

the vagina and pubic bone are referred to as the pubovaginalis muscle. These muscle fibres are responsible for elevating the urethra during pelvic floor muscle (PFM) contraction; this occurs because the muscle is connected to the fascia supporting the urethra, rather than because the muscle goes to the urethra itself (Fig. 2.4).

The iliococcygeal muscle is a sheet of muscle that spans the pelvis from the arcus tendineus levator ani on one side to the other, passing dorsal to the anorectum and anal sphincter. The pubococcygeus is the most cephalic portion of the levator and passes from the pubic bones to insert on the inner surface of the coccyx and comprises only a small portion of the overall levator complex. Some fibres also pass to the anal canal and behind the rectum. The term pubococcygeus is often used by gynaecologists to refer to the entire pubovisceral muscle and pubococcygeus muscle.

The levator ani muscles are composed of striated muscle. It is known that two-thirds of the fibres are type I (slow-twitch) muscle fibres[3] responsible for the resting tonus of the levator ani muscle. One-third of the fibres are type II (fast-twitch) fibres which are thought to act when a quick, powerful contraction is needed.

2.3.2 Perineal Membrane

The perineal membrane (urogenital diaphragm) is a relatively thin layer underneath the pelvic diaphragm. Triangular, with the tip directed anteriorly, it lies at the level of the hymenal ring, and attaches the urethra, vagina and perineal body to the ischiopubic rami. It mainly consists of a connective tissue membrane, with muscle lying immediately above.[17] The striated muscle fibres associated with the perineal membrane (compressor urethrae and urethrovaginal sphincter) act to constrict the distal urethra and have been discussed with that organ.

2.3.3 Bulbocavernous Muscles

The bulbocavernous muscles, the most distal muscular layer of the pelvic floor, merely have sexual function and do not provide pelvic floor support.

2.4 Anatomic Basis of Urinary Continence

The two factors important to urinary continence during increases in abdominal pressure are urethral constriction by the muscles of the urethral wall and urethral stabilisation by the PFM during stressful events. The urinary continence mechanism is complex, still not completely understood and based on the functional co-ordination of several parts of the pelvic floor.

The primary basis for continence is the urethra whose wall contains small muscles (striated urogenital sphincter and urethral smooth muscles) that are able to generate intraurethral pressure. The support of the urethra is determined by the surrounding suspending structures and by the state of relaxation or contraction of the levator ani muscle. Voluntary contraction of the levator ani muscle causes bladder neck elevation and voluntary relaxation causes it to be lowered – this is easily visualised on perineal ultrasound. The urethra and the levator ani muscle are connected to each other by the arcus tendineus levator ani.

The role of the urethral supportive tissue's connection to the levator ani is important for the following reasons:

- The resting position of the proximal urethra is high within the pelvis, some 3 cm above the inferior aspect of the pubic bones.[18] Maintenance of this position would best be explained by the constant muscular activity of the levator ani.[19]

- In addition, the upper two-thirds of the urethra is mobile[20-22] and under voluntary control.

- At the onset of micturition, relaxation of the levator ani muscles allows the urethra to descend, which obliterates the posterior urethrovesical angle. Resumption of the normal tonic contraction of the muscle at the end of micturition returns the vesical neck to its normal position. Some of the control of the proximal vesical neck's position and mobility, therefore, must come from activity of the levator ani muscles and connections of the periurethral tissues to the fibrous elements of the pelvic wall (ligaments and fasciae).

From these observations, it seems that the support of the urethra involves both voluntary muscle and inert elements.[23,24] Observations that patients with stress incontinence have neurological damage to the pelvic floor support the importance of the levator ani to urinary continence.[25] Functionally it has been shown that when the PFM are paralysed there is a decrease in continence.[26] There does not appear to be a one-to-one relationship between denervation and stress incontinence, and so the relative role of the muscular and fascial tissues in urethral support remains incompletely defined. The anterior vaginal wall and urethra arise from the urogenital sinus, and are intimately connected. The support of the urethra depends not on

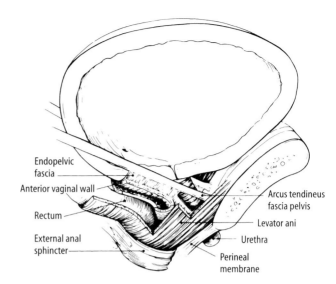

Endopelvic fascia

Anterior vaginal wall

Rectum

External anal sphincter

Arcus tendineus fascia pelvis

Levator ani

Urethra

Perineal membrane

Figure 2.5 Lateral view of the pelvic floor structures related to urethral support seen from the side in the standing position, cut just lateral to the midline. [DeLancey JOL. Structural support of the urethra as it relates to stress urinary incontinence: the hammock hypothesis. Am J Obstet Gynecol 1994; 170: 1713–23.]

attachments of the urethra itself to adjacent structures, but on the connection of the vagina and periurethral tissues to the muscles and fascia of the pelvic wall. On either side of the pelvis, the arcus tendineus fascia pelvis is a band of connective tissue attached at one end to the lower one-sixth of the pubic bone, 1 cm from the midline, and at the other end to the ischial spine. In its anterior portion this band lies on the inner surface of the levator ani muscle which arises some 3 cm above the arcus tendineus fasciae pelvis. Posteriorly, the levator ani arises from a second arcus, the arcus tendineus fasciae levatoris ani, which fuses with the arcus tendineus fasciae pelvis near the spine.

It is the urethral supportive structures rather than urethral position that is crucial for the maintenance of urinary continence. Simulated increases in abdominal pressure in anatomic specimens reveal that the urethra lies in a position where it can be compressed against the supporting hammock consisting of the connective tissue layer of the anterior vaginal wall and the lateral suspension structures connecting it to the levator ani muscle (Fig. 2.5).[24] In this model, it is the stability of this supporting layer rather than the height of the urethra that determines stress continence. In an individual with a firm supportive layer the urethra is compressed between abdominal pressure and pelvic fascia in much the same way that you can stop the flow of water through a garden hose by stepping on it and compressing it against an underlying concrete path. If, however, the layer under the urethra becomes unstable, the opposing force that causes closure is lost and the occlusive action is diminished. This is analogous to trying to stop the flow of water through a garden hose resting on soft soil.

2.5 Pelvic Organ Support

Pelvic floor function is understandable only through knowledge of the fascial connection between muscles and viscera. The ligaments and fascia of the pelvic floor are composed primarily of loose connective tissue, smooth muscle, elastic fibres, blood vessels and nerves. They resemble a mesentery more than a skeletal ligament. This is an important concept to keep in mind when the function of these structures is discussed.

The top layer of the pelvic floor is provided by the endopelvic fascia that attaches the pelvic organs to the pelvic walls thereby suspending the pelvic organs,[27–29] it will be referred to as the viscerofascial layer. The endopelvic fascia is a continuous mass of tissue with different thickened parts attaching the uterus and the vagina to the pelvic sidewall.

Withstanding constant forces is not the main function of ligaments. Connective tissue is not suited to withstanding gravitational forces over a long period of time. If the ligaments and fasciae within the pelvis were subjected to the continuous stress imposed on the pelvic floor by the great weight of abdominal pressure, they would stretch. It is therefore illogical to believe that pelvic floor ligaments are the primary factors that prevent the uterus and the vagina from prolapsing. The fact that these ligaments do not limit the downward movement of the uterus in normal healthy women is attested to by the observation that the cervix may be drawn down to the level of the hymen with little difficulty.[30] As in other parts of the body, it is the muscular tonus that holds the organs in place. The opening within the levator ani muscle through which the urethra and vagina pass (and through which prolapse occurs) is called the urogenital hiatus of the levator ani. The rectum also passes through this opening, but because the levator ani muscles attach directly to the anus and external anal sphincter it is not included in the name of the hiatus. The hiatus is therefore bounded ventrally (anteriorly) by the pubic bones, laterally by the levator ani muscles and dorsally (posteriorly) by the perineal body and external anal sphincter. The normal tonic activity of the levator ani muscle keeps the urogenital hiatus closed. On contraction, the levator ani squeeze the vagina, urethra and rectum closed by compressing them against the pubic bone, and lift the floor and organs in a cephalic direction.

The levator ani muscles constantly contract[19] and close the lumen of the vagina. This constant action eliminates any opening within the pelvic floor through which prolapse could occur, and forms a relatively horizontal shelf on which the pelvic organs are supported.[31,32] In the healthy female the vagina is directed posteriorly; the upper part of the vagina is therefore located above and on the levator ani muscle plate. Girls born with neurogenic deficits of pelvic floor innervation such as spina bifida are known to develop pelvic organ prolapse at a young age.[33]

This support of the uterus has been likened to a ship in its berth floating on the water attached by ropes on either side to a dock.[34] The ship is analogous to the uterus, the ropes to the ligaments, and the water to the supportive layer formed by the pelvic floor muscles. The ropes function to hold the ship (uterus) in the centre of its berth as it rests on the water (PFM). If, however, the water level were to fall far enough that the ropes would be required to hold the ship without the support of the water, the ropes would all break. The analogous situation in the pelvic floor involves the PFM supporting the uterus and vagina, which are stabilised in position by the ligaments and fascias. Once the PFM become damaged and no longer support the organs, the connective tissue fails because of overload.

2.6 Male Pelvic Anatomy

Urinary and faecal incontinence are frequent in females, but less common in males. Pelvic organ prolapse is virtually unknown in men. This might be explained by two basic anatomic differences. Men do not have the genital hiatus of the vagina through which pelvic organ prolapse occurs, and the male urethra is significantly longer and thereby better

able to provide continence. Male stress urinary incontinence mainly occurs when the urethral sphincter is damaged during prostatic surgery.

The male urethra extends from the bladder neck to the external meatus at the end of the penis and is divided into three portions: the prostatic, the membranous and the spongy. The prostatic portion is widest and passes through the prostate gland; the membranous part is the shortest and narrowest extending between the apex of the prostate and the bulb of the corpus spongiosum; the spongy portion is the longest section and is contained in the corpus spongiosum. The male urethra is composed of a continuous mucous membrane lined with transitional epithelium. The submucous tissue consists of a vascular erectile layer surrounded by a layer of circular smooth muscle separating the mucous membrane and submucous tissue from the tissue of the corpus spongiosum.

In terms of urinary incontinence the prostate gland plays an important role. Its enlargement (benign prostatic hypertrophy) causes voiding difficulties (obstructed voiding with poor flow, dribbling and overflow incontinence). Radical surgical excision of the prostate for prostate cancer can lead to stress urinary incontinence. The prostate gland is a firm, partly glandular, partly muscular body located immediately below the vesical neck and around the commencement of the urethra. In shape and size it resembles a chestnut. It is located in the pelvic cavity behind the lower part of the pubic symphysis and rests on the rectum. It is easily palpated through the rectum, especially when enlarged. The prostate is immediately enveloped by a thin but firm fibrous capsule. It is separated from the rectovesical fascia by a venous plexus. The prostate gland is perforated by the urethra and the ejaculatory ducts that open into the prostatic part of the urethra.

The two Cowper's glands are located behind the fore part of the membranous portion of the urethra: they are small, rounded bodies the size of a pea. The excretory duct of each gland opens into a minute orifice on the floor of the bulbous part of the urethra.

The penis consists of a root, body and extremity (the glans penis). The root is connected to the os pubis and ischium by two strong fibrous processes, the crura. The suspensory ligament is a strong fibrous band that passes from the front of the pubic symphysis to the upper surface of the root of the penis. The penis is composed of a mass of erectile tissue enclosed in three cylindrical compartments: the two corpora cavernosa side by side along the upper side of the organ, and the corpus spongiosum surrounding the urethra.

2.7 Neurogenic Basis of Continence and Micturition

Continence and micturition are naturally contrary conditions. Because of the bladder's dual function of storage and elimination of urine, many of the neural circuits controlling micturition demonstrate phasic or switch-like patterns of activity, unlike other viscera.[35] Their correct functioning reflects the summary of inhibitory and facilitative neural mechanisms which comprise highly complex central and peripheral, afferent (sensory) and efferent (motor) autonomic pathways that are integrated and coordinated by cephalic control centres, spinal cord nuclei and infra-spinal relay stations in peripheral ganglia.[36]

The following summary in mainly based on the work of Mahony et al., whose papers are highly recommended for further reading.[37–39]

The sacral micturition reflex centre is the important "steering centre" for the regulation of micturition and continence. If it is underfacilitated, voiding can be difficult to initiate or maintain. If it works properly, the patient can maintain continence and is able to void. If the sacral micturition reflex centre is overactive, this will result in detrusor instability and urgency. The ability to initiate micturition voluntarily, to empty the bladder completely and to maintain continence in situations when the pelvic floor is stressed is critically dependent on correct function of storage and voiding reflexes. The storage reflexes are responsible for the maintenance of continence, and the voiding reflexes initiate and support complete bladder emptying.

The neural reflex system is based on receptors that are located in the detrusor muscle, in the trigone, in the bladder neck, in the urethra and in the levator ani muscles. These receptors send afferent signals to the sacral micturition reflex centre or to the pontine micturition reflex centre (PMC) which is located in the brain stem. Cortical effects on these two centres are mainly facilitating.

Mahony and co-authors described 12 main reflexes, 4 of which are storage reflexes, 7 are micturition reflexes and 1 stops voiding and reinstalls the storage phase.

2.7.1 Storage Reflexes

Increasing mural tension of the bladder wall activates the sympathetic detrusor-inhibiting reflex and also the sympathetic sphincter constrictor reflex, leading to an increase in urethral pressure. The perineo-detrusor inhibiting reflex is activated by an increase of tension in the PFM, so a contraction of the levator ani muscles can induce an inhibition of the detrusor. Tension of the trigone or entrance of urine into the proximal urethra can activate the urethrosphincteric guarding reflex, resulting in an increase in tone of the external urethral sphincter.

2.7.2 Initation of Micturition and Continued Micturition

The perineobulbar detrusor facilitative reflex is activated by voluntary increase of intra-abdominal pressure through contraction of the diaphragm and the rectus abdominis muscles, and simultaneous relaxation of the pelvic floor muscles. This facilitates the sacral micturition reflex centre. Mural tension with increasing bladder volume activates the detruso-detrusor facilitative reflex, which has a strong facilitating impact on the pontine micturition reflex centre, which in turn facilitates the sacral micturition reflex centre.

2.7.3 Maintenance of Detrusor Pressure During Micturition

To secure complete bladder emptying, detrusor pressure has to be strong throughout micturition and the urethral sphincters have to remain relaxed. The latter is maintained by the detruso-urethral inhibitory reflex, which results in inhibitory impulses to the bladder neck and the proximal urethra. This is supported by the detruso-sphincteric inhibitory reflex inhibiting the striated sphincter. Both reflexes are activated by mural tension of the bladder wall. Receptors located in the urethra also contribute to complete bladder emptying. The urethro-detrusor facilitative reflex increases the excitability of the micturition reflexes. The urethro-sphincteric inhibition reflex is activated by urine passage through the urethra and results in further relaxation of the urethral sphincters.

2.7.4 Cessation of Micturition

When the voiding process is terminated, contraction of the PFM activates the perineobulbar detrusor inhibitory reflex.

In summary, the function of the lower urinary tract is regulated by a complex neural control system located in the brain and spinal cord. This control system performs a simple switching circuit to maintain a reciprocal relation between the reservoir (bladder) and outlet (urethra and urethral sphincter).[40]

References

1. Gil Vernet S (1968) Morphology and Function of the Vesico-Prostato-Urethral Musculature. Edizioni Canova, Treviso, Italy.

2. DeLancey JOL (1986) Correlative study of paraurethral anatomy. Obstet Gynecol 68: 91–7.

3. Gosling JA, Dixon JS, Critchley HOD, Thompson SA (1981) A comparative study of the human external sphincter and periurethral levator ani muscle. Br J Urol 53: 35–41.

4. Rud T, Andersson KE, Asmussen M, Hunting A, Ulmsten U (1980) Factors maintaining the intraurethral pressure in women. Invest Urol 17: 343–7.

5. Berkow SE (1953) The corpus spongiosum of the urethra: its possible role in urinary control and stress incontinence in women. Am J Obstet Gynecol 65: 346–351.

6. Schweiger M (1979) Method for determining individual contributions of voluntary and involuntary anal sphincters to resting tone. Dis Colon Rectum 22: 415–16.

7. Frenckner B, Euler CV (1975) Influence of pudendal block on the function of the anal sphincters. Gut 16: 482–9.

8. Oh C, Kark AE (1972) Anatomy of the external anal sphincter. Br J Surg 59: 717–23.

9. Ayoub SF (1979) Anatomy of the external anal sphincter in man. Acta Anat (Basel) 105: 25–36.

10. Milligan ETC, Morgan CN (1934) Surgical anatomy of the anal canal with special reference to ano-rectal fistula. Lancet 2: 150–6.

11. Aronson MP, Lee RA, Berquist TH (1990) Anatomy of anal sphincters and related structures in continent women studied with magnetic resonance imaging. Obstet Gynecol 76: 846–51.

12. Snooks SJ, Setchell M, Swash M, Henry MM (1984) Injury to innervation of pelvic floor sphincter musculature in childbirth. Lancet 2(8402): 546–50.

13. Snooks SJ, Swash M, Mathers SE, Henry MM (1990) Effect of vaginal delivery on the pelvic floor: a 5-year follow-up. Br J Surg 77: 1358–60.

14. Sultan AH, Kamm MA, Hudson CN, Thomas JM, Bartram CI (1993) Anal-sphincter disruption during vaginal delivery [see comments]. N. Engl J Med 329: 1905–11.

15. Haadem K, Dahlstrom JA, Ling L, Ohrlander S (1987) Anal sphincter function after delivery rupture. Obstet Gynecol 70: 53–6.

16. Lawson JO (1974) Pelvic anatomy. I. Pelvic floor muscles. Ann R Coll Surg Engl 54: 244–52.

17. Oelrich TM (1983) The striated urogenital sphincter muscle in the female. Anat Rec 205: 223–32.

18. Noll LE, Hutch JA (1969) The SCIPP line – an aid in interpreting the voiding lateral cystourethrogram. Obstet Gynecol 33: 680–9.

19. Parks AG, Porter NH, Melzak J (1962) Experimental study of the reflex mechanism controlling muscles of the pelvic floor. Dis Colon Rectum 5: 407–14.

20. Muellner SR (1951) Physiology of micturition. J Urol 65: 805–10.

21. Jeffcoate TNA, Roberts H (1952) Observations on stress incontinence of urine. Am J Obstet Gynecol 64: 721–38.

22. Westby M, Asmussen M, Ulmsten U (1982) Location of maximum intraurethral pressure related to urogenital diaphragm in the female subject as studied by simultaneous urethrocystometry and voiding urethrocystography. Am J Obstet Gynecol 144: 408–12.

23. DeLancey JOL (1988) Structural aspects of the extrinsic continence mechanism. Obstet Gynecol 72: 296–301.

24. DeLancey JOL (1994) Structural support of the urethra as it relates to stress urinary incontinence: the hammock hypothesis. Am J Obstet Gynecol 170: 1713–20.

25. Smith AR, Hosker GL, Warrell DW (1989) The role of pudendal nerve damage in the aetiology of genuine stress incontinence in women. Br. J Obstet Gynaecol 96: 29–32.

26. Bump RC, Huang KC, McClish DK et al (1991) Effect of narcotic anesthesia and skeletal muscle paralysis on passive dynamic urethral function in continent and stress incontinent women. Neurourol Urodynamics 10: 523–32.

27. Ricci JV, Thom CH (1954) The myth of a surgically useful fascia in vaginal plastic reconstructions. Q Rev Surg Obstet Gynecol 2: 261–3.

28. Uhlenhuth E, Nolley GW (1957) Vaginal fascia – a myth? Obstet Gynecol 10: 349–58.

29. DeLancey JOL (1992) Anatomic aspects of vaginal eversion after hysterectomy. Am J Obstet Gynecol 166: 1717–24.

30. Bartscht KD, DeLancey JOL (1988) A technique to study the passive supports of the uterus. Obstet Gynecol 72: 940–3.

31. Berglas G, Rubin IC (1953) Study of the supportive structures of the uterus by levator myography. Surg Obstet Gynecol 97: 677–92.

32. Nichols DH, Milley PS (1970) Surgical significance of the rectovaginal septum. Am J Obstet Gynecol 108: 215–220.

33. Mola J de, Carpenter SE (1996) Management of genital prolapse in neonates and young women. Obstet Gynecol Surv 51: 253–60.

34. Paramore RH (1918) The uterus as a floating organ. In: The Statics of the Female Pelvic Viscera. H.K. Lewis, London.

35. Chai TC, Steers WD (1996) Neurophysiology of micturition and continence. Urol Clin North Am 23: 221–36.

36. Elbadawi A (1996) Functional anatomy of the organs of micturition. Urol Clin North Am 23: 177–210.

37. Mahony DT, Laferte RO, Blais DJ (1977) Integral storage and voiding reflexes. Neurophysiologic concept of continence and micturition. Urology 9: 95–106.

38. Mahony DT, Laferte RO, Blais DJ (1980) Incontinence of urine due to instability of micturition reflexes: Part I. Detrusor reflex instability. Urology 15: 229–39.

39. Mahony DT, Laferte RO, Blais DJ (1980) Incontinence of urine due to instability of micturition reflexes. Part II. Pudendal nucleus instability. Urology 15: 379–88.

40. de Groat WC (1993) Anatomy and physiology of the lower urinary tract. Urol Clin North Am 20: 383–401.

3 Aetiology and Classification of Urinary Incontinence

V. Khullar, K. Boos and L. Cardozo

Many factors have been identified in the development of urinary incontinence, including childbirth, gender, age, race, the menopause, smoking, constipation, obesity and gynaecological surgery. Urinary incontinence is multifactorial, being the end result of many different pathological processes.

3.1 International Continence Society Standards

Central to all studies of incontinence is the common classification of lower urinary tract dysfunction provided by the standardisation committee of the International Continence Society (ICS).[1] These standards have been revised and extended to keep pace with improvements in urodynamic studies. Unless otherwise stated all methods, definitions and units referred to in this chapter conform to the standards recommended by the ICS.[2]

The complex symptomatology of lower urinary tract dysfunction and the common presentation of predominantly mixed symptoms mean that diagnosis based on urinary symptoms alone often correlates poorly with urodynamic findings.[3]

3.2 Risk Factors for Urinary Incontinence

Bladder function becomes less efficient with age, and Wagg and Malone Lee[4] have shown that elderly women have a reduced flow rate, an increased residual urine, a higher end filling cystometric pressure (and maximum filling pressure), reduced bladder capacity and lower maximum voiding pressures. Additionally, whereas younger women excrete the bulk of their daily fluid intake before bedtime, the pattern reverses with age, nocturia becoming more common with advancing age.

An important aspect of female ageing is the menopause. Oestrogen receptors are present in the bladder, urethra and pelvic floor, and fluctuations in oestrogen levels have been shown to result in symptomatic and urodynamic changes during pregnancy, the normal menstrual cycle and after the menopause. Falling oestrogen levels at the time of the climacteric are associated with an increased incidence of urinary symptoms including dysuria, frequency, nocturia, urgency and urinary incontinence. In addition, urinary tract infections become more frequent as a result of an alteration of vaginal pH and perineal flora.

The impaired physical status of elderly women results in additional causes of incontinence not fre-

---

Box 3.1

Additional causes of incontinence in the elderly

Dementia
Urinary tract infection
Faecal impaction
Decreased mobility
Acute illness/acute confusional state
Drugs (e.g. diuretics, hypnotics)
Change of environment (e.g. hospitalisation)
Heart failure
Oestrogen deficiency
Metabolic abnormalities
Endocrine abnormalities (e.g. diabetes)
Renal problems

---

quently encountered by younger women (Box 3.1). Many of these conditions are reversible and should be elicited by a thorough clinical history and physical examination.

3.2.1 Race

Very little epidemiological data is available regarding the racial differences of incontinence, although it appears to be least common amongst Chinese, Eskimo and black women. An anatomical study involving the dissection of Chinese female cadavers showed that the levator ani muscle bundles of the Chinese cadavers were judged to be thicker and to extend more laterally on the arcus tendineus than in white cadavers. Bump compared clinical and urodynamic parameters of 54 black and 146 white women.[5] The results showed the causes of urinary incontinence to be significantly different between the two groups (Table 3.1).

Table 3.1.   Cause of incontinence and racial origin.[5] All figures are percentages

Variable	Race	
	Black	White
Symptoms of incontinence		
Stress incontinence	7	31
Urge incontinence	56	28
Mixed incontinence	37	41
Cause of incontinence		
Genuine stress incontinence	27	61
Detrusor instability	56	28
Mixed incontinence	17	11

3.2.2 Childbirth

The association of parity and incontinence is mainly due to an increase in the incidence of stress incontinence, and postpartum detrusor instability appears to be little affected by pregnancy or childbirth. Cardozo and Cutner[6] have shown an increased incidence of detrusor instability during pregnancy, possibly a result of elevated serum progesterone levels, although it appears that these cases resolve postpartum.

Childbirth injury has been implicated as the major aetiologic factor in genuine stress incontinence, and there is histological[7] and electromyographic (EMG)[8,9] evidence of injury to the pelvic floor postpartum. Women delivered by caesarean section without labour have greater pelvic floor muscle strength postpartum. Urethral pressure profilometry has shown a reduction in functional urethral length, urethral closure

pressure and maximum urethral pressure following vaginal delivery, changes which are not observed following caesarean section. In addition Wilson et al.[10] have shown that a program of intensive postpartum pelvic floor exercises can reduce the incidence of stress incontinence 1 year after delivery.

3.2.3 Connective Tissue Factors

Bø et al. reported stress incontinence in 13/37 fit healthy nulliparous physical education students,[11] and demonstrated significantly lower resting urethral pressures and stress profiles in this group than in continent nulliparous controls.

Research has suggested that the collagen of women with prolapse and stress incontinence may be abnormal and predispose them to develop these conditions. Type I collagen forms thick, strong fibre units whereas type III collagen forms thin, weak and isolated fibres. Keane et al.[12] performed periurethral biopsies on 30 nulliparous women with urodynamically proven genuine stress incontinence and found a decrease in the ratio of type I to type III collagen, as well as a reduction in the total amount of collagen in the women with genuine stress incontinence compared to continent controls.

3.2.4 Smoking, Obesity and Chronic Constipation

Any condition resulting in a chronically elevated intra-abdominal pressure is likely to increase the risk of developing or exacerbating stress incontinence. Obesity, smoking, coughing and chronic constipation have been suggested as important predisposing factors in the causation of genuine stress incontinence, although insufficient data exists to refute or confirm these assumptions.

Carey and Dwyer[13] found that obesity (>20% above average weight for height and age) was significantly commoner in women with genuine stress incontinence and detrusor instability than in the normal population. There were, however, no significant differences between obese and non-obese incontinent women with respect to any urodynamic variables. Bump et al. studied 13 morbidly obese women before and after surgically induced weight loss.[14] Weight loss resulted in a significant improvement in incontinence, obviating the need for treatment of incontinence in the majority of women.

In a large case-controlled study Bump and McClish noted a 2–3-fold increase in the incidence of all forms of urinary incontinence amongst cigarette smokers.[15] Although the increased incidence of chronic chest complaints is likely to exacerbate stress incontinence, the effects of nicotine on the bladder require further evaluation.

Spence Jones et al. investigated 23 women with stress incontinence, 23 with uterovaginal prolapse and 27 control women.[16] Straining at stool and an increased frequency of bowel opening was significantly commoner for women with stress incontinence and prolapse than for controls.

3.2.5 Hysterectomy and Urinary Incontinence

Incontinence may be a complication of hysterectomy. In a review of 131 women after abdominal hysterectomy, Petri found postoperative urinary incontinence in 68% of patients, all of whom were previously asymptomatic.[17] Stress incontinence (37%) was more common than urge incontinence (29%). Unfortunately this study was retrospective, and in two prospective studies there was no evidence to suggest increased bladder dysfunction after abdominal hysterectomy.[18,19] There are many potential mechanisms of incontinence following hysterectomy: derangement of the bladder supports,[20] pelvic nerve damage,[21,22] and oestrogen deficiency resulting from concomitant oophorectomy. In addition, postoperative catheter care may be suboptimal and prolonged overdistension of the bladder resulting from urinary retention can lead to chronic bladder hypotonicity.

At present the evidence is inconclusive, and large detailed prospective studies are required.

3.2.6 Prolapse and Anterior Repair

Genital prolapse and urinary incontinence are common conditions and it is therefore not surprising to find both in some women. Cystocele may be the cause of voiding difficulties. Romanzi et al.[23] found almost 60% of women with severe genital prolapse and no symptoms of incontinence have underlying urinary incontinence revealed by urodynamic testing: 41% of their patients had genuine stress incontinence following reduction of the prolapse with a ring pessary; 30% of women with either small or large cystoceles had detrusor instability on urodynamic testing, and a higher percentage had symptoms of urge incontinence.

3.2.7 Radiotherapy and Urinary Incontinence

Radiotherapy is still frequently used for the treatment of locally invasive bladder cancer, and subsequent frequency and urgency of micturition affects as many as

50% of patients.[24] This is partly attributable to fibrotic bladder damage, and partly to denervation supersensitivity.[25] The characteristic urodynamic findings are a reduced bladder capacity and low compliance.

3.2.8 Urinary Tract Infection

Many factors contribute to the frequency of urinary tract infection (UTI) including structural and functional abnormalities of the urinary tract and nephropathies associated with various diseases such as diabetes. Although the risk of UTI is relatively low for intermittent and short-term catheterisation, it is a common consequence of long-term catheterisation with reports of up to 98% bacteriuria rates (77% polymicrobial).[26] UTIs are common in postmenopausal women because oestrogen deficiency results in an alteration of the vaginal flora and subsequent increase in vaginal pH resulting in colonisation by gram-negative uropathogens.

Sexual intercourse is commonly implicated in the causation of UTIs, and several behavioural factors have been shown to enhance the risk of recurrent UTIs. These include deferred voiding after sexual intercourse, frequency of intercourse, low fluid intake and deferred voiding after the initial urge to micturate.[27–29]

Contraceptive diaphragms increase urethral pressure, reduce urinary flow and may result in incomplete bladder emptying. Research has shown that the risk of referral to hospital for urinary tract infection was 2–3 times higher amongst diaphragm users than among well-matched controls.[29] Additionally, spermicidal cream containing nonoxynol 9 can kill lactobacilli and other vaginal flora, but most uropathogens and candida thrive in its presence.[30]

3.2.9 Nocturnal Enuresis

By 4 years of age 20–40% of normal children still wet the bed, with a spontaneous resolution rate of approximately 15% of cases each year. However, 1–2% retain the problem until adulthood, and in many cases lifelong. Boys are more commonly affected than girls, and heredity seems to be important.[31]

Rittig et al.[32] investigated 15 enuretic children and 11 controls without nocturnal enuresis. Enuretic patients were found to lack the normal diurnal rhythm of vasopressin secretion and therefore suffered nocturnal polyuria. Bladder capacities of normal and enuretic children were similar, and sleep patterns as judged by EEGs were similar in the two groups. Clinical trials of DDAVP (desmopressin) have revealed a second pathology, namely a nephrogenic receptor failure in which the renal collecting system is unresponsive to endogenous ADH or exogenous DDAVP. What is unclear is why the enuretic child does not wake up when their bladder is full and needs emptying.

3.3 Classification of Urinary Tract Dysfunction

Assuming the absence of inflammation, infection and neoplasm, lower urinary tract dysfunction can be caused by:

- disturbances of neurological or psychological control
- disorders of muscle function
- structural abnormalities.

The ICS[2] classifies lower urinary tract dysfunction into disorders of the storage and voiding phases of the micturition cycle (Tables 3.2 and 3.3).

3.4 Urinary Incontinence

3.4.1 Definition

The ICS definition of incontinence is "The involuntary loss of urine which is a social or hygienic

Table 3.2. Lower urinary tract dysfunction during the storage phase of the micturition cycle[2]

Bladder	
Detrusor activity	Normal
	Overactive (detrusor instability/ hyperreflexia)
Bladder sensation	Normal
	Increased (hypersensitive)
	Reduced (hyposensitive)
	Absent
Bladder capacity	Normal adult 400 ml s^{-1}
Bladder compliance	V/P (normally $\leqslant$15 cm H$_2$O pressure rise for filled volume $\leqslant$500 ml)
Urethra	
Urethral function	Normal
	Incompetent (urethral sphincter incompetence)

Table 3.3. Lower urinary tract dysfunction during the voiding phase of the micturition cycle

Detrusor	Acontractile (atonic bladder)
	Underactive (hypotonic bladder)
Urethra	Obstructive (mechanical;urethral stricture)
	Overactive (detrusor sphincter dyssynergia)

problem and objectively demonstrable".[33] The loss of urine through channels other than the urethra is termed extraurethral incontinence. Urinary incontinence denotes either the symptom of involuntary urine loss, the objective demonstration of urinary leakage or the urodynamic diagnosis of the causative condition.

3.4.2 Symptoms

- *Stress incontinence* is the commonest symptom with which women present, and indicates the involuntary loss of urine during physical exertion.
- *Urge incontinence* is the involuntary loss of urine associated with a strong desire to void.
- *Unconscious incontinence* denotes urinary leakage in the absence of urgency and without conscious recognition of the urine loss.
- *Enuresis* means any involuntary loss of urine, although it is usually used to denote incontinence during sleep (nocturnal enuresis).
- *Post-micturition dribble* and *continuous incontinence* denote other symptomatic forms of urinary leakage often associated with prolapse or urethral diverticulae and urinary fistulae respectively.

The major types and causes of urinary incontinence are listed in Table 3.4.

3.4.3 Genuine Stress Incontinence

Genuine stress incontinence (GSI) is a diagnosis made by urodynamic assessment. It is defined as the involuntary loss of urine occurring when, in the absence of detrusor contraction, the intravesical pressure exceeds the maximum urethral pressure. It is the commonest cause of urinary incontinence among women, accounting for about 50% of cases. Stress incontinence is most commonly caused by coughing, sneezing or, in severe cases, by only minimal activity such as walking. It mainly occurs in parous women and is exacerbated by lifting, straining and constipation.

Table 3.4. The causes and types of urinary incontinence

Genuine stress incontinence (GSI)
Detrusor instability (DI) (detrusor hyperreflexia)
Overflow incontinence
Fistulae (vesicovaginal, ureterovaginal, urethrovaginal)
Congenital
Urethral diverticulae
Temporary (e.g. urinary tract infection, faecal impaction, drugs)
Functional (e.g. immobility)

3.4.4 Detrusor Instability (DI)

Detrusor instability (DI) is the second commonest cause of incontinence, accounting for 20–40% of referrals for urodynamic investigation. The incidence increases with age. and DI is the commonest cause of urinary incontinence in elderly people.[4] The condition is termed *detrusor hyperreflexia* if there is associated overt neurological pathology.

An unstable bladder is one that contracts involuntarily, either spontaneously or on provocation, during the filling phase of cystometry whilst the patient is attempting to inhibit micturition. Urodynamic assessment is required to make a diagnosis. A list of the common causes of frequency and urgency of micturition is shown in Table 3.5.

Table 3.5. The causes of frequency and urgency of micturition

Type	Example
Gynaecological/urological	Urinary tract infection Detrusor instability Inflammation (e.g. interstitial cystitis) Fibrosis (radiation) Atrophy (menopause) Intravesical lesion (e.g. calculus) Urethral pathology (e.g. urethral syndrome) External pressure (e.g. pelvic mass or fibroids) Pregnancy
Medical/psychological	Drugs (e.g. diuretics) Diabetes Neurological disease (e.g. multiple sclerosis) Excessive fluid intake Habit

3.4.5 Sensory Urgency

This is diagnosed when there are intense irritative bladder symptoms in the absence of unstable detrusor contractions. Patients have a reduced functional bladder capacity, daytime frequency, nocturia and sometimes incontinence. It may be caused by inflammatory conditions of the bladder or urethra (e.g. interstitial cystitis, atrophic urethritis), and can be diagnosed by cystoscopy and bladder biopsy.

3.4.6 Overflow Incontinence

Overflow incontinence secondary to chronic retention of urine is characterised by voiding difficulties, impaired bladder sensation, recurrent

Table 3.6. Causes of overflow incontinence

Cause	Examples
Outflow obstruction	Following bladder neck surgery, urethral stricture, cystocele
Myogenic bladder damage	Following acute retention of urine
Anticholinergic medication	Oxybutynin
Painful perineal conditions	Genital herpes, postpartum vaginal tears
Neurological conditions	Detrusor sphincter dyssynergia, lower motor neuron lesions
Pelvic mass	Ovarian cyst, gravid uterus.
Blocked catheter	
Epidural anaesthesia	

urinary tract infections, and the frequent leakage of small amounts of urine. Common causes are listed in Table 3.6.

3.5 Conclusion

Urinary incontinence has a high prevalence in the community and this impairs the patient's quality of life. There are many causes of urinary incontinence, and the treatments may vary greatly according to the aetiology.

References

1 International Continence Society (1976) First report on the standardisation of terminology of lower urinary tract function. Br J Urol 48: 39–42.
2 International Continence Society (1988) The standardisation of terminology of the lower urinary tract function. Scand J Nephrol Suppl 114: 5–19.
3. Farrar DJ, Whiteside CG, Osborne JL, Turner-Warwick RT (1975) A urodynamic analysis of micturition symptoms in the female. Surg Gynecol Obstet 141: 875–881.
4. Wagg A, Malone-Lee J (1998) The management of urinary incontinence in the elderly. Br J Urol 82 (Suppl 1): 11–17.
5. Bump RC (1993) Racial comparisons and contrasts in urinary incontinence and pelvic organ prolapse. Obstet Gynecol 81: 421–5.
6. Cardozo L, Cutner A (1997) Lower urinary tract symptoms in pregnancy. Br J Urol 80 (Suppl)(1): 14–23.
7. Gilpin SA, Gosling JA, Smith AR, Warrell DW (1989) The pathogenesis of genitourinary prolapse and stress incontinence of urine. A histological and histochemical study. Br J Obstet Gynaecol 96: 15–23.
8. Laurberg S, Swash M, Snooks SJ, Henry MM (1988) Neurologic cause of idiopathic incontinence. Arch Neurol 45: 1250–3.
9. Smith AR, Hosker GL, Warrell DW (1989) The role of partial denervation of the pelvic floor in the aetiology of genitourinary prolapse and stress incontinence of urine. A neurophysiological study. Br J Obstet Gynaecol 96: 24–8.

10. Wilson PD, Herbison GP (1988) A randomised controlled trial of pelvic floor muscle exerise to treat postnatal urinary incontinence. Int Urogynecol J 9: 257–4.

11. Bø K, Stien R, Kulseng Hanssen S, Kristofferson M (1994) Clinical and urodynamic assessment of nulliparous young women with and without stress incontinence symptoms: a case-control study. Obstet Gynecol 84: 1028–32.

12. Keane DP, Sims TJ, Abrams P, Bailey AJ (1997) Analysis of collagen status in premenopausal nulliparous women with genuine stress incontinence. Br J Obstet Gynaecol 104: 994–8.

13. Carey MP, Dwyer PL (1991) Position and mobility of the urethrovesical junction in continent and stress incontinent women before and after successful surgery. Aust NZ J Obstet Gynaecol 31: 279–84.

14. Bump RC, Sugerman HJ, Fantl JA, McClish DK (1992) Obesity and lower urinary tract function in women: Effect of surgically induced weight loss. Am J Obstet Gynecol 167: 122–8.

15. Bump RC, McClish DM (1994) Cigarette smoking and pure genuine stress incontinence of urine: a comparison of risk factors and determinants between smokers and non-smokers. Am J Obstet Gynecol 170: 579–82.

16. Spence Jones C, Kamm MA, Henry MM, Hudson CN (1994) Bowel dysfunction: a pathogenic factor in uterovaginal prolapse and urinary stress incontinence. Br J Obstet Gynaecol 101: 147–52.

17. Petri E (1999) Urological trauma in gynaecological surgery: diagnosis and management. Curr Opin Obstet Gynecol 11: 495–8.

18. Parys BT, Haylen BT, Hutton JL, Parsons KF (1990) Urodynamic evaluation of lower urinary tract function in relation to total hysterectomy. N Z J Obstet Gynaecol 30: 161–5.

19. Langer R, Neuman M, Ron-el R, Golan A, Bukovsky I, Caspi, E (1989) The effect of total abdominal hysterectomy on bladder function in asymptomatic women. Obstet Gynecol 74: 205–7.

20. Morgan JL, O'Connell HE, McGuire EJ (2000) Is intrinsic sphincter deficiency a complication of simple hysterectomy? J Urol 164: 767–769.

21. Mundy AR (1982) An anatomical explanation for bladder dysfunction following rectal and uterine surgery. Br J Urol 54: 501–4.

22. Parys BT, Woolfenden KA, Parsons KF (1990b) Bladder ysfunction after simple hysterectomy: urodynamic and neurological evaluation. Eur Urol 17: 129–33.

23. Romanzi LJ, Chaikin DC, Blaivas JG (1999) The effect of genital prolapse on voiding. J Urol 161: 581–6.

24. Hanfmann B, Engels M, Dorr W (1998) Radiation-induced impairment of urinary bladder function. Assessment of micturition volumes. Strahlenther Onkol 174 (Suppl)(3): 96–8.

25. Crook J, Esche B, Futter N (1996) Effect of pelvic radiotherapy for prostate cancer on bowel, bladder, and sexual function: the patient's perspective. Urology 47: 387–94.

26. Tambyah PA, Maki DG (2000) Catheter-associated urinary tract infection is rarely symptomatic: a prospective study of 1,497 catheterized patients. Arch Int Med 160: 678–82.

27. Ronald A (1996) Sex and urinary tract infections. New Eng J Med 335: 511–12.

28. Hooton TM, Roberts PL, Stamm WE (1994) Effects of recent sexual activity and use of a diaphragm on the vaginal microflora. Clin Infect Dis 19: 274–8.

29. Hooton TM, Scholes D, Hughes JP et al. (1996) A prospective study of risk factors for symptomatic urinary tract infection in young women. New Eng J Med 335: 468–474.

30. McGroarty JA, Soboh F, Bruce AW, Reid G (1990) The spermicidal compound nonoxynol-9 increases adhesion of Candida species to human epithelial cells in vitro. Infect Immun 58: 2005–7.

31. Rodriguez LM, Marugan JM, Lapena S (2000) Therapeutic strategy in nocturnal enuresis. Acta Paediatr 89: 498–9.

32. Rittig S, Knudsen UB, Norgaard JP, Pedersen EB, Djurhuus JC (1989) Abnormal diurnal rhythm of plasma vasopressin and urinary output in patients with enuresis. Am J Physiol 256: F664–71.

33. Abrams P, Blaivas JG, Stanton SL, Andersen JT (1990) The standardisation of terminology of lower urinary tract function. Br J Obstet Gynaecol Suppl 6: 1–16.

4 Assessment and Treatment of Urinary Incontinence in Neurologically Impaired Patients

S. Islam and C.D. Betts

This chapter is mainly concerned with the neurogenic bladder dysfunction in multiple sclerosis (MS), following a cerebrovascular accident (CVA) and in idiopathic Parkinsons' disease (IPD). In recent years, a good deal has been learnt about the bladder disorder in multiple system atrophy (MSA) and about urinary retention in premenopausal women; sections about these problems have been included.

For some patients with neurologic disease the bladder symptoms can be the most distressing feature of the disorder. In a patient with neurological impairment, the combination of urinary urgency and frequency is likely to have a highly adverse effect upon their well-being. In MS, CVA and IPD it is extremely uncommon for the neurogenic bladder disorder to result in serious upper urinary tract problems and kidney failure. Patients with spinal bifida or spinal cord injury are at risk from renal impairment and the management of these patients has not been included in this chapter.

4.1 Prevalence

The central neural pathways, which are important in bladder control, extend from the frontal lobes to the sacral spinal cord, lesions at many levels of the neuraxis may cause neurogenic bladder dysfunction.

4.1.1 Multiple Sclerosis

The high incidence of bladder symptoms in MS has been recognised for more than 100 years. Oppenheim[1] found urinary symptoms in 80% of patients with MS, and most investigators since have reported that approximately 75% of all patients with MS develop urinary symptoms. A few studies have reported a lower incidence of bladder problems in

MS,[2] but this is almost certainly because the patients included in these studies had mild degrees of disability. Miller et al.[3] found bladder symptoms in 75% of patients with MS (Table 4.1)

In the past, urinary symptoms alone were thought to be the first symptoms of MS in a small number of patients. Miller et al.[3] and Goldstein et al.[4] stated that bladder symptoms were the sole presenting feature of MS in 2% and 2.3% of patients, respectively. In a more recent study[5] of 170 patients with MS and urinary symptoms, none of the patients had first presented with urinary symptoms alone. In earlier times, urinary retention in women was often said to be due to MS and this could account for the reports that patients with MS had first presented with bladder problems. An alternative cause for retention in young women is now recognised, and retention without other neurological features should not be regarded as a symptom of MS.[5-8]

4.1.2 Idiopathic Parkinson's Disease

Parkinsonism is a disturbance of motor function named after James Parkinson, who first described a case of paralysis agitans in 1817.[9] There are several causes of Parkinsonism; the commonest is idiopathic Parkinson's disease, followed by multiple system atrophy (MSA), the Steele–Richardson–Olskowski syndrome and certain drugs. The diagnosis of IPD disease is based largely on clinical features. Recent postmortem studies suggest that the other causes of Parkinsonism, especially MSA, have been underdiagnosed.[10,11]

The neurodegeneration in IPD involves the neural mechanisms that are important in the central control of bladder function. Frequency and urgency of micturition are common urinary symptoms in IPD.[12] In elderly men with IPD it is often difficult to

Table 4.1. Urinary symptoms in multiple sclerosis

First author and year	Reference	Number of patients with MS	MS patients first presenting with only urinary symptoms (%)	MS patients first presenting with urinary and other neurological symptoms (%)	Overall % of patients with MS and urinary symptoms.
Oppenheim (1889)	1	30	–	–	80
Kahleyss (1890)	2	35	–	–	88
Sachs (1921)	3	141	–	–	40
Brickner (1936)	4	62	–	10	85
Langworthy (1938)	5	157	–	–	62
Muller (1949)	6	582	–	5	62
Carter (1950)	7	47	–	11	78
Adams (1950)	8	389	–	2.8	44.5
Moore (1960)	9	604	–	–	42
Ivers (1963)	10	144	–	1	10
Miller (1965)	11	297	2[a]	12	78
Goldstein (1982)	12	86	2.3[a]	14	97
Betts (1993)	13	170	0	2.3	100

[a] See text for explanation.
–; no value reported.

Table 4.2. Urinary symptoms in 11 studies of patients with MS and bladder dysfunction

First author and year	Reference	Number of patients	% with urgency	% with frequency	% with urge incontinence	% with hesitancy	% with retention[a]
Sachs (1921)	3	57	31%	–	37%	49%	–
Langworthy (1938)	5	97	54%	33%	34%	40%	–
Carter (1950)	7	36	24%	17%	50%	–	17%
Moore (1960)	9	254	–	67%	16%	29%	5%
Miller (1965)	11	231	60%	50%	36%	33%	2%
Bradley (1973)	41	90	86%	60%	–	28%	20%
Philp (1981)	42	52	61%	59%	47%	25%	8%
Goldstein (1982)	12	86	32%	32%	49%	–	–
Awad (1984)	43	47	85%	65%	72%	36%	–
Gonor (1985)	44	64	70%	48%	56%	30%	–
Betts (1993)	23	170	85%	82%	63%	49%	–

–; no value reported.
[a] See text for explanation.

distinguish between the bladder symptoms due to the neurological disorder and the urinary problems resulting from benign prostatic hypertrophy (BPH).[13] In many, it is likely that the urinary symptoms arise from a combination of BPH and the neurogenic bladder dysfunction.

The prevalence of urinary symptoms in patients diagnosed as having IPD has been reported to be between 37–71%.[12,14–16] Figures for the incidence of urinary symptoms in IPD need to be interpreted with some caution since there may be uncertainty about the neurological diagnosis.

4.1.3 Cerebrovascular Accident

Bladder dysfunction is an important complication of a stroke, and in addition to affecting morale it can adversely affect rehabilitation, discharge from hospital and the long-term outcome from the stroke.[17]

Brocklehurst et al.[18] reported urinary continence problems in 52 of 135 consecutive stoke patients during the first 2 weeks after the CVA. The authors concluded that incontinence after a CVA was largely a result of immobility and was usually a transient problem.[18] In a prospective study of 151 patients following a stroke, 60%, 42% and 29% of those surviving the CVA had problems with urinary incontinence at 1 week, 4 weeks and 12 weeks, respectively. At 4 weeks, the factors that were significantly associated with urinary incontinence were; moderate or severe motor deficit, impaired mobility and mental impairment; 66% of patients who were said to have mild incontinence at 4 weeks were continent by 12 weeks. In several studies of urinary incontinence after stroke, the investigators conclude that bladder incontinence occurring shortly after a CVA is a specific indicator of a poor prognosis.[19–22]

The long-term prevalence of bladder dysfunction in patients who have had a CVA is uncertain since the population at risk from strokes are also likely to have symptoms from prostatic disease, bladder stones, bladder cancer and idiopathic detrusor instability.

4.2 Aetiology and Pathophysiology of the Neural Control of Bladder Function

The neural pathways that are important in bladder function traverse the whole length of the spinal cord between the pons and the sacral spinal cord, and are particularly likely to be affected by diseases involving the spinal cord. Knowledge of the areas in the central nervous system that are important in bladder control may be helpful in predicting the bladder dysfunction in central neurologic disease. In humans, the exact location of the central neural pathways for bladder control remains uncertain.

4.2.1 The External Urethral Sphincter and the Nucleus of Onuf

The external urethral sphincter, the rhabdosphincter, is made up of circularly orientated, predominately type I (slow-twitch) striated muscle fibres.[23] In men the external sphincter is just distal to the prostate gland; in women it surrounds much of the shorter urethra. The striated muscle of the urethral sphincter is the only part of the urinary tract to receive a somatic innervation. Onufrowicz, in 1899,[24] described a nucleus in the ventral horn of the spinal cord at S2, S3 and S4. Onuf's nucleus contains the cell bodies of the motor neurons that innervate the urethral and anal sphincters. Motor fibres from Onuf's nucleus pass into the pudendal nerves, giving branches to the anal and urethral sphincters.

4.2.2 Detrusor Muscle Innervation

The main motor supply of the detrusor muscle of the bladder comes from parasympathetic preganglionic neurons with cell bodies in the intermediolateral columns of the cord between S2 and S4. The preganglionic parasympathetic nerve fibres pass by way of the pelvic nerves to the pelvic plexus and then by short postganglionic nerves to innervate the detrusor muscle. The bladder neck in males has a rich noradrenergic innervation; sympathetic activity during ejaculation causes closure of the bladder neck and antegrade ejaculation.

4.2.3 The Pons and the Frontal Regions in Bladder Function

The importance of the pons for the control of micturition was first recognised by Barrington, working on decerebrate cats at University College London.[25] A nucleus in the dorsal tegmentum of the pons has been identified as a centre important in coordinating micturition. This nucleus in the pons has been referred to as "Barrington's nucleus",[26] and it is also known as the pontine micturition centre (PMC). In 1964, Andrew and Nathan[27] first drew attention to the importance of the frontal regions of the brain in bladder control.[28] Furthermore, de Groat has proposed that higher centers control the PMC, which acts as a "switch" on a long reflex, alternating the bladder's storage and voiding phases.[29,30]

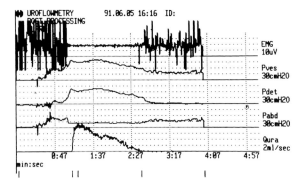

Figure 4.1 Urodynamic study during voiding. External urethral sphincter activity is recorded with an electromyographic needle positioned in the striated sphincter muscle. Sphincter activity deceases (EMG) when the detrusor muscle contracts (pdet) and voiding occurs (Qura).

In recent years there have been some interesting Positron Emission Tomography (PET) studies in humans, which have shown that the neural control in humans is similar to that described in cats and other animals.[31,32] For a description of these studies the reader is referred to an editorial by Fowler.[33] The evidence supports a "bimodal control" of the bladder; suprapontine centres and particularly areas in the frontal lobes are involved in the decision as to when to switch the PMC between the storage and voiding states.

Higher centres, particularly the medial frontal lobes, act on the PMC in a mainly inhibitory manner. When the bladder is full and voiding is socially acceptable, higher centres, particularly the medial frontal lobes, facilitate the micturition reflex through the PMC. Pelvic nerve activity increases, resulting in contraction of the detrusor muscle. At the same time the nervous innervation of the external urethral sphincter muscle is inhibited and this relaxes to allow voiding.

In normal circumstances the detrusor muscle contracts only when a person wishes to empty their bladder. The external urethral sphincter normally relaxes at the same time as bladder contraction and the PMC is known to play a key role in this coordinated action (Fig. 4.1).

4.3 Bladder Dysfunction in Multiple Sclerosis

4.3.1 Urinary Symptoms in Multiple Sclerosis

The most common urinary symptom in MS is urgency of micturition, followed by frequency and

urge incontinence. In the literature concerning MS and the bladder, the term "retention" has been used to describe a complete inability to void and also hesitancy, this means that the true incidence of complete retention is unclear. A complete inability to void from a failure of detrusor muscle contraction is unusual (Table 4.2).

4.3.2 Urodynamic Studies in Multiple Sclerosis

There have been a large number of papers concerned with urodynamic studies in MS and the data can appear confusing (Table 4.3).

Bladder hyperreflexia[34] has been the commonest urodynamic finding in patients with MS and urinary symptoms (Fig. 4.2). In this disorder the bladder contracts in an abnormal involuntary manner, often when the urinary volume is low.

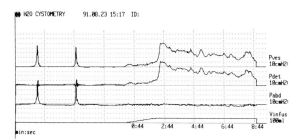

Figure 4.2 Urodynamic study during bladder filling in a patient with MS and urge incontinence. The trace shows detrusor hyperreflexia. At about 100 ml (Vinfus) of filling the detrusor (Pdet) and intravesical (Pves) pressure rise because of an involuntary contraction of the bladder muscle. As the pressure rises the patient experiences the sense of urinary urgency. If the pressure is high then urethral leakage will occur despite the patient trying to resist this, by strongly contracting the pelvic floor muscles.

At the onset of one of these bladder contractions the patient will usually experience the sensation that they are about to empty their bladder. They may be able to avoid an episode of incontinence by tightly contracting their pelvic floor muscles until they reach a toilet, or sometimes the involuntary bladder contraction will abate and the sensation will fade away. Often the pressure within the bladder during one of these involuntary detrusor contractions can be so great that urine escapes from the bladder and incontinence occurs (urge incontinence).

In our study[5] the urodynamic finding of hyperreflexia correlated well with the symptoms of urgency, frequency and urge incontinence. All of the patients who had moderate or severe pyramidal dysfunction in their legs (Kurtzke pyramidal scores 3 or

Table 4.3. Summary of the urodynamic findings in 20 studies of the bladder dysfunction in MS. Detrusor hyperreflexia is the most common urodynamic abnormality

First author and year	Reference	Number of patients	Detrusor function (%)		
			Hyperreflexia	Hypo/areflexia	Normal
Bradley (1973)	41	99	59	40	0
Andersen (1976)	45	52	63	33	4
Bradley (1978)	46	302	62	34	4
Summers (1978)	47	50	52	12	18
Schoenburg (1979)	48	39	69	5	15
Piazza (1979)	49	31	74	6	9
Blaivas (1979)	50	41	56	40	4
Philp (1981)	42	52	99	0	1
Goldstein (1982)	12	86	76	19	–
Van Poppel (1983)	51	160	66	24	10
Awad (1984)	43	57	66	21	12
Hassouna (1984)	52	37	70	18	11
Petersen (1984)	53	88	83	16	1
McGuire (1984)	54	46	72	28	0
Gonor (1985)	44	64	78	20	2
Weinstein (1988)	55	91	70	16	12
Betts (1993)	13	70	91	0	9
Sirls (1994)	56	113	70	15	6
Hinson (1997)	57	70	63	28	9
Barbalias (1998)	58	90	58	16	–

–; no value reported.

higher) and complained of frequency, urgency or urge incontinence were found to have detrusor hyperreflexia on urodynamic testing.

In MS the spinal cord lesions interrupt the neural pathways from the pons to the sacral cord, causing detrusor hyperreflexia. The spinal lesions may also result in a loss of the coordinated action of the detrusor muscle and the external urethral sphincter; this is known as detrusor sphincter dyssynergia (DSD). Bladder hyperreflexia and DSD often occur in the same patient.[35–37]

DSD occurs when the external sphincter contacts in an involuntary manner at the same time as contraction of the detrusor muscle. The symptoms suggestive of DSD include hesitancy of micturition, an interrupted urinary flow and a failure to empty the bladder completely. The demonstration of DSD is difficult because it involves the simultaneous measurement of bladder pressure, urinary flow and urethral sphincter electromyography (Fig. 4.3). DSD is likely to be present in a patient with spinal cord disease who has a significant postmicturition residual.

The occurrence of bladder areflexia[34] in MS remains a controversial issue. It has been suggested that early studies of the bladder function in MS may have included patients who did not actually have MS.[5,38] There is little doubt that bladder hyperreflexia, with or without DSD, is the most common urodynamic finding in MS patients with urinary symptoms.

4.3.2 Genitourinary Dysfunction and the Neurological Features of Multiple Sclerosis

Several authors have reported a correlation between bladder symptoms and the presence of pyramidal tract signs in the patients' lower limbs.[3,5,39] Also, the severity of the urinary symptoms has been shown to be related to the degree of pyramidal tract dysfunction in the lower limbs.[3,5,39] In our study the majority of patients with MS and moderately severe paraparesis experienced urge incontinence, at least to some extent[5].

In men with MS it is known that there is a strong association between urinary symptoms, erectile dysfunction and neurological impairment in the lower limbs.[3,40–42] In women with MS, little is known about

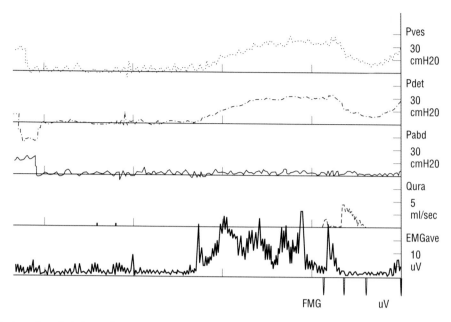

Figure 4.3 Urodynamic study during voiding in a patient with MS and complaining of hesitancy and an interrupted flow. The trace shows detrusor sphincter dyssynergia (DSD). Sphincter activity is recorded by an EMG needle in the external sphincter (EMG). Sphincter activity increases when the detrusor contracts and voiding (Qura) takes place only when the sphincter activity reduces.

the relationships between abnormalities of the bladder and sexual function.[42]

4.4 Bladder Dysfunction in Idiopathic Parkinson's Disease

4.4.1 Urinary Symptoms in Idiopathic Parkinson's Disease

Frequency and urgency of micturition are common in patients with IPD.[12] The problem of distinguishing neurogenic bladder symptoms from prostatic symptoms in elderly men with IPD has been discussed earlier.

4.4.2 Urodynamic Studies in Idiopathic Parkinson's Disease

Urodynamic studies in patients with IPD and urinary symptoms have shown a high incidence of detrusor hyperreflexia.[43,44] In neurologically intact humans, the basal ganglia are thought to exert an inhibitory influence on the PMC and the micturition reflex. In IPD it is often proposed that with loss of cells in the substantia nigra the inhibitory effect of

the basal ganglia on the micturition reflex is reduced and detrusor hyperreflexia is the result.[45,46]

Investigators have undertaken urodynamic tests in patients with IPD and studied the effect of administering L-dopa or apomorphine.[47–50] The overall results have been inconclusive; in some patients with IPD there has been a lessening of the hyperreflexia after L-dopa and in others a worsening of the bladder disorder.

4.5 Multiple System Atrophy

Graham and Oppenheimer[51] introduced the term multiple system atrophy (MSA) to cover several related conditions. The condition is probably more common than previously believed, and in recent postmortem studies 10–15% of patients diagnosed in life as having IPD were actually found, on pathological examination of the nervous system, to have had MSA. It is beyond the scope of this chapter to give a detailed account of this neurologic disease and the reader is referred to Quinn,[10,11] Wenning[52] and Chandiramani and Fowler.[53]

Clinically there are various subtypes of MSA with varying degrees of extrapyramidal, pyramidal, cerebellar and autonomic dysfunction. It is possible to consider two main forms of MSA: an atypical form of

Parkinson's disease which is often poorly responsive to the usual dopaminergic medication, and a brainstem and cerebellar form with loss of coordination, gait ataxia and dysarthria. Postural hypotension is an important feature of MSA and well described in the neurological texts.

In MSA pathological studies show cell loss and gliosis in several "at risk" central nervous system structures.[54] Many of these sites are important in the nervous control of the bladder, so disturbances of micturition and sexual function are common in MSA.[55]

In MSA, there is often cell loss in Onuf's nucleus resulting in denervation of the striated muscle of the urethral and anal sphincters.[56,57] Also, there is degeneration of cells in the midbrain and this may result in detrusor hyperreflexia. As the disease progresses, many patients develop a failure of the detrusor muscle and this probably results from cell loss in areas of the sacral cord containing the parasympathetic neurons to the bladder. In MSA the degree of urinary incontinence often becomes very marked and this is probably due to the combination of a denervated urethral sphincter and abnormal bladder function, either hyperreflexia or an underactive detrusor muscle.

4.5.1 Urinary Symptoms in Multiple System Atrophy

Studies have shown that about 60% of patients with MSA develop urinary symptoms before or at the same time as they present with Parkinsonism.[55,58] Many patients with MSA are referred to a urologist with urinary symptoms or erectile dysfunction at an early stage in the disease, very often before the neurological disorder is fully apparent[55]. Patients presenting to urologists in this way are frequently thought to have prostatic disease or (in women) to have uncomplicated stress urinary incontinence. Urinary control in patients with MSA is often made worse by surgical intervention. In one study all of the men were incontinent either immediately after prostate surgery or within 1 year of the operation.[55]

In the early stages of the disease urgency, frequency and nocturia are the most common urinary symptoms; in women, stress incontinence may be a feature. The majority of men develop erectile failure. As the neurological disorder progresses, urinary incontinence and nocturia become very prominent symptoms.

4.5.2 Urodynamic Studies in Multiple System Atrophy

Detrusor hyperreflexia is common in the earlier stages of the disease but as the neurological disorder

advances detrusor failure develops with incomplete bladder emptying.[55,59] Many patients develop large postmicturition residual volumes: in one study of 57 patients with suspected MSA; the average residual was 275 ml.[55] It is probably this tendency to high residual volumes that results in a significant number of men undergoing prostate surgery, before the neurological diagnosis is realised. As described earlier, the results of surgery are invariably poor.

4.5.3 Sphincter Electromyography in Multiple System Atrophy

In MSA, the degeneration in Onuf's nucleus results in denervation of the striated muscle in the anal and urethral sphincters. The changes of chronic reinnervation have been well demonstrated by electromyography (EMG) in the sphincter muscles of patients with probable MSA.[55–57,60] In Parkinson's disease, Onuf's nucleus is not affected and there is no denervation in the sphincter muscles. Sphincter EMG can be helpful in distinguishing between MSA and Parkinsons's disease.[61]

In sphincter electromyography, the most important measurement for detecting chronic reinnervation is the duration of individual motor units. The mean motor unit duration for the anal and urethral sphincters is normally less than 10 ms.[61] In a study, 82% of patients who were eventually diagnosed as having MSA had an abnormal sphincter EMG.[60] EMG may test the anal or urethral sphincters, and the duration of at least 10 individual motor units is measured.

Erectile dysfunction is frequently the first symptom of MSA, and may occur several years before the onset of any other neurological symptom.

The diagnosis of MSA may not be apparent to the doctor who is managing a patient with Parkinsonism, and the clinicians investigating the genitourinary symptoms may need to question the neurological diagnosis. The likelihood of a diagnosis of MSA in a patient with Parkinsonism and urinary symptoms is important because the results of urological procedures are known to be poor in MSA.

4.6 Cerebrovascular Accident

This section is concerned with bladder function in patients who have had CVA. Bladder problems occurring after brainstem strokes or vascular accidents involving the spinal cord have not been included. In the literature, there is information about urodynamic tests in patients following a stroke and some investigators have concentrated on the prevalence of urinary incontinence after a cerebrovascular accident.

4.6.1 Urodynamic Studies in Cerebrovascular Accident

Khan et al. undertook two studies of bladder dysfunction after stroke and correlated the computed tomography (CT) findings with the urodynamic results.[62,63] In the first study 20 CVA patients were studied, of whom 19 had detrusor hyperreflexia. The second study demonstrated again that detrusor hyperreflexia was the most common urodynamic abnormality, present in 26 of 33 patients who had urinary symptoms after a stroke.[63] The authors concluded that it was not possible to correlate the area of brain injury with bladder dysfunction. The findings were similar in another study, urge incontinence and detrusor hyperreflexia being the most common problem.[64]

In a further investigation,[65] 53% of patients had significant urinary symptoms at 3 months after a stroke: 36% had nocturnal frequency, 29% had urge incontinence and 25% difficulty in voiding. In 6% urinary retention occurred in the acute phase after the stroke. CT and magnetic resonance imaging (MRI) studies were undertaken and there was a positive correlation between urinary symptoms and hemiparesis.[65] The findings from the studies of stroke patients indicate that lesions in the anteromedial frontal lobe and its descending pathway are most important in the aetiology of bladder dysfunction after stroke. Frequency, urgency and urge incontinence are the most common urinary symptoms after a stroke, and bladder hyperreflexia is the most frequent urodynamic finding.

A stroke may result in urinary symptoms and incontinence by causing a true neurogenic dysfunction of the bladder. Also, a CVA may cause dementia and an impairment of normal social behaviour with respect to micturition.

4.7 Urinary Retention in Premenopausal Women

Retention of urine in young women is not an uncommon clinical problem for the urologist; neurological disease is part of the differential diagnosis. In the past, the problem was often said to be due to demyelination in the sacral cord, but since the introduction of MRI scanning it is relatively easy to exclude MS as a diagnosis. In the absence of finding an obvious urological or neurological cause

for the inability to void, the problem in young women is often said to be "hysterical" or psychogenic.[66-69]

Fowler et al.[7] described an abnormality of the striated muscle of the urethral sphincter in young women with retention, and this disorder is thought to impair relaxation of the sphincter. The abnormality described by Fowler has a very characteristic EMG signal[7] and consists of complex repetitive discharges (CRDs) and decelerating bursts (DBs)[61,70,71]. The work undertaken by Fowler has been supported by reports from other centres.[72,73] Approximately half of the patients with the abnormal EMG finding have polycystic ovaries, and it has been suggested that there may be an underlying hormonal basis for the abnormal EMG activity and voiding dysfunction.[70]

4.8 Evaluation of Urinary Symptoms in Patients with Neurological Disease

In patients with neurological disease and urinary symptoms it is necessary to establish whether there is neurogenic bladder dysfunction or urological pathology in addition to the nervous system disorder. In some patients there may be urological disease and neurogenic bladder dysfunction. The likelihood of coexisting conditions will, at least in part, be determined by the age and sex of the patient. In a young women with MS and urge incontinence it is extremely likely the symptom will be due to detrusor hyperreflexia, whereas in an elderly man with IPD, a combination of BPH and bladder hyperreflexia is quite probable.[13]

4.9 History and Examination

There are many factors to take into account before deciding the most appropriate management of the bladder dysfunction in a patient with a neurological disease. It is necessary to learn about the patient's disabilities, their home circumstances, work and daily routine. With the patients' consent, their carers and family members should be involved in the evaluation process.

It is important to obtain accurate information about the patient's urinary symptoms (urgency, frequency, nocturia, urge incontinence, stress leakage, enuresis, hesitancy, strength or weakness of the urinary flow, interruption of the flow, sensation of incomplete bladder emptying) the severity of the complaints and the effect on their lives. The completion of a chart, recording the urinary frequency and the number of incontinent episodes, is most valuable. Haematuria may indicate serious disease, and the patient should be investigated to exclude urological malignancy. In patients with spinal cord disease, bladder and sexual dysfunction often coexist. Asking about urinary symptoms may provide an appropriate opportunity to enquire about problems with sexual function.[74,75]

General examination should include an assessment of hand function, vision and neurological impairment in the lower limbs. If there are fixed deformities or marked adductor spasm then intermittent catheterisation may be difficult. The lower limbs should be examined for pyramidal tract signs, particularly in patients with MS.[5,42]

The bladder may be palpable on abdominal examination because of incomplete emptying, and inspection of the external genitalia may be helpful in assessing the degree of soiling, in detecting skin problems and in determining if there is a rectal or uterine prolapse.

4.9.1 Bladder Emptying

Measurement of the residual volume in the bladder after micturition is the single most important test in a patient with a neurological disease and urinary symptoms.[76,77] An ultrasound scan of the bladder immediately after voiding or passing a catheter is the usual means of measuring the residual urine (Fig. 4.4).

4.9.2 Urinary Flow

This is one of the simplest of urodynamic studies (Fig. 4.5). If the urinary flow test is good and there is no residual then it is likely there is no obstruction to the urinary flow from the bladder.

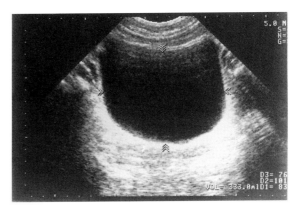

Figure 4.4 Post micturition ultrasound scan of the bladder in a women with MS. The residual was calculated to be 333 ml.

A very prolonged tracing with a low maximum flow rate suggests obstruction and in men this may be due to prostatic disease or a urethral stricture (Fig. 4.6).

An interrupted flow pattern in a patient with spinal cord disease is likely to be due to detrusor sphincter dyssynergia.

4.9.3 Cystometry

Intravesical pressure can be measured during bladder filling and during voiding. Normally, the pressure in the bladder rises little above zero as the bladder fills and to a moderate level when the detrusor contracts during voiding. There has been considerable debate about the indications for cystometry in patients with central nervous system disease and urinary symptoms.[5,42,78] Some authors recommend cystometry in every patient with urinary symptoms; others suggest that treatment may be commenced on the basis of symptoms

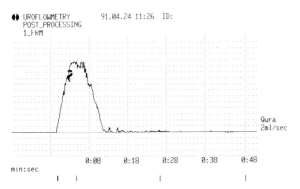

Figure 4.5 Normal urine flow test (uroflometry). The maximum flow rate was 22 ml s^{-1}.

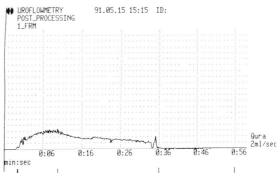

Figure 4.6 An abnormal urine flow test as a result of prostatic hypertrophy. The maximum flow rate was 6 ml s^{-1}.

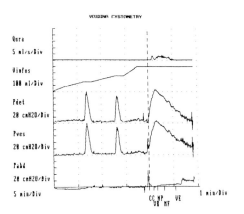

Figure 4.7 A filling and voiding urodynamic study in a man with IPD. During filling there was marked bladder instability as shown by the rises in Pdet and Pves. At the dotted line the patient was asked to void; there was a strong detrusor contraction resulting in an intra-vesical pressure of 100 cm H_2O but the urinary flow rate was poor (Qura); indicating some form of bladder outflow obstruction. The man gained considerable improvement in his symptoms following resection of the prostate gland and anticholinergic medication to suppress the detrusor hyperreflexia.

and measurement of the residual volume.[79] In MS, detrusor hyperreflexia will invariably be present in patients with irritative urinary symptoms (frequency, urgency, urge incontinence) and pyramidal

tract signs in their legs.[5] For patients with MS and bladder dysfunction, treatment can be often instituted on the basis of the symptoms and the residual.

In IPD and cerebrovascular disease, detrusor hyperreflexia is the most common finding during filling Cystometrogram (CMG). However, patients with IPD or cerebrovascular disease are often at an age in which urological disease is common. Voiding CMG may help establish if there is bladder outflow obstruction due to prostatic enlargement in men with neurological disease and urinary symptoms (Fig 4.7).

4.9.4 Sphincter EMG

In the literature, the term "sphincter EMG" is often applied to two different tests. A concentric needle electrode can be positioned in the external sphincter and analysis of individual motor units undertaken.[61,80] This form of detailed EMG study enables changes within the muscle due to denervation and reinnervation to be investigated.[61] Sphincter EMG can also be performed to examine the pattern of activity of the sphincter muscle. This type of EMG test is performed in conjunction with urodynamic studies to examine the activity of the urethral sphincter in relation to detrusor function (see Figs 4.1 and 4.3)

592

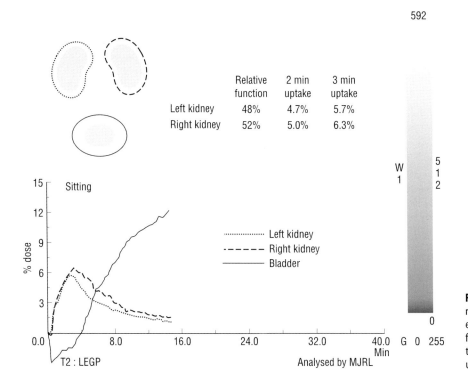

Figure 4.8 A normal MAG3 renogram. There is almost equal (48% and 52%) renal function in both kidneys, and the graph indicates a normal urine flow from the kidneys.

4.9.5 "Urological" Investigations

If the clinician suspects pathology such as BPH then the relevant urological investigation is required. Neurogenic bladder dysfunction may result in urinary tract complications, including infection, stones and dilatation of the upper urinary tracts. A plain radiograph of the abdomen may reveal stones in the urinary tract. The anatomical condition of the urinary tracts may be investigated by intravenous pyelography and ultrasonography. Isotopic renography provides a means of assessing drainage from the kidneys and split renal function (Fig. 4.8).

Endoscopic examination of the bladder by flexible cystoscopy, under local anaesthesia, is particularly useful in detecting strictures, bladder tumours and stones.

4.10 Treatment of Bladder Dysfunction in Neurological Disease

This section deals with the conservative treatment of bladder dysfunction in neurological disease. Treatment must be modified according to the patient's disabilities and wishes, cognitive function and nature of the underlying neurological disorder. Conditions such as MS and MSA are very likely to progress, and this must be taken into account in deciding on treatment. In patients with neurologic disease, the inconvenience and occasional complications of treatment should be measured against the possible benefits.

Suprasacral and suprapontine lesions tend to result in detrusor hyperreflexia because the normal inhibitory control of the higher centres on the micturition reflex is diminished or absent. Lesions between the PMC and the sacral cord, in addition to bladder hyperreflexia, may also cause detrusor sphincter dyssynergia with incomplete bladder emptying.

For many patients with neurological disease and urinary symptoms, conservative treatment is directed towards controlling the detrusor hyperreflexia with anticholinergic medication and instituting intermittent cathetcrisation if there is incomplete emptying.

Patients with diseases involving the spinal cord often have difficulty understanding the vesicourethral function: overactivity of the bladder, but incomplete emptying due to a failure of external urethral sphincter relaxation. Patients will benefit from an explanation of the abnormal bladder function in relation to their neurological disease.

Renal failure due to neurogenic bladder dysfunction is unusual in patients with neurologic disease but it is an important problem after spinal cord injury and in those with congenital spinal cord abnormalities.

4.10.1 Intermittent Catheterisation

Frankel and Guttmann, in 1966, first proposed intermittent catheterisation as an alternative to long-term catheterisation in patients with spinal cord injury.[67] In this procedure a catheter is passed into the bladder to drain the residual urine and then removed. Intermittent catheterisation has transformed the management of patients with neurogenic bladder disorders. At first, it was carried out as an aseptic procedure[81] but later it was shown to be safe when undertaken in a clean manner.[82] Clean intermittent self-catheterisation is a well-established technique for improving bladder emptying and has been successfully practised by children and adults.[83] In general, only patients with residual volumes of more than 100 ml are likely to benefit from intermittent catheterisation. If detrusor hyperreflexia is present, then the full benefit from intermittent catheterisation will only be obtained if the hyperreflexia is managed by anticholinergic medication.

Intermittent catheterisation is undertaken 1–6 times a day; it is often best if the patient determines the frequency of catheterisation for him- or herself. A continence advisor or a urology nurse specialist will teach the technique; women usually need the aid of a mirror to learn the procedure. Manual dexterity, motivation, mobility and cognitive function are important factors in determining a patient's ability to carry out clean intermittent catheterisation.

Various types of catheter are available for intermittent catheterisation; the usual size is 10–12Ch for women and 12–14Ch for men. The catheters are available in female and male lengths. Some catheters are made from polyvinyl chloride and if they are washed after each use the catheter may be used for up to 7 days. Some single-use catheters have a hydrophilic coating, which is activated after immersing in water.

UTI is a surprisingly infrequent complication of clean intermittent catheterisation. If recurrent infections occur then using a new catheter for each catheterisation may reduce the problem and low-dose antibiotic prophylaxis might be indicated.

4.11 Therapy for Detrusor Hyperreflexia

4.11.1 Anticholinergic Agents

Detrusor hyperreflexia is most usually managed by drug therapy. Many pharmacological agents have been used for hyperreflexia; the most effective have been those with predominately anticholinergic action, which act by blocking the effect of acetylcholine on muscarinic receptors. Oxybutinin is probably the most common non-specific antimuscarinic in use today for detrusor hyperreflexia, and the drug also has some direct smooth muscle relaxant properties.[84] Oxybutinin has been used in clinical practice for over 30 years and remains a very useful part of the uroneurologists armamentarium. The dosage of oxybutinin is limited by the anticholinergic side-effects: dry mouth, constipation and blurred vision are the most frequent problems. In recent years drugs have been developed which are said to be more specific to bladder antimuscarinics.[85,86]

All of the agents with anticholinergic action may exacerbate the tendency to incomplete bladder emptying and urinary retention. The residual volume should be measured before commencing therapy, and if it is more than 100 ml then intermittent catheterisation should be instituted. If the residual is less than 100 ml then the patient should be prepared for the possibility of needing intermittent catheterisation; this will depend upon the effect of the anticholinergic on bladder emptying.

4.11.2 Capsaicin

Capsaicin is the pungent ingredient in red-hot chilli peppers. The first use of intravesical capsaicin in human bladders was reported in 1989.[87] Capsaicin blocks the C-fibre-mediated long latency micturition reflex in cats.[88] In humans, intravesical capsaicin can increase bladder capacity and decrease hyperreflexic contractions. The beneficial effect may last for up to 3 months.[89–91]

4.11.3 Desmopressin

In neurogenic bladder dysfunction, nocturnal urinary frequency may be a problem and some patients may benefit from DDAVP (desmopressin), a synthetic antidiuretic hormone.[92,93] Desmopressin is available as a nasal spray or tablets and when taken before going to bed reduces urine output for 6–8 h. It increases the reabsorption of water in the collecting tubule of the kidney and should be used with caution in patients over the age of 65 years. It is reasonable for some patients to use desmopressin on a very occasional basis in the daytime for an important event such as attending a wedding.[94]

4.11.4 Chronic Indwelling Catheter

In some circumstances an indwelling catheter may be the best option to ensure personal hygiene and adequate bladder drainage. Despite the disadvantages of a long-term indwelling catheter, there are times when the insertion of a catheter can provide the patient with a welcome relief from incontinence.

The complications of long-term catheterisation include blockage of the catheter, leakage alongside the catheter, urethral erosion, infection and stone formation. Bypassing around a urethral catheter is a common problem, resulting usually from uninhibited detrusor contractions. It may be resolved by anticholinergic medication. Suprapubic catheterisation has several benefits over long-term urethral catheterisation, including avoidance of urethral destruction, ease of changing, improved catheter hygiene and facilitation of sexual activity.[95,96] The initial insertion of a suprapubic catheter is not without complications, and an experienced urologist should undertake it. The first catheter change is often performed in a hospital clinic, but thereafter is usually undertaken in the patient's home by a qualified nurse. If a patient with a suprapubic catheter has very marked bladder hyperreflexia, which is not controlled with anticholinergics, then urethral leakage may continue to be a problem.

If the bladder is of good capacity then it may be possible for the patient to use a catheter valve rather than attaching the tube to a free drainage bag. The catheter valve enables the bladder to fill and be emptied at a convenient time. A certain degree of manual dexterity is required to operate the valve mechanism; alternatively, a carer may undertake this. The catheter valve can be used with either a urethral or a suprapubic catheter.

4.11.5 Appliances

The most commonly used appliances for containing urinary leakage are penile sheaths and absorbent pads. The penile sheath fits over the penis and connects to a drainage bag. In women, there is no widely used external appliance for the containment of urinary leakage.

Absorbent pads are widely used by patients and there is a considerable range of products available. The continence advisor or specialist urology nurse is the best professional to advise about the most suitable appliance or absorbent product for a patient.

4.12 Summary

In neurologic disease, the urinary symptoms can be the most distressing aspect of the disorder for the patient, carers and family. Explanation of the cause of the bladder dysfunction in relation to the neurological disease process is likely to be of great benefit to the patient and those concerned with providing care. The main forms of conservative treatment are pharmacotherapy for control of detrusor hyperreflexia and intermittent catheterisation to ensure satisfactory bladder emptying. Effective therapy is available for many patients with central nervous system disease and urinary symptoms. It is important that the professionals involved in the care of patients with neurological impairment have a good knowledge of the modern management of the bladder dysfunction in neurological disease.

References

1. Oppenheim H (1889) Weitre notizen zur pathologie der disseminerten sklerose. Charite-ann 14: 412–18.
2. Ivers RR, Goldstein NP (1963) Multiple sclerosis: a current appraisal of symptoms and signs. Proc Mayo Clin 38: 457–66.
3. Miller H, Simpson CA, Yeates WF (1965) Bladder dysfunction in multiple sclerosis. BMJ 1: 1265–9.
4. Goldstein I, Siroky MB, Sax S et al. (1982) Neurogenic abnormalities in multiple sclerosis. J Urol 128: 541–5.
5. Betts CD, D'Mellow MT, Fowler CJ et al. (1993) Urinary symptoms and the neurological features of bladder dysfunction in multiple sclerosis. J Neurol Neurosurg Psychiat 56: 245–250.
6. Betts CD (1999) Bladder and sexual dysfunction in multiple sclerosis. In: Fowler CJ (ed) Neurology of Bladder, Bowel and Sexual Dysfunction. Butterworth-Heinemann, Boston, pp. 289–308.
7. Fowler CJ, Kirby RS (1985) Abnormal electromyographic activity (decelerating bursts and complex repetitive discharges) in the striated muscle of the urethral sphincter in 5 women in urinary retention. Br J Urol 57: 67–70.
8. Betts CD (1997) Multiple sclerosis presenting solely with bladder disturbance (letter). Br J Urol 80: 513–14.
9. Parkinson J (1817) An essay on the shaking palsy. Whittingham and Rowland, London.
10. Quinn N (1989) Multiple system atrophy – the nature of the beast. J Neurol Neurosurg Psychiat Suppl: 78–89.
11. Quinn N (1995) Parkinsonism – recognition and differential diagnosis. BMJ 310: 447–52.
12. Murnaghan GF (1961) Neurogenic disorders of the bladder in Parkinsonism. Br J Urol 33: 403–9.
13. Moore T (1960) The neurogenic bladder in a general hospital. Proc R Soc Med 53: 266–72.
14. Andersen JT, Hebjorn S, Frimodt-Moller C et al. (1976) Disturbances of micturition in Parkinson's disease. Acta Neurol Scand 53: 161–70.
15. Greenberg M, Gordon HL, McCutchen JJ (1972) Neurogenic bladder in Parkinson's disease. South Med J 65: 446.
16. Porter RW, Bors E (1971) Neurogenic bladder in Parkinsonism: effect of thalamotomy. J Neurosurg 34: 27.
17. Borrie MJ, Campbell AJ, Caradoc-Davies TH, Spears GFS (1986) Urinary incontinence after stroke: a prospective study. Age Ageing 15: 177–181.
18. Brocklehurst JC, Andrews K, Richards B, Laycock PJ (1985) Incidence and correlates of incontinence in stroke patients. J Am Geriatr Soc 33: 540–2.
19. Wade D, Langton-Hewer R (1985) Outlook after an acute stroke: urinary incontinence and loss of consciousness compared in 532 patients. Q J Med 56: 601–8.
20. Barer D, Mitchell J (1989) Predicting the outcome of acute stroke: do multivariate models help? Q J Med 70: 27–39.
21. Barer D (1989) Continence after stroke: useful predictor or goal therapy. Age Ageing 18: 183–91.
22. Sakakibara R, Fowler CJ (1999) Cerebral control of bladder, bowel and sexual function and effects of brain disease. In: Fowler CJ (ed) Neurology of Bladder, Bowel and Sexual Dysfunction. Butterworth-Heinemann, Boston, pp. 229–43.
23. Gosling JA, Dixon JS, Critchley HOD et al. (1981) A comparative study of the human external sphincter and periurethral levator ani muscles. Br J Urol 53: 35–41.
24. Onufrowicz B (1899) Notes on the arrangement and function of the cell groups in the sacral region of the spinal cord. J Nerv Ment Dis 26: 498–504.
25. Barrington FJF (1921) The relation of the hind-brain micturition. Brain 44: 23–53.
26. Kuru M, Yamamoto H (1964) Fiber connections of the pontine detrusor nucleus (Barrington). J Comp Neurol 123: 161–85.
27. Andrew J, Nathan PW (1964) Lesions of the anterior frontal lobes and disturbances of micturition and defaecation. Brain 87: 233–62.
28. Betts CD (1996) Neurogenic bladder induced by brain abscess (letter). Br J Urol 77: 932–3.
29. de Groat WC (1975) Nervous control of the urinary bladder of the cat. Brain Res 87: 201–11.
30. de Groat WC (1990) Central neural control of the lower urinary tract. In: Bock G, Whelan J (eds) Neurobiology of Incontinence. Wiley, Chichester, pp. 27–42.
31. Blok BFM, Willemsen AT, Holstege G (1997) A PET study on brain control of micturition in humans. Brain 120: 111–121.
32. Blok BFM, Sturms LM, Holstege G (1998) Brain activation during micturition in women. Brain 121: 2033–42.
33. Fowler CJ (1998) Brain activation during micturition. Brain 121: 2031–2.

34. International Continence Society Committee (1988) The standardisation of terminology of lower urinary tract function. Scand J Urol Nephrol 114: 5–19.

35. Piazza DH, Diokno AC (1979) Review of neurogenic bladder in multiple sclerosis. Urology 14: 33–5.

36. Blaivas JG, Bhimani G, Labib KB (1979) Vesicourethral dysfunction in multiple sclerosis. J Urol 122: 342–7.

37. Poppel H Van, Vereecken RL, Leruitte A (1983) Neuromuscular abnormalities multiple sclerosis. Paraplegia 21: 374–9.

38. Philp T, Read DJ, Higson RH (1981) The urodynamic characteristics of multiple sclerosis. Brit J Urol 53: 672–5.

39. Awad SA, Gajewski JB, Sogbein SK et al. (1984) Relationship between neurological and urological status in multiple sclerosis. J Urol 132: 499–502.

40. Vas CJ (1969) Sexual impotence and some autonomic disturbances in men with multiple sclerosis. Acta Neurol Scand 45: 166–84.

41. Betts CD, D'Mellow MT, Fowler CJ (1994) Erectile dysfunction in multiple sclerosis: associated neurological and neurophysiological deficits, and treatment of the condition. Brain 117: 1303–10.

42. Litwiller SE, Frohman EM, Zimmern PE (1999) Multiple sclerosis and the urologist. J Urol 161(3): 743–57.

43. Andersen JT, Bradley WE (1976) Cystometric, sphincter and electromyelographic abnormalities in Parkinson's disease. J Urol 116: 75–8.

44. Pavlakis AJ, Siroky MB, Goldstein I, Krane RJ (1983) Neurourologic findings in Parkinson's disease. J Urol (1): 80–83.

45. Lewin RJ, Dillard GV, Porter RW (1967) Extrapyramidal inhibition of the urinary bladder. Brain Res 4: 301–7.

46. Yoshimura N, Sas M, Yoshida O, Takaori S (1992) Dopamine D1 receptor-mediated inhibition of micturition reflex by central dopamine from the substantia nigra. Neurourol Urodyn 11: 535–45.

47. Fitzmaurice H, Fowler CJ, Rickards D et al. (1985) Micturition disturbance in Parkinson's disease. Br J Urol 57: 652–6.

48. Christmas TJ, Chapple CR, Lees AJ et al. (1988) Role of subcutaneous apomorphine in parkinsonian voiding dysfunction. Lancet 2: 1451–3.

49. Aranda B, Cramer P (1993) Effect of apomorphine and L-dopa on the parkinsonian bladder. Neurourol Urodyn 12(3): 203–9.

50. Galloway NTM (1983) Urethral sphincter abnormalities in Parkinsonism. Br J Urol 55(6): 691–3.

51. Graham JG, Oppenheimer DR (1969) Orthostatic hypotension and nicotine sensitivity in a case of multiple system atrophy. J Neurol Neurosurg Psychiat 32: 28–34.

52. Wenning GK, Ben Shlomo Y, Magalhaes M et al. (1994) Clinical features and natural history of multiple system atrophy – an analysis of 100 cases. Brain 117: 835–45.

53. Chandiramani VA, Fowler CJ (1999) Urogenital disorders in Parkinson's disease and multiple system atrophy. In: Fowler CJ (ed) Neurology of bladder, bowel and sexual dysfunction. Butterworth-Heinemann, Oxford, pp. 245–53.

54. Oppenheimer DR (1988) Neuropathology of autonomic failure. In: Bannister R (ed) Autonomic failure. A textbook of Clinical Disorders of the Autonomic Nervous System. Oxford University Press, Oxford, pp. 451–64.

55. Beck RO, Betts CD, Fowler CJ (1994) Genitourinary dysfunction in multiple system atrophy: clinical features and treatment in 62 cases. J Urol 151: 1336–41.

56. Sakuta MS, Nakanishi T, Tohokura Y (1978) Anal muscle electromyograms differ in amyotrophic lateral sclerosis and Shy-Drager syndrome. Neurology 28(12): 1289–93.

57. Eardley I, Quinn NP, Fowler CJ et al. (1989) The value of urethral sphincter electromyography in the differential diagnosis of parkinsonism. Br J Urol 64(4): 360–2.

58. Chandiramani VA, Palace J, Fowler CJ (1997) How to recognize patients with parkinsonism who should not have urological surgery. Br J Urol 80(1): 100–4.

59. Berger Y, Salinas JN, Blaivas JG (1990) Urodynamic differentiation of Parkinson's disease and the Shy Drager syndrome. Neurourol Urodyn 9: 117–21.

60. Palace J, Chandiramani VA, Fowler CJ (1997) Value of sphincter electromyography in the diagnosis of multiple system atrophy. Muscle Nerve 20: 1396–1403.

61. Vodusek DB, Fowler CJ (1999) Clinical neurophysiology. In: Fowler CJ (ed) Neurology of Bladder, Bowel, and Sexual Dysfunction. Butterworth-Heinemann, Oxford, pp. 109–43.

62. Khan Z, Hertanu J, Yang W et al. (1981) Predictive correlation of urodynamic dysfunction and brain injury after cerebrovascular accident. J Urol 126: 86–8.

63. Khan Z, Starer P, Yang W, Bhola A (1990) Analysis of voiding disorders in patients with cerebrovascular accidents. Urology 35: 263–70.

64. Tsuchida S, Noto H, Yamaguchi O, Itoh M (1983) Urodynamic studies on hemiplegic patients after cerebrovascular accidents. Urology 21: 315–18.

65. Sakakibara R, Hattori T, Yasuda K, Yamanishi T (1996) Micturitional disturbance after acute hemispheric stroke: analysis of the lesion by CT and MRI. J Neurol Sci 137: 47–56.

66. Larson JW, Swenson WM, Utz DC, Steinhilber RM (1963) Psychogenic urinary retention in women. JAMA 184: 697–700.

67. Margolis G (1965) A review of the literature on psychogenic urinary retention. J Urol 94: 257–8.

68. Bird P (1980) Psychogenic urinary retention. Psychother Psychosom 34: 45–51.

69. Bassi P, Zattoni F, Aragona F et al. (1988) Psychogenic urinary retention in women. Diagnostic and therapeutic aspects. J Urol 94: 159–62.

70. Swinn MJ, Fowler CJ (1999) Nonpsychogenic urinary retention in young women. In: Fowler CJ (ed) Neurology of bladder, bowel and sexual dysfunction. Butterworth-Heinemann, Oxford, pp. 367–71.

71. Fowler CJ (1995) Pelvic Floor Neurophysiology. In: Osselton JW, Binnie CD, Cooper R et al. (eds) Clinical neurophysiology: EMG, Nerve conduction and Evoked Potentials. Butterworth-Heinemann, Oxford, pp. 233–52.

72. Jensen D, Stein R (1996) The importance of complex repetitive discharges in the striated female urethral and male bulbocavernosus muscle. Scand J Urol Nephrol Suppl 179: 69–73.

73. Webb RJ, Fawcett PRW, Neal DE (1992) Electromyographic abnormalities in the urethral sphincter and anal sphincters of women with idiopathic retention of urine. Br J Urol 70: 22–25.

74. Chandler BJ (1999) Impact of Neurologic Disability on Sex and Relationships. In: Fowler CJ (ed) Neurology of bladder, bowel and sexual dysfunction. Butterworth-Heinemann, Oxford, pp. 69–93.

75. Hatzichristou DG (1999) Treatment of Sexual Dysfunction and Infertility in Patients with Neurologic Diseases. In: Fowler CJ (ed) Neurology of bladder, bowel and sexual dysfunction. Butterworth-Heinemann, Oxford, pp. 209–25.

76. Fowler CJ (1996) Investigation of the neurogenic bladder. J Neurol Neurosurg Psychiat 60: 6–13.

77. Kornhuber H, Schulz A (1990) Efficient treatment of neurogenic bladder disorders in multiple sclerosis with initial intermittent catheterisation and ultrasound-controlled training. Eur J Neurol 30: 260.

78. Fowler CJ (1999) Neurological disorders of micturition and their treatment. Brain 122(7): 1213–31.

79. Fowler CJ, Kerrebroeck PE van, Nordenbo A, Poppel H Van (1992) Treatment of lower urinary tract dysfunction in patients with multiple sclerosis. Committee of the European Study Group of SUDIMS. J Neurol Neurosurg Psychiat 55: 986–9.
80. Fowler CJ, Betts CD (1994) Clinical value of Electrophysiological Investigations of Patients with Urinary Symptoms. In: Mundy AR, Stephenson TP, Wein AJ (eds) Urodynamics; Principles, Practice and Application. Churchill Livingstone, Edinburgh, UK, pp. 165–81.
81. Guttmann L, Frankel H (1966) The value of intermittent catheterisation in the early management of traumatic paraplegia and tetraplegia. Paraplegia 4: 63–84.
82. Lapides J, Diokno AC, Lowe BS et al. (1974) Follow up on unsterile, intermittent self catheterisation. J Urol 111: 184–7.
83. Webb RJ, Lawson AL, Neal DE (1990) Clean intermittent self-catheterisation in 172 adults. Br J Urol 65: 20–3.
84. Gajewski JB, Awad SA (1986) Oxybutinin versus probantheline in patients with multiple sclerosis and detrusor hyperreflexia. J Urol 135: 966–8.
85. Nilvebrant L, Glas G, Jonsson A, Sparf B (1994) The in vitro pharmacological profile of tolterodine – a new agent for the treatment of urinary urge incontinence. Neurourol Urodyn 13: 433–5.
86. Rentzhog L, Stanton SL, Cardozo L et al. (1998) Efficacy and safety of tolterodine in patients with detrusor hyperreflexia: a dose ranging study. Br J Urol 81: 42–8.
87. Maggi CA, Barbanti G, Santicioli P et al. (1989) Cystometric evidence that capsaicin-sensitive nerves modulate the afferent branch of the micturition reflex in humans. J Urol 142: 150–4.
88. Groat WC de, Kawatani M, Hisamitsu T et al. (1990) Mechanisms underlying the recovery of urinary bladder function following spinal cord injury. J Auton Nerv Syst 30 (Suppl): S71–8.
89. Fowler CJ, Beck RO, Gerrard S et al. (1994) Intravesical capsaicin for treatment of detrusor hyperreflexia. J Neurol Neurosurg Psychiat 57: 585–9.
90. Dasgupta P, Chandiramani V, Fowler CJ et al. (1996) Intravesical capsaicin: its effects on nerve densities in the human bladder. Neurol Urodyn 15: 373–4.
91. Cruz F, Guimaraes M, Silva C, Reis M (1997) Suppression of bladder hyperreflexia by intravesical resiniferotoxin. Lancet 350: 640–1.
92. Hilton P, Hertogs G, Wall H de, Dalm E (1983) The use of desmopressin (DDAVP) for nocturia in women with multiple sclerosis. J Neurol Neurosurg Pyschiat 46: 854–5.
93. Kinn A-C, Larsson P (1990) Desmopressin: a new principle for symptomatic treatment of urgency and incontinence in patients with multiple sclerosis. Scand J Urol Nephrol 24: 109–12.
94. Hoverd PA, Fowler CJ (1998) Desmopressin in the treatment of daytime urinary frequency in patients with multiple sclerosis. J Neurol Neurosurg Psychiat 65(5): 778–80.
95. MacDiarmid SA, Arnold EP, Palmer NB, Anthony A (1995) Management of spinal cord injured patients by indwelling suprapubic catheterisation. J Urol 154: 492–4.
96. Sheriff MK, Foley S, McFarlane J et al. (1998) Long-term suprapubic catheterisation: clinical outcome and satisfaction survey. Spinal Cord 36(3): 171–6.

5 The Ageing Lower Urinary Tract

A. Wagg

The major problem defining the changes in lower urinary tract function associated with age, especially in humans, has been that of ascribing causality. Studies in elderly people have been typified by a lack of age-matched controls and it is only recently that this has, to an extent, been rectified. This chapter summarises what is currently understood about age-related changes in lower urinary tract function, drawing upon human data. The limitations of these data are discussed and areas of current debate are highlighted.

5.1 Basic Architecture

The bladder muscle, the detrusor, is made up of smooth muscle cells in bundles surrounded by a matrix of collagen and elastin. The smooth muscle fibres are not arranged in any particular orientation; each is sheathed by a collagen sheet. These join loosely to unite the muscle bundles. Each individual myocyte is enclosed within its own collagenous matrix. This linkage enables the tension generated by myocytes to be transmitted across the entire muscle. Elastin fibres appear to be arranged in a loose network around these muscle fascicles.[1]

Most studies concerned with age-associated changes in the bladder are derived from cross-sectional analysis of human bladder specimens, so ascribing the reported changes to ageing is difficult. Most have noted an increase in bladder weight,[2,3] and an increase in the ratio of collagen to smooth muscle of the order of 20–30% in elderly people when compared to younger controls. The absolute increase in collagen appears to be greater for women.[4] There appears to be a change in the predominant form of collagen from type I to type III. This type forms more cross-linkages and con-

tributes to an increased stiffness, resulting in the decreased compliance of the elderly bladder. These findings, once thought to be due to the influence of prostatic outflow tract obstruction, have been described both in the presence and absence of such obstruction and are described in age-matched women.[5] Outflow tract obstruction is rare in women.[6]

A reduction in the number of acetylcholinesterase-containing nerves in association with increasing age has been seen, but available data are conflicting[5,7] and the conclusions of studies must be considered in the light of the limitations of the analytical methods used. The appearance of bladder wall trabeculation, originally associated with increasing age and the development of prostatic hypertrophy and outflow tract obstruction, is now almost invariably associated with detrusor instability.[8,9] An increase in muscle cell size in association with outflow tract obstruction is generally described.[10] Electron microscopy studies of bladder from elderly people have reported a tight association between structural abnormality, detrusor contractile function and urodynamic diagnosis.[11] These abnormalities are common to elderly men and women, and are reflected in the detrusor muscle, its interstitium and in the surrounding nerves.[12,13] However, other studies using a similar method have reported a random occurrence of these same ultrastructural changes throughout the elderly population, regardless of underlying diagnosis.[14] It is difficult to reach a firm conclusion regarding the relevance of such described changes, and there is clearly room for more work in this area. However, given that disease is likely to occur along a continuum, it is unlikely that such a clear distinction between ultrastructural abnormality and pathological diagnosis can be made.

5.2 Functional Studies

Much of the data regarding changes in lower urinary tract function are derived from studies of individuals with lower urinary tract symptoms who have undergone urodynamic studies. Data from community-dwelling, continent individuals are sparse, but, where they do exist, tend to confirm the associations identified by other means. There is, as ever, an inadequate definition of "normal" in later life. When compared to norms from younger individuals only 18% of normal community-dwelling elderly men and women have been reported as having normal lower urinary tract function.[15] There is an increase in the prevalence of people with urinary frequency in later life.[16] Significant features are a reduced bladder capacity, an increased incidence of detrusor instability, an increased incidence of outflow tract obstruction, and alterations in renal function and water and solute excretion. Factors unrelated to the function of the lower urinary tract include concomitant cardiovascular, neurological and musculoskeletal disease and the effects of drug therapy and environmental change, all of which promote an increased frequency of micturition in an attempt to avoid incontinence.

Detrusor contractile function as measured in vivo by an index of maximal speed of muscle shortening (Fig. 5.1), bladder capacity (Fig. 5.2) and urinary flow rates (Fig. 5.3) all appear to decline in association with greater age in both sexes, although the decline in contractile function is not so apparent in men.[17]

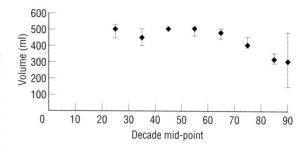

Figure 5.2 Increased age is associated with a reduction in bladder capacity.[17]

Studies of contractile function of the bladder using urodynamic variables rely on measures using bladder pressures.[18,19] The relationship between pressure and flow depends on bladder volume and variation during voiding, owing to the interaction of flow with the properties of the outflow tract. There are data suggesting that Q*, a measure of isotonic contractile function,[20] is able to differentiate "fast" from "slow" contracting bladders and may accurately predict the occurrence of voiding difficulty following colposuspension for stress incontinence.[21] However, the relationship between urodynamic measures and contractility of the bladder has not been established.

There is also an increase in the prevalence of incomplete emptying, as demonstrated by the existence of a significant post-micturition residual volume of urine[22] (Fig. 5.4). In men, the progressive enlargement of the prostate with age tends to dominate the

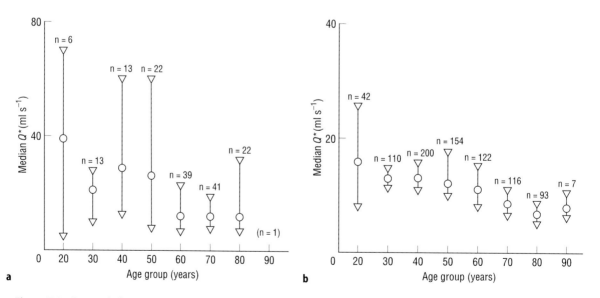

Figure 5.1 Contractile function as measured by Q* in association with greater age in men (**a**) and women (**b**) with lower urinary tract symptoms, n = 157.[17]

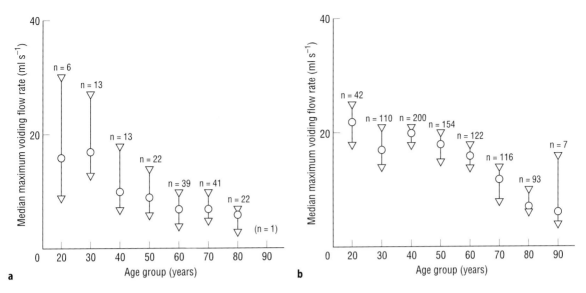

Figure 5.3   Median (95% CI) maximum flow rate for men (**a**) and women (**b**) with lower urinary tract symptoms in relation to greater age.[17]

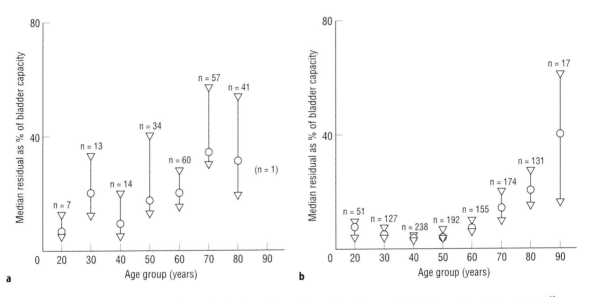

Figure 5.4   Post void residual volume of urine related to increasing age in men (**a**) and women (**b**) with lower urinary tract symptoms.[17]

behaviour of the urinary outflow tract, up to half of all men suffering from outflow tract obstruction.[15] As obstruction increases, the bladder requires a greater contractile effort to overcome the effects of the obstruction, this eventually leads to a chronically overdistended bladder, which fails to empty effectively. In others acute urinary retention may develop. In women, the prevalence of ineffective voiding is much lower.[23]

Detrusor instability is conventionally thought to be associated with the development of outflow tract obstruction and is present in 43–86% of patients.[24]

This viewpoint has been reinforced by the fact that relief of the obstruction leads to bladder stability in a significant proportion.[25] However, once again, the incidence of detrusor instability increases in association with age per se, and is similar in women. In men with lower urinary tract symptoms, the likelihood of detrusor instability being the cause of these reaches 85% in the eighth decade, regardless of outflow tract obstruction.[17] The true incidence of symptomatic detrusor instability is unknown because of the inherent problem of under-reporting, but is estimated at 10–15% of men and women

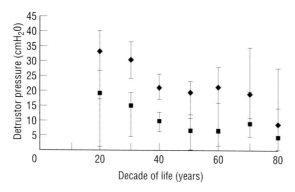

Figure 5.5 Detrusor pressures at urethral opening and closure for women with stable bladders in association with greater age.[31] Black diamonds (♦), detrusor pressure at urethral opening; black squares (■), detrusor pressure at urethral closure.

between 10 and 50 years, rising to 35% of those aged >75 years[26].

There are also age-associated changes in the sensory function of the bladder. The bladder capacity at first desire to void, as a proportion of bladder capacity, rises significantly in association with increasing age in women.[27] This suggests a decreasing sensitivity of the bladder to filling and this, coupled with the reduced maximal bladder capacity, tends to reduce the time that an individual has available to void successfully and appropriately. There may be an influence of higher centres accounting for this observation.[28]

5.3 Urethral Function

Studies using the urethral pressure profile[29,30] or detrusor closure pressures[31] have both described a reduction in urethral function in later life. There is evidence of an increased collagen content in the urethra of elderly women.[32] There is also a loss of striated muscle cells in the aged female urethral sphincter.[33]

5.4 Nocturia

There is an increase in nocturnal frequency in elderly people.[34] This is due to a combination of factors:

In later life the majority of urine production occurs nocturnally.[35]

- In older individuals, renal concentrating ability falls[36,37] and glomerular filtration rate increases in the supine position.

- There is a redistribution of fluid at night, particularly if the individual has venous insufficiency or is on medication that predisposes to the development of peripheral oedema, such as calcium channel blockers or non-steroidal anti-inflammatory agents.

- In addition, some older adults have a delayed diuresis in response to a fluid load and lose their diurnal rhythm of ADH secretion,[38] although there are studies in other groups showing no such loss.[39]

All in all, this means that the kidneys are working harder overnight to produce greater quantities of more dilute urine, the amount of which may be in excess of a smaller functional bladder capacity. The presence of nocturnal frequency (two or more episodes per night) has been reported as 13–29%, the latter figure from an older age group.[40,41] There is evidence for the efficacy of DDAVP[42] and early evening diuretic,[43] and limited evidence for daytime recumbence[44] in treating nocturia, but these are not well tolerated by all. In particular, the usefulness of DDAVP may be limited to patients with true nocturnal polyuria rather than urinary frequency,[45] and its use may be hampered by drug–drug interactions predisposing to hyponatraemia.

Primary nocturnal enuresis may persist into adulthood. This affects approximately 0.6–1% of all adults, and 50% of sufferers had never sought help for the problem.[46] Most men with persistent nocturnal enuresis, up to the age of 65 years, appear to have underlying detrusor instability.[47-49] Treatment with imipramine has shown a marked antidiuretic effect on patients with nocturnal polyuria.[50] A study comparing the use of DDAVP with the antimuscarinic medication oxybutynin showed no difference in improvement between the DDAVP group and combination treatment. The incidence of nocturnal incontinence also increases linearly in association with greater age. This incidence is increased in the presence of concomitant urinary storage disorders.[51] Once the relative contributions of associated conditions can be established, intervention studies may be better planned.

5.5 Conclusion

The changes in urinary tract structure and function identified in association with greater age enable the generation of hypotheses which will enable prospective, longitudinal studies to be undertaken. The interrelationship of urinary tract symptoms, co-existent diseases and their treatment make the conclusions from studies conducted in elderly people more difficult to interpret, and there is a continued need for studies utilising younger controls. The lack of normal data in elderly people makes the identification of abnormal function more problematic. However, it is becoming clearer that the changes in the bladder once thought to be associated with prostatic outflow tract obstruction are apparently just as common in women. The incidence of detrusor instability also follows a similar pattern, regardless of outflow tract obstruction. Knowledge is accumulating, but there is still much to learn.

References

1. Murakumo M, Ushiki T, Abe K et al. (1995) Three-dimensional arrangement of collagen and elastin in the human urinary bladder: a scanning electron microscopic study. J Urol 154: 251–6.
2. Bercovich E, Barabino G, Pirozzi-Farina F, Deriu M (1999) A multivariate analysis of lower urinary tract ageing and urinary symptoms: the role of fibrosis. Arch Ital Urol Androl Dec 71(5): 287–92.
3. Susset JG, Servot-Viguier D, Lamy F, Madernas P, Black R (1978) Collagen in 155 human bladders. Invest Urol 16: 204–6.
4. Lepor H, Sunaryadi I, Hartano V, Shapiro E (1992) Quantitative morphometry of the adult human bladder. J Urol 148: 414–17.
5. Holm NR, Horn T, Hald T (1995) Detrusor in ageing and obstruction. Scand J Urol Nephrol 29: 45–49.
6. Resnick NM (1988) Voiding dysfunction in the elderly. In: Yalla SV, McGurie EJ, Elbadawi A, Blaivas JG (eds) Neurology and Urodynamics. Principles and practice. Macmillan, New York, pp. 303–30.
7. Gilpin SA, Gilpin CJ, Dixon JA, Kirby RS (1986) The effect of age on the autonomic innervation of the urinary bladder. Br J Urol 58: 378–81.
8. Leriche A (1989) Mécanisme des symptômes fonctionnels de l'hypertrophie bénigne de la prostate. Pathophysiologie et symptômes. In: Prostate et alpha bloquants. Exerpta Medica, Amsterdam, pp. 76–98.
9. Levy BJ, Wight NT (1990) Structural changes in the ageing submucosa: new morphologic criteria for the evaluation of the unstable human bladder. J Urol 144: 1044–55.
10. Gilpin SA, Gosling JA, Barnard JA (1985) Morphological and morphometric studies of the human obstructed, trabeculated urinary bladder. Br J Urol 57: 525–9.
11. Elbadawi A, Yalla SV, Resnick NM (1993) Structural basis of geriatric voiding dysfunction I. Method of a prospective ultrastructural urodynamic study and an overview of the findings. J Urol 150: 1650–6.
12. Elbadawi A, Yalla SV, Resnick NM (1993) Structural basis of geriatric voiding dysfunction III. Detrusor overactivity. J Urol 150: 1668–80.
13. Elbadawi A, Yalla SV, Resnick NM (1993) Structural basis of geriatric voiding dysfunction IV. Bladder outlet obstruction. J Urol 150: 1681–95.
14. Carey M, Jong S de, Moran P et al. (1997) The unstable bladder: Is there an ultrastructural basis? Neurourol Urodyn 16: 423–4.
15. Resnick NM, Elbadawi A, Yalla SV (1995) Age and the lower urinary tract: what is normal? Neurourol Urodyn 14: 577–9.
16. Saito M, Kondo A, Kato T, Yamada Y (1993) Frequency-volume charts: Comparison of frequency between elderly and adult patients. Br J Urol 72: 38–41.
17. Malone-Lee JG, Wahedna I (1993) Characterisation of detrusor contractile function in relation to old age. Br J Urol 72: 873–80.
18. Griffiths D, Mastrigt R van, Bosch R (1989) Quantification of urethral resistance and bladder function during voiding with special reference to the effects of prostate size reduction on urethral obstruction due to benign prostatic hyperplasia. Neurourol Urodyn 8: 17–27.
19. Schäfer W (1983) The contribution of the bladder outlet to the relation between pressure and flow rate during micturition. In Hinman FJr (Ed): Benign Prostatic Hypertrophy. Springer, New York, pp. 470–96.
20. Griffiths DJ (1980) Urodynamics: The mechanics and hydrodynamics of the lower urinary tract. Medical Physics Handbooks. Adam Hilger, Bristol.
21. Boos K, Cardozo L, Anders K, Malone-Lee JG (1996) The calculation of detrusor muscle velocity to explain voiding difficulties after Burch colposuspension. In: Proceedings of the International Continence Society Annual Meeting, Abstr 281.
22. Bonde HV, Sejr D, Erdmann L et al. (1996) Residual urine in 75 year old men and women. A normative population study. Scand J Urol Nephrol 30: 89–91.
23. Wagg AS, Malone-Lee JG (1997) Pressure flow plot analysis and voiding inefficiency in women with lower urinary tract symptoms. Neurourology Urodynamics 16: 435–7.
24. Cockett ATK, Khoury S, Aso Y et al. (1993) The effects of obstruction and ageing on the function of the lower urinary tract. In: Proceedings: The second International Consultation on Benign Prostatic Hyperplasia, 1993. Scientific Communication International, Jersey, Channel Islands.
25. Abrams PH, Farrar DJ, Turner-Warwick R, Whiteside CG, Fenely RCL (1979) The results of prostatectomy: a symptomatic and urodynamic analysis of 152 patients. J Urol 121(131): 640–2.
26. Abrams PH (1984) Bladder instability: Concept, clinical associations and treatment. Scand J Urol Nephrol 87 (Suppl 7).
27. Collas DM, Malone-Lee JG (1996) Age-associated changes in detrusor sensory function in women with lower urinary tract symptoms. Int Urogynecol J 7: 24–9.
28. Griffiths DJ, McCracken PN, Harrison GM, Gormley EA (1994) Cerebral aetiology of geriatric urge incontinence. Age Ageing 23: 246–50.
29. Rud T (1980) Urethral pressure profile in continent women from childhood to old age. Acta Obstetr Obstet Gynecol Scand 59: 331–5.
30. Wijma J, Tinga DJ, Visser GHA (1992) Compensatory mechanisms which prevent urinary incontinence in ageing women. Gynecol Obstet Invest 33: 102–4.
31. Wagg AS, Lieu PK, Ding YY, Malone-Lee JG (1996) A urodynamic analysis of age associated changes in urethral function in women with lower urinary tract symptoms. J Urol 156: 1984–8.
32. Susset J, Plante P (1980) Studies of female urethral pressure profile. Part II Urethral pressure profile in female incontinence. J Urol 123: 70–4.
33. Strasser H, Tiefenthaler M, Steinlechner M, Bartsch G, Konwalinka G (1999) Urinary incontinence in the elderly and age-dependent apoptosis of rhabdosphincter cells. Lancet Sep 11(354): 918–19.
34. Fultz HL, Herzog AR (1996) Epidemiology of urinary symptoms in the geriatric population. Urol Clin North Am 23: 1–10.
35. Kirkland JL, Lye M, Banerjee AK (1983) Patterns of urine flow and electrolyte excretion in healthy elderly people. BMJ 287: 1665–1667.
36. Rowe JW, Andres R, Tobin JD, Norri AH, Shock NW (1976) Age-adjusted standards for creatinine clearance. Ann Intern Med 84: 567–9.

37. Lewis WH, Alving AS (1938) Changes with age in the renal function of adult men. Am J Physiol 123: 500–15.

38. Asplund R, Aberg H (1993) Diurnal variation in the levels of antidiuretic hormone in the elderly. J Intern Med 229: 131.

39. Johnson AG, Crawford GA, Kelly D, Nguyen TV, Cyory AZ (1994) Arginine vasopressin and osmolality in the elderly. J Amer Geriatr Soc 42: 399–404.

40. Britton JP, Dowell AC, Whelan P (1990) Prevalence of urinary symptoms in men aged over 60. Br J Urol 66: 175–6.

41. Minors DS, Waterhouse JM (1981) Circadian Rhythms and the Human. Wright, Bristol, p. 182.

42. Hilton P, Stanton SL (1982) The use of desmopressin (DDAVP) in nocturnal frequency in the female. Br J Urol 54: 252–5.

43. Reynard JM, Cannon A, Yang Q, Abrams P (1998) A novel therapy for nocturnal polyuria: a double-blind randomized trial of frusemide against placebo. Br J Urol 81(2): 215–18.

44. O'Donnell PD, Beck C, Walls RC (1990) Serial incontinence assessment in elderly inpatient men. J Rehab Res Dev 27: 1–9.

45. Asplund R, A[o]berg H (1993) Desmopressin in elderly subjects with increased nocturnal diuresis. Scand J Urol Nephrol 27: 77–82.

46. Hirasing RA, van Leerdam FJ, Bolk-Bennink L, Janknegt RA (1997) Enuresis nocturna in adults. Scand J Urol Nephrol 31: 533–6.

47. Torrens MJ, Collins CD (1975) The urodynamic assessment of adult enuresis. Br J Urol 47: 433–40.

48. McGuire EJ, Savastano JA (1984) Urodynamic studies in enuresis and the non-neurogenic, neurogenic bladder. J Urol 132: 299–302.

49. Fidas A, Galloway NTM, McInnes A, Chisholm GD (1985) Neurophysiological measurements in primary adult enuretics. Br J Urol 57: 635–40.

50. Hunsballe JM, Rittig S, Pedersen EB, Olesen OV, Djurhuus JC (1997) Single dose imipramine reduces nocturnal urine output in patients with nocturnal enuresis and nocturnal polyuria. J Urol 158: 830–6.

51. Swithinbank LV, Donovan JL, Rogers CA, Abrams P (2000) Nocturnal incontinence in women: A hidden problem. J Urol 164: 764–6.

6 Patient Assessment

J. Laycock

6.1 Lower Urinary Tract Dysfunction

Bladder and bowel symptoms rarely occur in isolation and many are due to adaptive strategies; furthermore, multipathology often exists. To fully understand the pathophysiology of lower urinary tract (LUT) disorders, information is required about any problems during bladder filling and emptying, and the character, onset and duration of symptoms. Furthermore, all past and present obstetric, gynaecological, urological, medical and relevant surgical history should be documented, along with current drug therapy, including over-the-counter (OTC) medication. Finally, a physical examination is carried out, examining the abdomen, external genitalia and pelvic floor muscles.

In simple terms, LUT dysfunction can be considered to be a pathology of the bladder, e.g. overactive/underactive detrusor, small functional bladder capacity, sensory/motor urgency; or a problem of the outlet e.g. outlet obstruction or weakness of the sphincters and pelvic floor muscles (PFM), or a combination of all these storage and voiding factors.

6.2 Frequency/Volume Chart

The normal adult fluid output from the kidneys varies between 1 and 3 litres/24 h, with approximately 80% excreted during waking hours, obviating the need to empty the bladder at night, and the average adult bladder capacity is in the range 300–600 ml.[1]

Probably the most useful assessment tool is the frequency/volume chart (bladder diary); this chart is a means of self-recording the time and quantity of drinks and urine output and the time of incontinent episodes, over a period of 4–7 days (a 4-day chart is shown in Appendix 1). Ideally, the chart should be mailed to the patient prior to the first appointment, and completed by the patient or carer; consequently, the instructions must be easily understood.

Further questioning will be necessary to identify the types of drinks taken and the severity of incontinence; this can be measured by recording how often incontinence generally occurs, how much urine is lost at each incontinent episode, and the size and number of incontinence pads used per day or week. An assessment form is shown in Appendix 2.

In addition, it is important to identify what caused the incontinence; for example, was urine leakage caused by an increase in abdominal pressure, e.g. coughing, or was it caused by not getting to the toilet in time?

From the chart, the following information can be recorded:

6.2.1 Frequency of Voiding

Normal diurnal frequency is 6–8 voids/24 h. Increased frequency may be caused by increased fluid input, habit, medication (e.g. diuretics), reduced bladder capacity, detrusor instability and a number of medical conditions such as diabetes.

6.2.2 Nocturia

Nocturia is defined as being awakened each night by the need to urinate. More than one episode per night is bothersome and nocturia tends to increase with age. Nocturia may be due to the same causes as diurnal frequency, and often improves as daytime frequency reduces.

6.2.3 Frequency of Incontinence

Frequency of incontinent episodes should be recorded on the frequency/volume chart. However, the chart may not always represent the patient's problem, if a typical week is not recorded. Further questioning should elicit the actual frequency of incontinence episodes.

6.2.4 Voided Volume

Maximum and minimum voided volumes, and total volume voided over 24 h, give an indication of fluid intake, functional bladder capacity and bladder habits. However, fluid loss due to respiration, sweating in hot climates and activity will obviously reduce the fluid excreted by the kidneys. The first void of the day is generally the largest, unless a patient has nocturia.

6.3 Assessment Forms

An assessment form enables the health professional to compile present and past history relevant to the presenting problem, including the urological symptoms, in an orderly and systematic way. The form shown in Appendix 2 is designed to facilitate an audit of clinical outcomes, by recording at the initial visit and on discharge, the presence and severity of LUT symptoms, in addition to information gained from the frequency/volume chart and other investigations. Various items on the form are discussed below.

6.3.1 Activities

Any lifestyle activities, occupation or hobbies that may cause incontinence should be discussed.

6.3.2 Stress Incontinence

Stress incontinence is the involuntary loss of urine during increases in intra-abdominal pressure, e.g. coughing or sneezing. It may be due to urethral hypermobility, an incompetent bladder neck, an incompetent urethral sphincter mechanism or a combination of all three.

6.3.3 Urgency

This is the term applied to a strong desire to void which may be due to a hypersensitive bladder (sensory urgency) or an unstable bladder (motor urgency).

6.3.4 Urge Incontinence

This describes incontinence associated with a strong desire to void and is related to an overactive bladder. Urge incontinence can be triggered in a variety of ways; for example, running water, coughing, "key-in-the-door" syndrome, or simply entering the bathroom.

6.3.5 Urinary flow

Patients should be questioned about hesitancy, or any change in their flow rate or time taken to complete voiding. It may not be abnormal to have hesitancy when trying to void less than 100 ml or very large amounts (>700 ml).

6.3.6 Incomplete Bladder Emptying

The bladder is intended to be compliant and relaxed during the storage of urine and to contract during the voiding phase, emptying to completion. Failure to empty completely may be due to a number of factors, including outflow obstruction, inability to relax the pelvic PFM and external urethral sphincter, or detrusor hypotonia/atonia. In many centres, an asymptomatic residual urine (RU) of 100 ml or less is often monitored, but not necessarily treated; however, it is important to view a post-void residual (PVR) in light of the functional bladder capacity.

6.3.7 Post-Micturition Dribble

Leakage after voiding is completed may be caused by failure of the detrusor to relax after urination, or failure of the PFM to contract and empty the penile urethra (in men) or failure of the normal milk-back mechanism returning urine in the proximal urethra to the bladder (men and women), or a combination of these problems (see Chapter 7).

6.3.8 Bladder Pain

Bladder pain during the storage phase, or dysuria (pain on voiding), should always be investigated. Pain may be due to a number of pathologies, including inflammatory conditions of the bladder and urethra, urethral syndrome and idiopathic hypersensitive bladder. Furthermore, tumours and stones may cause pain, in addition to pain following trauma and pelvic surgery. It is important that pain is distinguished from urgency or bladder fullness.

6.3.9 Haematuria

Evidence of blood in the urine should be investigated. Haematuria results from bleeding from the upper or lower urinary tract. Possible causes include kidney damage due to trauma, glomerulonephritis, pyelonephritis, strenuous activity, cystitis, urethritis, calculi and tumours.

6.3.10 Childhood Problems

It is always useful to ascertain whether a patient had urinary problems after the age of 5 years, including nocturnal enuresis and "giggle incontinence", as this may give a clue to the present condition.

6.3.11 Family History

It is not uncommon for LUT symptoms to be familial. This may be due to variation in collagen types, an underlying pathology or bladder habits, and may give a clue to prognosis.

6.3.12 Incontinence During Sexual Activity

Female patients should be questioned on the presence of coital incontinence. Incontinence on penetration is more likely to be due to stress incontinence, associated with pressure of the penis on the bladder base, whereas incontinence accompanying orgasm is more likely to be due to detrusor instability provoked by rhythmical parasympathetic discharge; both may be exacerbated by the woman lying supine under her partner.[2,3] Patients who report a considerable volume of urine leakage may be harbouring a large residual urine.

6.3 13 Severity of Incontinence

This can be measured by recording the frequency of incontinence, the amount of urine lost at each incontinence episode, or the number and size of pads used daily or weekly. However, the degree of wetness is a very personal affair and it is difficult to assess objectively, although 1-h and 24-h pad tests have been usefully used in research as an objective measurement of change.

6.3.14 Obstetric History

It is recognised that several factors connected with vaginal delivery may contribute to the increased risk of urinary incontinence[4] (also see Chapter 1):

- injury to connective tissue supports
- vascular damage to the pelvic structures
- damage to the pelvic nerves or muscles
- direct injury to the urinary tract.

6.3.15 Gynaecological History

It is important to enquire into the patient's menstrual and menopausal status, as the continence mechanisms are greatly influenced by hormonal changes. Many patients report worse symptoms during pregnancy and the week before their period, due to an increase in progesterone. Reduction in oestrogen levels in post menopausal women may produce an increase in irritative symptoms (see Chapter 3).

6.3.16 Surgical History

Patients often report the onset of incontinence after a surgical procedure, such as hysterectomy or spinal surgery. More research is required to ascertain the causes of this phenomenon, but intraoperative damage to neuromuscular and supporting structures has been proposed. Previous incontinence surgery should be noted.

6.3.17 Bowel History

Faecal incontinence or constipation may co-exist with LUT problems, and information on bowel habits and any dysfunction should be identified. An impacted rectum pressing on the urethra may cause outflow obstruction and difficult voiding, or constant pressure on the bladder, resulting in urgency. The complete assessment and treatment of bowel dysfunction is described in Chapters 20–22.

6.3.18 Medical History

Systemic disease processes which influence the LUT may be due to interference with innervation, for example multiple sclerosis, diabetes mellitus or degenerative disease of the spine. Chronic respiratory disease, respiratory allergies and smoking, causing repeated coughing or sneezing, should be documented, and appropriate treatment and advice given. Enquiries should be made of the history and frequency of urinary tract infection (UTI), as this may explain some irritative symptoms. The height and weight of all patients should be recorded, and counselling on obesity and its possible adverse effect on bladder control should be explained.

6.3.19 Drug Therapy

Present and past medication, including OTC remedies, should be recorded and evaluated, and enquiries should be made as to the use of hormone replacement therapy (HRT).

6.3.20 Previous Therapy

Previous surgery and drug therapies, including dose and length of treatment, should be recorded. Previous PFM re-education may have been ineffective, and enquiries should be made to ascertain the treatment received.

6.3.21 Urinalysis

This is an essential test for all patients complaining of LUT problems, especially those with irritative symptoms. See Chapter 7.12.

6.4 Investigations

The results of urodynamics and other upper and lower tract studies should be recorded (see Chapter 7).

6.4.1 Stop Test

Historically, health professionals have proposed that patients should exercise their PFM during micturition, by repeatedly stopping and starting the flow of urine. However, many respected clinicians believe that this is inappropriate[5] for the following reasons:

- possible reflux of urine to the kidneys with subsequent damage
- interference with the micturition reflexes, aimed at continuous contraction of the detrusor to completely empty the bladder, may cause the development of abnormal reflex activity
- patients unable to re-start urine flow may develop residual urine
- patients unable to stop the flow may become disillusioned

The stop test should be discouraged for all patients.

6.4.2 Physical Examination

It is advisable to have a department or hospital policy on consent procedures before any intimate examination. In all cases, it is necessary to obtain verbal, informed consent from the patient; in some institutions, written consent may be required. The Royal College of Obstetricians and Gynaecologists (RCOG) London, through the General Medical Council (GMC), have published the following guidelines for intimate examinations[6]:

- Explain that an intimate examination needs to be done and why.
- Explain what the examination will involve.
- Obtain the patient's permission.
- Whenever possible, offer a chaperone or invite the patient to bring a relative or friend.
- Give the patient privacy to undress and dress.
- Keep discussion relevant and avoid unnecessary personal comments.
- Encourage questions and discussion.

6.4.2.1 Neurological Examination

Testing of sacral dermatomes (Fig. 6.1) and myotomes supplied by S2–4 will give information on the integrity of these nerves; activation of dermatomes and myotomes supplied by S2–4 is thought to have an inhibitory effect on the sacral micturition reflex centre.[7]

Myotomes supplied by S2–4 include the PFM, external urethral and anal sphincters, and hip extensors and lateral rotators. In addition, the plantar flexors and the small muscles of the foot, (lumbricals and interossei) all derive some innervation from S2. If abnormalities are noted, or patients are

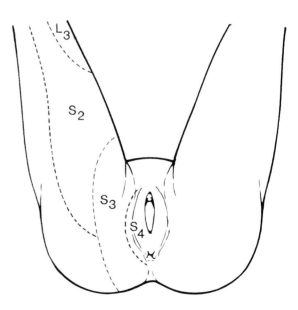

Figure 6.1 S_{2-4} Dermatomes

suspected of having neurological problems, an extended examination should be performed, which will include lumbosacral dermatomes, myotomes and reflexes. If the history and subsequent simple tests arouse suspicions of a neurological problem, the patient should be seen by the appropriate specialist.[8]

6.4.2.2 Abdominal Examination

The abdomen should be evaluated for skin condition and surgical incisions and palpated to identify any abnormal pelvic mass, hernias or full bladder.

6.4.2.3 Vaginal Examination

This part of the assessment should take place with the patient in a good light, supine, with knees bent and feet apart. A department infection control policy should be drawn up to cover this examination and the use of any instruments used during the assessment or treatment (see Chapter 37).

Findings will be described under information observed and information gained from palpation. Many of these findings can be recorded on the "ring of continence" (ROC) as depicted in Figs 6.2–6.6, or simply written in the patient's notes. The rectal examination is described in Chapters 16 and 22. The large ROC represents the vagina, with 12 o'clock denoting the anterior portion and 6 o'clock the pos-

terior segment; 9 o'clock represents the patient's right lateral wall and 3 o'clock the left (see Fig. 6.2); the smaller "ring" represents the anus.

6.5 Observations

6.5.1 Skin and Vaginal Mucosa

Red and excoriated skin on the upper thighs and vulva is generally indicative of severe incontinence or sensitive skin. The labia should be parted and the vaginal mucosa inspected. A well-oestrogenised vagina has a moist, pink, thickened epithelium, with transverse rugae in the lower two-thirds, whereas a poorly oestrogenised vagina appears red, dry and sore, with thinned epithelium and absence of transverse rugae.[9] Atrophic vaginitis is generally mirrored in the urethra, and atrophic urethritis may give rise to irritative symptoms during both the storage and the voiding phase of the micturition cycle.

6.5.2 Scars

Scars following childbirth or surgery should be recorded on the ring of continence (Fig. 6.2).

6.5.3 Prolapse

Vaginal wall laxity may give rise to a prolapse, and this is described in greater detail in Chapters 28 –30. This present section provides a simple explanation of the different types and degrees of prolapse, and an easy way to record the information. The labia are parted, and the patient is asked to cough or bear down. A well-supported anterior vaginal wall should not cross the longitudinal axis of the vaginal canal. Bulging in this area is indicative of an anterior vaginal wall defect, described as a cystocele or urethrocele (cystourethrocele if both the urethra and bladder are bulging into the vagina). Likewise, a well-supported posterior vaginal wall should not cross the longitudinal axis of the vaginal canal. A rectocele is the term given to a posterior vaginal wall defect, presuming that the rectum is bulging through the posterior vaginal wall, and an enterocele describes some segment of bowel bulging through the upper (proximal) posterior vaginal wall. These protrusions are commonly caused by defects in the rectovaginal fascia. Uterine prolapse describes descent of the uterine cervix caused by defective uterine and vaginal suspension mechanisms.

A simple method of grading prolapse is described below and describes the position of the vaginal walls

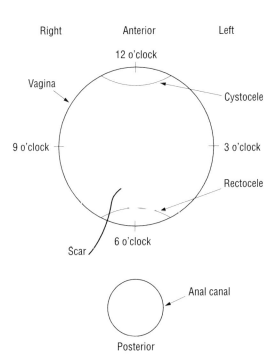

Figure 6.2 Rings of continence showing orientation, cystocele, rectocele and scar.

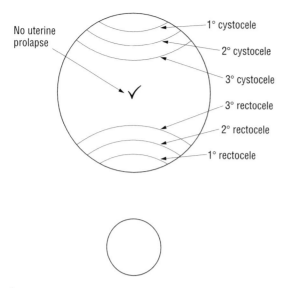

Figure 6.3 Rings of continence showing grades of cystocele and rectocele; a central tick (√) indicates no descent of the cervix or vaginal vault.

during coughing or straining, and illustrated in Figs 6.3 and 6.4.

- A mild (1°) prolapse is not visible at the introitus, but bulging may be palpated. This is usually asymptomatic.
- A moderate (2°) prolapse is visible at the introitus and may be asymptomatic, or give rise to symptoms of "dragging down" or "bulging" in the vagina.

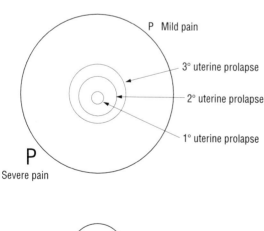

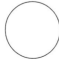

Figure 6.4 Rings of continence showing grades of uterine prolapse and areas of pain.

- A severe (3°) prolapse protrudes outside the body and is symptomatic.

Figure 6.3 shows a way of recording the different grades of cystocele and rectocele, and the degree of prolapse is labelled accordingly. Figure 6.4 shows how to record different grades of uterine or vaginal vault prolapse.

6.5.4 Pelvic Floor Muscle Assessment

During a maximum voluntary contraction (MVC) of the pelvic floor muscles, the following observations can be observed:

- the anus retracts
- the perineum is drawn inwards
- the posterior vaginal wall moves towards the anterior wall.

If a vaginal digital assessment is inappropriate, it is useful to be able to observe the perineum and assess the correct muscle action.

6.5.5 Accessory Muscle Activity

There is growing evidence to support the synergistic action of the transversus abdominis and pelvic floor muscles (for details, see Chapter 8.2). This infers that co-contraction of the transversus abdominis will take place during an MVC of the pelvic floor muscles.

6.6 Internal Palpation Results

6.6.1 Digital Vaginal Palpation

The examiner should enquire if the patient is allergic to latex or lubricating gel; if so, alternatives should be used. The labia are held apart with the thumb and middle finger, and the lubricated index finger of the examining hand is introduced into the vagina. The muscle fibres of the pelvic floor can be palpated through the vaginal walls, from 2 o'clock clockwise round to 10 o'clock; posteriorly, the rectum (and its contents) can be palpated. Anteriorly, the urethra is identified as it lies between the examining finger and the symphysis pubis.

6.6.2 Vaginal Size

This refers to the vaginal capacity, and is important if cones or vaginal probes are used. A narrowing of the vagina may be seen in women who have had vaginal surgery, or postmenopausal women who are not sexually active. It is important that vaginal size is determined before any device is inserted.

6.6.3 Prolapse

The location of the cervix (which feels like the tip of the nose) and the support of the vaginal walls indicates the degree, if any, of vaginal laxity and prolapse (see Chapters 28–30).

6.6.4 Sensitivity and Pain

The examiner should apply gentle pressure on all the vaginal walls and record symmetry of sensation. This is then repeated with firm pressure, and any pain recorded on the ROC; severe pain can be indicated by a large "P" and mild pain by a small "p".

6.7 Muscle Bulk, Symmetry and Contractility

The symmetry, bulk and contractility of the pelvic floor muscles can be determined by palpation, and areas of muscle atrophy can often be felt as "valleys" between muscle bundles. These areas are thought to

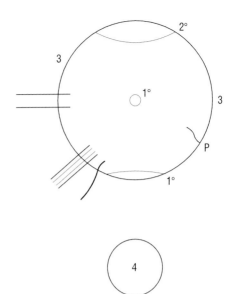

Figure 6.6 Example of completed rings of continence for a patient with 2° cystocele, 1° uterine prolapse and 1° rectocele. Pubovisceralis muscle contraction grade 3 at right and left. An area of muscle atrophy at 9 o'clock, decreased muscle bulk at 7 o'clock. Scars at 7 o'clock and 4 o'clock with pain at 4 o'clock. Anorectal examination revealed grade 4 for external anal sphincter and puborectalis.

be either regions of total or partial denervation, scar tissue, or possibly sections of the muscle whose origin or insertion has been torn from the pelvic fascia during childbirth.[10] MRI studies[11] found evidence of levator ani muscle degeneration in 45% of incontinent women, and this can be shown on the ROC (see Fig. 6.5). Figure 6.6 shows a completed ROC.

With the index finger inserted into the vagina and bent over to rest on the pelvic floor at 8 o'clock, contraction of the levator ani (the deep muscles) will be felt on the distal pad of the finger. In Chapter 2, Peschers and DeLancey propose that, for descriptive purposes, the levator ani be divided into the medially located pubovisceralis (which has several components) and laterally, the iliococcygeus, which forms a shelf on which the organs may rest. It is postulated that contraction of the pubovisceralis is identified as a "squeeze" on the examining finger, and as a "lift" of the rectum and vagina in a cephalad direction. The superficial pelvic floor muscles can be palpated externally, lateral to the labia majora.

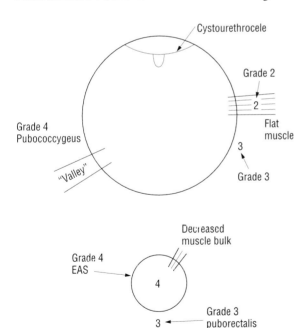

Figure 6.5 Rings of continence showing cystourethrocele, muscle power grade 4 (right side), grade 3 (left side) and area of reduced muscle bulk, graded 2 (left side). Muscle power (Modified Oxford Scale) graded during maximum voluntary contraction. The "valley" represents an area of muscle atrophy. EAS, external anal sphincter.

6.7.1 Muscle Contractility: The PERFECT Scheme

The acronym PERFECT (see Table 6.1) was developed and validated[4] to assess PFM contractility and

Table 6.1. The PERFECT assessment scheme

P	Power
E	Endurance
R	Repetitions
F	Fast
E	Every
C	Contraction
T	Timed

enable the planning of patient-specific muscle training regimens, identifying the number and hold time of MVCs required to train (overload) the pelvic floor muscles (see Chapter 8).

6.7.1.1 Power (P)

Having established that the correct pelvic floor muscle contraction is being performed, the examiner now grades the power (or pressure) P of the contraction, using a modified Oxford scale (see Table 6.2). Actually, one is assessing "strength" not power, but the original study utilised pressure measurements and so P was established as the symbol of strength. Both the right side and the left are graded and recorded on the ROC (see Figs 6.5 and 6.6), and the strongest side is then assessed for endurance, repetitions and fast contractions (see below). The non-examining hand palpates the lower abdominals.

- *Grade 0* indicates no discernible PFM contraction.
- *Grade 1* feels like a flicker or a pulsation under the examining finger, and represents a very weak contraction.
- *Grade 2*, a weak contraction, is detected as an increase in tension in the muscle, without any discernible lift or squeeze.
- *Grade 3* is a moderate contraction, and is characterised by a degree of lifting of the posterior vaginal wall and squeezing on the finger (pubovisceralis) and in-drawing of the perineum. A grade 3 (and grade 4 and 5) contraction is generally discernible on visual perineal inspection.

Table 6.2. Modified Oxford scale

0	Nil
1	Flicker
2	Weak
3	Moderate
4	Good
5	Strong

- *Grade 4* represents a good PFM contraction which produces elevation of the posterior vaginal wall against resistance (applied as pressure to the posterior vaginal wall) and in-drawing of the perineum. If two fingers (index and middle) are placed laterally in the vagina and separated, a grade 4 contraction can squeeze them together against resistance.
- *Grade 5* is the result of a strong contraction of the PFM; strong resistance can be given against elevation of the posterior vaginal wall and approximation of the index and middle fingers.

Careful palpation can identify weakness in different portions of pubovisceralis. For example, good lift but poor squeeze, and so muscle training should be directed to the relevant muscle dysfunction. See Chapter 2 for further description of anatomy of the pelvic floor musculature.

6.7.1.2 Endurance (E)

This is the time, up to 10 s, that the maximum contraction is held, before a reduction in power of 50% or more, is detected. In other words, the contraction is timed until the muscle fatigues. This will be different for all patients; some patients may hold a contraction for several seconds, others for only 1–2 s.

6.7.1.3 Repetitions (R)

The number of repetitions (up to 10) of the MVC is recorded, allowing 4 s rest between contractions. Different "rest" periods have been tested, and 4 s allows easily fatiguable muscles chance to recover, without permitting excessive rest periods for stronger muscles.

6.7.1.4 Fast (F)

After a short rest of at least 1 min, the number of fast (up to 10), 1-s MVC's is assessed, with the patient instructed to "contract–relax" as quickly and strongly as possible, in her own time, until the muscles fatigue.

6.7.1.5 Every Contraction Timed (ECT)

This completes the acronym, and reminds the examiner that the PERFECT scheme assesses the contractility of the PFM by timing and recording each contraction; this enables the planning of a patient-specific exercise programme. Below are examples of PERFECT assessments.

Example 1

P E R F

3 5 4 7   This assessment describes a patient with a moderate (grade 3) contraction, held for 5 seconds and repeated 4 times, followed, after a rest, by 7 fast contractions.

Example 2

P E R F

2 2 3 –   This patient has weak, fatigueable muscles: a grade 2 contraction, held for 2 seconds and repeated 3 times. Inappropriate to assess fast contractions.

Obviously, patients with such different PERFECT assessments will require different exercise programmes (see Chapter 8).

In addition to maximum contractions to promote strength gains, submaximal pelvic floor contractions should be assessed and practised to increase endurance; these submaximal contractions, up to 3 min, should also be practised daily.

The PERFECT assessment can be adapted for use with a perineometer (either EMG or pressure) and applied to the levator ani via the vaginal or the anal route.

6.7.2 Specificity/Function

The PFM have to be further assessed depending on the patients' particular needs. For example, the reflex response to coughing should be tested, especially for a patient with stress incontinence on coughing. This can be detected by visual inspection of the perineum or tested by palpating the pubovisceralis on each side during a cough, and recording the presence or absence of a reflex contraction. Following on from this test, it is important to determine whether a patient can hold a contraction during a cough, progressing to holding a contraction for up to 6 coughs. This effective technique, known as "the knack",[12] helps to brace the pelvic floor before and during a cough, or any activity causing incontinence.

Once a PFM contraction has been monitored by digital palpation, the PERFECT scheme and all functional tests can be carried out using EMG biofeedback, and all the tests should be repeated in sitting and standing. Many patients produce a weaker, shorter contraction when standing than when lying.

6.7.3 Perineometer

This is an instrument that monitors changes in activity in the perineum, and can consist of a pres-

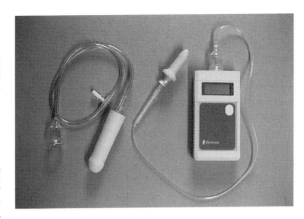

Figure 6.7   Peritron perineometer with vaginal and anal pressure probes.

sure or an EMG monitoring device, or the Periform, which works on a modified Q-tip test.[8]

The Peritron (Cardio Design, Australia; Neen HealthCare, UK) is illustrated in Fig. 6.7. This is an electronic (battery-operated) pressure device, for use with vaginal and anal probes.

The Periform (Neen Health Care, UK) is a vaginal electrode which enables simple monitoring of a pelvic floor contraction and can also be used for EMG biofeedback and electrical stimulation. As a simple biofeedback device, downward (posterior) movement of the indicator signifies a correct PFM contraction; the indicator moves upwards (anteriorly) during a cough or incorrect contraction (Fig. 6.8).

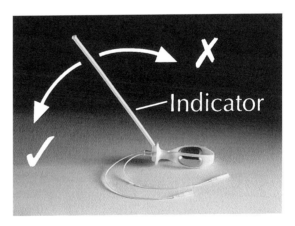

Figure 6.8   Periform vaginal electrode with indicator. A correct voluntary contraction of the pelvic floor muscles produces downward (posterior) movement of the indicator; an incorrect voluntary muscle contraction or cough produces upward (anterior) movement of the indicator.

6.8 Quality of Life

There are many validated quality of life questionnaires,[13] often used in research. It is important to ascertain which activities, if any, are denied the patient because of a bladder problem. In addition, many patients report that frequency and nocturia are more bothersome than occasional incontinence, and treatment should be directed at the most troublesome symptoms.

References

1. Abrams P, Feneley R, Torrens M (1983) Patient assessment. In: Abrams P, Feneley R, Torrens M (ed) Urodynamics. Springer, Berlin, pp. 6–27.
2. Cardozo L (1988) Sex and the bladder. Br Med J 296: 587–8.
3. Hilton P (1988) Urinary incontinence during sexual intercourse: a common, but rarely volunteered symptom. Br J Obstet Gynaecol 95: 377–81.
4. Laycock J, Jerwood D (2001) Pelvic floor assessment; the PERFECT scheme. Physiotherapy. 87: 12: 631–642.
5. Bump RC, Hurt W, Fantl A, Wyman JF (1991) Assessment of Kegel pelvic muscle performance after brief verbal instruction. Am J Obstet Gynecol 165: 322–9.
6. RCOG (1997)Intimate Examinations. Report of a Working Party. Royal College of Obstetricians and Gynaecologists Press, London.
7. De Groat WC and committee (1999) Basic neurophysiology and neuropharmacology. In: Abrams P, Khoury A, Wein A (ed) Incontinence. Plymbridge Distributors, UK, pp. 107–19.
8. Shull B L and committee (1999) Physical examination. In: Abrams P, Khoury A , Wein A (ed) Incontinence. Plymbridge Distributors, UK, pp. 335–49.
9. Fantl A, Cardozo L McClish D and the Hormones and Urogenital Therapy Committee (1994) Estrogen therapy in the management of urinary incontinence in postmenopausal women: a meta-analysis. Obstet Gynecol 83: 12–18.
10. DeLancey JOL and committee (1999) Pregnancy, childbirth and the pelvic floor. In: Abrams P, Khoury A, Wein A (ed) Incontinence. Plymbridge Distributors, UK, pp. 287–94.
11. Kirschner-Hermanns R, Wein B, Niehaus S et al. (1993) The contribution of magnetic resonance imaging of the pelvic floor to the understanding of urinary incontinence. Br J Urol 72: 715.
12. Miller J, Ashton-Miller JA, DeLancey JOL (1996) The Knack: use of precisely-timed pelvic muscle contraction can reduce leakage in SUI. Neurourol Urodynamics 15(4): 392–3.
13. Donovan J and committee (1999) Symptom and quality of life assessment. In: Abrams P, Khoury A, Wein A (ed) Incontinence. Plymbridge Distributors, UK, pp. 295–332.

7 Investigations

V. Khullar , K. Boos and L. Cardozo

Urodynamic studies assess the function of the lower urinary tract rather than its structure. This allows diagnoses to be made, and the classification of lower urinary tract disorders is based on urodynamic parameters. Investigations of lower urinary tract dysfunction range from simple procedures performed in the general practitioner's surgery, e.g. frequency/volume chart, urinalysis, to sophisticated investigations only available in tertiary referral centres. Each investigation has its own appropriate place in the assessment of lower urinary tract dysfunction, and investigations should be tailored to the individual patient's needs. Often the results of a number of tests are required to adequately diagnose a lower urinary tract problem. The various tests that are available are shown in Table 7.1. Urodynamic studies are recommended for all patients with lower urinary tract dysfunction before irreversible or costly treatments, but conservative measures may be initiated without them.

The initial assessment of patients with lower urinary tract dysfunction is a thorough history and physical examination, and this is covered in Chapter 6. This alone has been found to be inadequate, only correctly diagnosing up to half the women with disorders of the lower urinary tract, particularly urinary incontinence.[1,2]

7.1 Pad Test

This simple non-invasive investigation enables objective measurement of urine loss under standard and reproducible conditions. Over a 1h period, with a full bladder, a series of standard activities are performed e.g. walking, jumping, coughing, hand-washing, with the patient wearing a pre-weighed absorbent perineal pad.[3] The duration of the test can be extended to 24 or 48 h when appropriate. The amount of urine lost during the test is determined by the increase in weight of the pad in grams. A weight gain of greater than 1 g signifies incontinence. This test will confirm that the patient is, in fact, incontinent and may give a guide as to the severity of that involuntary urine loss.[4] Although between 13 and 36% of incontinent patients do not leak during the 1h pad test,[5-7] it is of value in research to evaluate the efficacy of conservative and surgical treatments for genuine stress incontinence and in patients who complain of incontinence but do not have any abnormality demonstrated during urodynamic studies.

Table 7.1. Investigations for lower urinary tract dysfunction

Non-specialist investigations	Mid-stream specimen of urine for urinalysis
	Frequency–volume chart
	Pad test
Specialist investigations	Uroflowmetry
	Cystometry
	Videocystourethrography
	Ambulatory urodynamics
	Urethral pressure profilometry
	Intravenous urography
	Micturating cystography
	Ultrasonography
	Magnetic resonance imaging
	Electromyography

7.2 Uroflowmetry

Measurement of urine flow provides objective evidence of voiding ability. First described by von Garrelts in 1956[8] it requires only simple equipment including a commode and flowmeter. Uroflowmetry enables measurement of maximum flow rate, volume voided, average flow rate, flow time and time to maximum flow. A flow rate is only interpretable if the patient voids more than 150 ml and the patient feels that the void was representative of how he or she normally voids. However, uroflowmetry alone cannot differentiate between outflow obstruction with a normal detrusor generating pressure during a void and detrusor hypotonia where the poor flow rate is due to an inability of the detrusor to contract.

The major value of uroflowmetry is in the prediction of postoperative voiding difficulties in patients with genuine stress incontinence, by identifying women with a poor peak flow rate.

7.3 Cystometry

Cystometry involves the measurement of the intravesical (bladder) pressure while the bladder is filled and as the bladder empties. When the abdominal pressure, measured intrarectally or intravaginally, is subtracted from the intravesical pressure, the resulting pressure represents the detrusor pressure.

7.3.1 Filling Phase

This is the single most useful investigation for the diagnosis of detrusor instability and allows classification of detrusor contractions into normal, hyperreflexic or hyporeflexic.[3]

During cystometry the pressure–volume relationship of the bladder is measured and detrusor contractility, bladder sensation, capacity and compliance are assessed. Intra-abdominal pressure and intravesical pressure are measured by using fluid-filled lines or microtransducers and the (subtracted) detrusor pressure is then calculated as the bladder volume increases. Usually the bladder is filled through a catheter at 10–100 ml/min. Fast filling (>100 ml/min) is a provocative test for patients with detrusor instability. The patient should assume a standing position at some stage during the test and provocation such as coughing or heel-bouncing should occur. Detrusor instability is diagnosed where a rise in detrusor pressure is associated with urgency or urinary leakage. In addition, the volume at which the patient first desires to void and the maximum cystometric capacity are noted.

The usual filling medium is sterile saline but a radio-opaque medium is used during video-cystourethrography (VCU) – see below.

7.3.2 Voiding Phase

At the end of filling the patient is asked to void into a flowmeter. The maximum voiding pressure and flow rate are noted and obstructed voiding (high pressure, low flow) can be differentiated from detrusor hypotonia (low pressure, low flow). After voiding it is usual to measure the post-void residual urine volume.

7.4 Videocystourethrography

In VCU the lower urinary tract is screened radiologically while there is synchronous recording of bladder function by urodynamic techniques i.e. cystometry, flow rate, etc. Although VCU is the 'gold standard' of urodynamic investigations, it is not needed to differentiate between genuine stress incontinence and detrusor instability in simple cases. It is useful in patients for whom previous surgery has failed, as the position and mobility of the bladder neck can be assessed at rest and on straining; VCU readily diagnoses morphological abnormalities such as bladder or urethral diverticulae, urethral stenosis or vesicoureteric reflux.

7.5 Ambulatory Urodynamics

Dual-channel subtracted cystometry is known to be unphysiological as the bladder is filled through a catheter at a volume per minute greater than the physiological 6 ml/min. Ambulatory urodynamic monitoring uses natural bladder filling and allows the patient to perform activities of normal daily living while pressure transducers (fine catheters) measure the intra-abdominal and intravesical pressure, as in standard cystometry.

Over a 4 h period the patient drinks a prescribed volume of fluid every 30 min. and keeps a detailed diary of symptoms and events. The catheters are checked periodically to ensure they remain in position. Provocative manoeuvres are carried out with a full bladder for the last 30 min. of the test.

Ambulatory urodynamics are more sensitive in diagnosing detrusor instability than are laboratory urodynamics,[9] but the former have been criticised for overdiagnosing detrusor instability. Before ambulatory urodynamics can become a standard clinical investigation it needs to be refined further and strict criteria on its methodology, definitions and interpretation are urgently required.

7.6 Urethral Pressure Profilometry

In urethral pressure profilometry (UPP) a soft silicone catheter, with two transducers 6 cm apart, is gradually withdrawn at a constant rate along the urethra. This enables simultaneous recording of the intravesical and intraurethral pressures. Electronic subtraction of these recordings gives a measure of urethral function at rest and during stress conditions.

While the UPP is helpful in understanding the pathophysiology of GSI, it is of no use clinically in the diagnosis, as there is an overlap in urethral pressure measurements between continent and incontinent patients.

7.7 Radiology of the Lower Urinary Tract

A plain film of the abdomen can be used to screen for urinary calculi or as the first film in an intravenous urogram. The intravenous urogram (IVU) remains the primary modality for visualising the kidneys, pelvicalyceal system and ureters and for assessing calculi and renal infection.

7.8 Ultrasound

The role of ultrasound in the detection of structural abnormalities such as duplex, ectopic or horseshoe kidneys, dilatation of the pelvicalyceal system or bladder diverticula is undisputed. In addition, trans-abdominal ultrasound is useful in the estimation of post-micturition residual urine volumes and is preferable to urethral catheterisation for this purpose. Various methods of calculating this volume have been proposed,[10] but inaccuracy can be around 20%.

Ultrasound has been advocated as a non-invasive, inexpensive alternative to VCU. Although trans-abdominal scanning is not useful in visualising the bladder neck owing to its position behind the symphysis pubis, transvaginal ultrasound images the urethral anatomy and the urethrovesical junction.[11,12] However the presence of a vaginal probe compresses the urethra and distorts the anatomy of the bladder neck, limiting its use as a means of assessment in incontinent women.[13] It may be more appropriate to use a transrectal or translabial probe in incontinent women, and pressure measurements are still required to make a urodynamic diagnosis.

Transvaginal ultrasound remains the imaging modality of choice for visualising urethral diverticula and their relation to the urethra and rhabdosphincter.[14] One final important use of transvaginal ultrasound is the measurement of bladder wall thickness when the bladder is empty.[15] This is a reproducible sensitive method of screening for detrusor instability.[16]

7.9 Magnetic Resonance Imaging

Magnetic resonance imaging (MRI) of the lower urinary tract has so far been limited to research (see Chapter 2). The advantage over ultrasound lies in its ability to provide good soft tissue differentiation. The test is expensive, limited to static studies and at present cannot be considered a practical aid to the diagnosis of female urinary incontinence.

7.10 Electromyography

Three main techniques of electromyography (EMG) measurement have been used in the investigation of lower urinary tract dysfunction: surface electrodes, needle electrodes and nerve conduction studies. Surface electrodes are relatively non-invasive and well tolerated; they give quantitative information about muscle activity rather than data for qualitative analysis. They are useful for timing of muscle activity in relation to pelvic floor exercises or voiding and can detect a stimulus applied to a distant site when measuring sensorimotor nerve latencies.

There are two types of needle electrodes, single-fibre and concentric. Single-fibre EMG involves recording of the fibre density within a muscle under study. This can be used to measure re-innervation of motor units. Concentric needle EMG has been used as a qualitative method of assessing motor units and can be used to diagnose detrusor-sphincter dyssynergia.

There are many different types of nerve conduction studies and the underlying principle is that the neurological lesion in the pathway being tested causes a delay in the conduction time. The main types of studies are the sacral reflex arc, distal motor latencies, spinal stimulation, cortical evoked responses and cerebral stimulation. EMG is most useful when a neurological abnormality is suspected.

7.11 Conclusion

Urodynamic techniques can provide useful information allowing the diagnosis of complex lower urinary tract dysfunction. Accurate diagnosis results in appropriate treatment. There is no perfect test of urethrovesical function, but much information can be obtained from the appropriate use of the available investigations.

7.12 Urinalysis

Ray Addison

Urinalysis using reagent strips has become a standard investigation carried out by healthcare professionals and is an essential part of a continence assessment.[17–19]

- Urinalysis should take place within 1 h of obtaining the specimen, and the urine allowed to warm to room temperature before testing.
- Clean containers should be used to collect specimens; alternatively, the strip can be passed through the urine stream.
- It is important to immerse the strip completely in the urine, then take it out and remove any excess urine.
- The strip should be read horizontal to the coloured segments on the bottle, following the times indicated on the label.

The appearance and smell of a urine specimen can indicate abnormalities which may be confirmed by urinalysis. However, many drugs and foods can change the colour of urine. Generally, clear urine is not usually infected.

7.12.1 Glucose

Glucose is not normally present in urine. Its presence may indicate diabetes mellitus, Cushing's syndrome, glucagonoma, the effects of a general anaesthetic, stress, shock, burns, steroid consumption, hyperthyroidism, acromegaly, trauma, stroke, myocardial infarction or circulatory collapse.[17,18]

7.12.2 Ketones

Ketones are not normally present in urine. Their presence may indicate uncontrolled diabetes, starvation, high fat diets, vomiting, diarrhoea, febrile states, hyperthyroidism or pregnancy.[17]

7.12.3 Specific Gravity

The specific gravity of urine indicates the hydration status of the body; the normal range is 1002–1035. A higher figure may indicate dehydration and a lower figure may indicate a high fluid intake.[17]

7.12.4 Blood

Some red blood cells are normally present in urine. Unusually high levels may indicate a number of conditions, including upper or lower urinary tract infection, disease or trauma (including instrumentation), stones, transfusion reaction, coagulopathy, menstruation, tumour within the urinary tract, patients with indwelling Foley catheters, sickle cell disease and collagen disorders.[17,18,20]

7.12.5 pH

The pH indicates the acidity or alkalinity of the urine: the lower the pH, the more acid the sample. The normal range is 4.5–8. Prolonged alkalinity may indicate certain urinary tract infections, renal failure or vomiting. Acidic urine may indicate acidosis, diarrhoea, dehydration, starvation, fever or certain infections.[17,18,20]

7.12.6 Protein

Very small amounts of protein are normally found in urine. The first morning sample is best to detect the presence of protein. The presence of high levels of protein may indicate renal disease, urinary tract infections, hypertension, pre-eclampsia, heart failure, myeloma or malignancies of the lower urinary tract.[17,18,20]

7.12.7 Urobilinogen

Small amounts of urobilinogen may be present in urine. The presence of higher levels may indicate cirrhosis, hepatic congestion, hepatitis or hyperthyroidism.

7.12.8 Nitrite

Nitrite is not normally present in urine. Its presence may indicate a (gram-negative) urinary tract infection. If the infection is caused by gram-positive bacteria, the urine will test negative for nitrite. Urine that has been in the bladder for some time (>3 h or overnight) is best to show a positive nitrite reaction. A positive leucocyte and nitrite result is highly indicative of a urinary tract infection. A negative result to both is also indicative that no infection is present in about 97% of cases. In the diagnosis of urinary tract infections, combined results of urinalysis are more significant than single findings.

7.12.9 Leucocytes

If pus cells are present in the urinary tract, esterase is released and this reacts with the reagent strip to confirm the presence of leucocytes. This may be indicative of urinary tract infection.[18,20]

7.12.10 Conclusions

Urinalysis using reagent strips is a quick and easy method of analysing samples of urine. If patients have not had their urine tested, and especially if they have irritative symptoms of urgency and frequency, then this test should be carried out. If the test reveals any abnormalities, the general practitioner should be notified.

References

1. Cardozo LD, Stanton SL (1980) Genuine stress incontinence and detrusor instability, a review of 200 patients. Br J Obstet Gynaecol 87: 184–90.
2. Cundiff GW, Harris RL, Coates KW, Bump RC (1997) Clinical predictors of urinary incontinence in women. Am J Obstet Gynecol 177: 262–7.
3. Abrams P, Blaivas JG, Stanton SL, Anderson JT (1989) The standardisation of terminology of lower urinary tract function. Scand J Urol Nephrol (Suppl) 114: 5–19.
4. Sutherst J, Brown M, Shawler M (1981) Assessing the severity of urinary incontinence in women by weighing perineal pads. Lancet 1: 1128–30.
5. Walters MD, Dombrowski RA, Prihoda TJ (1990) Perineal pad testing in the quantitation of urinary incontinence. Int Urogynaecol J 1: 3–6.
6. Jorgenson L, Lose G, Thunedborg B (1987) One hour pad weighing test for objective assessment of female urinary incontinence. Obstet Gynaecol 69: 39–41.
7. Richmond DH, Sutherst JR, Brown MC (1987) Quantification of urine loss by weighing perineal pads. Observation on the exercise regime. Br J Urol 59: 224–227.
8. Garrelts B von (1956) Analysis of micturition: a new method of recording the voiding of the bladder. Acta Chir Scand 112: 326–40.
9. Hill S, Khullar V, Cardozo L, Anders K, Yip A (1995) Ambulatory urodynamics versus videocystometrogram: a test-retest analysis. Neurourol Urodynamics 14: 528–9.
10. Hartnell CG, Kiely EA, Williams G, Gibson RN (1987) Real-time ultrasound measurement of bladder volume : a comparitive study of three methods. Br J Radiol 60: 1063–5.
11. Quinn MJ, Beynon J (1988) McC. Mortensen, Smith PJB. Transvaginal endosonography: a new method to study the anatomy of the lower urinary tract in urinary stress incontinence. Br J Urol 62: 414–418.
12. Weil EHJ, Waalwijk Doorn ESC van, Heesakkers JPFA, Meguid T, Janknegt RA (1993) Transvaginal ultrasonography: a study with healthy volunteers and women with genuine stress incontinence. Eur Urol 24: 226–30.
13. Wise BG, Burton G, Cutner A, Cardozo LD (1992) Effect of vaginal ultrasound probe on lower urinary tract function. Br J Urol 70: 12–16.
14. Keefe B, Warshauer DM, Tucker MS, Mittelstaedt CA (1991) Diverticula of the female urethra: diagnosis by endovaginal and transperineal sonography. AJR 156: 1195–97.
15. Khullar V, Salvatore S, Cardozo LD, Kelleher CJ, Bourne TH (1994) A novel technique for measuring bladder wall thickness in women using transvaginal ultrasound. Ultra Obstet Gynecol 4: 220–3.
16. Khullar V, Salvatore S, Cardozo LD, Hill S, Kelleher CJ (1994) Ultrasound bladder wall measurement–a non-invasive sensitive screening test for detrusor instability. Neurourol Urodynam 13: 461–2.
17. Getliffe K, Dolman M (1997) Promoting Continence, A Clinical and Research Perspective. Baillière Tindall, London.
18. Heywood-Jones I (1993) Skills update. Undertaking urinalysis. Community Outlook n: 26–27.
19. US Department of Health and Human Services (1992) Clinical Practice Guideline, Urinary Incontinence in Adults. Agency for Health Care Policy and Research, Rockville, MD.
20. Laker C (1994) Urological investigations. In: Urological Nursing. Scutari Press, London.

II Treatment of Urinary Incontinence

8 Pelvic Floor Muscle Exercise in the Treatment of Urinary Incontinence

J. Haslam

8.1 Specific Pelvic Floor Muscle Re-education

8.1.1 Effectiveness of Pelvic Floor Muscle Exercises

Pelvic floor muscle (PFM) re-education is an effective, low-risk intervention that can reduce incontinence significantly in varied populations and should be initially considered.[1] Many studies[2-5] have demonstrated the effectiveness of pelvic floor muscle exercises (PFME). A systematic review of randomised controlled trials (RCT) on the conservative treatment of stress urinary incontinence[6] revealed strong evidence to support PFME as being effective in reducing the symptoms of stress urinary incontinence. This corresponds well with the findings that vaginal and urethral pressures correlate significantly with PFM contractions.[7]

For PFME to be effective, a person must have an ability to contract the correct muscles and comply with a specific exercise regimen. It is not possible to establish whether or not a woman will be able to perform an adequate pelvic muscle contraction on clinical evaluation, merely by considering her age, clinical severity, urethral support or urethral profilometry.[7] Only by vaginal assessment can an active contraction be recognised and an appropriate exercise regimen be determined.[8,9] The assessment of male patients poses particular problems (see Chapter 16).

8.1.2 Exercise Physiology

It is only by a comprehension of both muscle physiology and exercise theory that the therapist will gain an understanding and ability to prescribe appropriate exercise.

The number of motor units recruited depends on the effort of the person exercising; the greater the effort, the greater the frequency of excitation and the greater the number of motor units recruited. The muscle fibre type is determined by the nerve fibre supplying it. Slow oxidative muscle fibres (tonic, type 1) sustain activity, whereas fast glycolytic muscle fibres (phasic, type 2) are involved in bursts of activity. In asymptomatic women, the PFM are approximately 33% fast fibres and 67% slow fibres.[10] Endurance is developed by slow-speed contractions with low repetitions; power is developed by high-speed contractions and repetitions. According to Henneman's size principle of recruitment, when a striated muscle contracts, slow motor units are initially recruited; as greater effort and load are placed on the muscle, the fast motor units are recruited.[11] A muscle contraction must be greater than that of its ordinary everyday activity in order to increase in force, and longer-lasting to increase the endurance capability. For muscle contractility to improve, the initial muscle strength, power, endurance, repetitions and fatigue must be considered together with a heed

Table 8.1. Muscle training considerations

Strength	The maximum force or tension that a muscle can generate
Power	The rate at which the work can be done. The ratio between the maximum force and the time taken to achieve that force
Endurance	The length of time over which a contraction can be maintained or repeated
Repetitions	The number of times that contractions of equal force can be repeated
Fatigue	Failure to maintain the required or expected force

to the principles of muscle training; overload, specificity, maintenance and reversibility (Table 8.1).

8.1.2.1 Overload and Specificity

To overload the PFM, the aim is to perform maximum contractions by lengthening the holding period, increasing repetitions, reducing rest intervals or a mixture of all three. This has shown an average improvement of 25–50% strength in skeletal muscle over a period of 6 months training.[12] A minimum period of 15–20 weeks exercise has been recommended.[13] It is believed that the first 6–8 weeks' effects are due to neural adaptation; muscle hypertrophy takes longer and continues over many months. PFME have been shown to have long-term effects 5 years after the cessation of training.[14]

To improve performance, muscles are best trained with movements as similar as possible to the desired activity. Therefore, exercise is most appropriate in a functional position. Although muscles work in patterns of movement, it is essential to ensure that the pattern of movement is neither detrimental nor masks activity in the target group. When aiming to strengthen the PFM it has been shown in a small study[15] that contraction of the transversus abdominis (TrA) results in a PFM contraction in healthy subjects. However, gross contraction of the abdominals, especially the rectus abdominus, results in raised intra-abdominal pressure and is inappropriate when re-educating the PFM. Pelvic floor stability and trunk muscle co-activation are considered in greater depth in section 8.2.

8.1.2.2 Maintenance and Reversibility

Muscle training can succeed in improving strength, power and endurance; to maintain improvement the exercise needs to be continued on a regular basis.[16] A reduced exercise programme can maintain moderate levels of strength and endurance,[17] but if training ceases the oxidative capacity of the muscles diminishes in 4–6 weeks,[18] the endurance ability declining more quickly than the ability to exert maximal power.[19]

8.1.3 Exercise Regimen

It has been suggested that the recommended exercise regimen to develop strength in skeletal muscle is to practise 3–4 sets of 8–12 high-resistance, slow-velocity contractions 3 times a week.[17] The 3 component parts to achieve this strength training are:

- sufficient effort of a suitable duration
- adequate frequency of exercise
- over a sufficient length of time.

A review of 16 papers[12] concerned with strength training of the PFM found great variety in the PFME regimens. However, all agreed that subjects should receive individual instructions, vaginal palpation, feedback and close follow-up. The self-reported cure and success rates varied between 17 and 84%.

The PFM should be able not only to generate force but also to work in a co-ordinated fashion at the time of need. There is a greater chance of success by teaching PFM awareness, an exercise regimen and the ability to contract the pelvic floor at the time of need. It has been shown that by teaching patients to contract the pelvic floor before and during a cough ('the knack'), stress urinary loss can be reduced by an average of 73.3% after 1 week of practice.[20] This can be taught and monitored during a digital examination.

8.1.3.1 Response to PFME

Many studies have shown the effectiveness of PFME related to childbirth.[21–24] Awareness, education and compliance are the three main factors for success.

Although bladder function and striated muscle alter with age, this does not necessarily mean that the elderly are incapable of improving their PFM function. A holistic assesment of the patient should be made including mobility, possible polypharmacy and any relevant behavioural considerations.

Researchers have attempted to identify patients likely to succeed with treatment. It has been shown that the best responders were older (mean age 48 years), had a longer history of incontinence (mean of 13 years), more severe incontinence on a visual analogue score, were more motivated and had stronger PFM at the commencement of the study.[25] It has also been shown that support by a physiotherapist, together with patient motivation and compliance is necessary for good results.[26] However, there is little evidence to identify which PFME regimen is the most effective, as studies have used different parameters.[6] Until there is a randomised controlled trial comparing different exercise programmes, no conclusions can be made regarding the most effective exercise protocol.

Before embarking on an exercise regimen, the patient must be thoroughly assessed (see Chapter 6). They may dislike undressing for a vaginal assessment and must be treated with great sensitivity at all times. As a patient may have suffered previous abuse or trauma, the clinician must have adequate skills to deal with any presenting problems and know to whom the patient can be referred for further help if necessary. There may be delicate tissues from postmenopausal oestrogen deficiency or recent childbirth trauma; also past surgery or childbirth injury may have resulted in nerve damage or scar tissue. These issues need consideration when prescribing any exercise regimen.

8.1.4 Teaching Pelvic Floor Muscle Exercise

In order to elicit a contraction and for the patient to work maximally, a careful explanation of what is expected should be given. If vaginal assessment is not possible, observation of perineal body movement inwardly denotes at least a grade 3 Oxford scale contraction (see Chapter 6). Any bulging indicates a lack of PFM contraction, and an increase in intra-abdominal pressure and must be discouraged. If no contraction is observed, extra proprioception by pressure on the perineal body with the instruction to 'try and lift away' may be helpful. During digital assessment extra encouragement can be given by using such phrases as 'squeeze and lift in' or 'try and pull your tail bone forwards' or 'try and stop me removing my examining finger'. The proprioceptors of the perineum and vagina transmit the information to higher centres to effect increased awareness, helping to increase voluntary effort.

8.1.4.1 Practical Application of PFME

Grade 0–2 If there is little or no discernible contraction, the examiner may be able to elicit a better contraction by stretching the PFM by hooking the index finger over the PFM and stretching in a posterolateral direction. If the vagina is capacious enough for two digits to be introduced in an 'east–west' direction, both sides can be put on the stretch simultaneously. The stretching movement increases proprioception and stimulates the stretch receptors in the muscle. If this together with verbal encouragement results in an improved contraction, the patient is assessed for muscle strength, duration of contraction, ability to repeat that contraction and the number of fast contractions possible. If the contraction is still grade 2 or less, neuromuscular electrical stimulation (NMES) or biofeedback should be considered.

For muscles of a low grade the rest phase should be 4 s or the same as the length of the contraction, whichever is the greater. People with less ability may find it easier to practise their PFME in lying, eliminating the effects of gravity; others find it easier to exercise with a pillow under their hips to have

gravity-assisted exercise. As ability increases, the aim must be to assume more functional positions.

Grades 3 and Over A baseline assessment will determine the specific exercise programme for the individual. Although initially PFME may be easiest in sitting, with a neutral lumbar spine and forearms resting on knees (stimulating the dermatome of S4), PFME must be developed more functionally and suitably for daily living activities.. Strengthening regimens should always be patient specific and progressed by consideration of the length of contractions, the number of repetitions of both slow and fast contractions and the length of the rest periods. Further objectives also need to be given, e.g. a patient with an assessment of 3/6/4/6 (grade 3/ endurance of 6 seconds/4 slow contractions/6 fast contractions) may have the new objective of increasing to 3/6/6/10. When this is accomplished, the length of contractions can then be increased.

Submaximal contractions of up to 3 min should also be practised daily.

Advanced Pelvic Floor Muscle Activity Different body positions with abducted legs are suggested to ensure maximal PFM fitness.[27] These positions may include standing, supine lying, prone lying and prone kneeling. It has been further shown that intensive group exercising once a week is more beneficial than exercising alone over a period of 6 months.[27] If classes can be incorporated as well as individual assessment, the patient will receive increased motivational input, peer support and an opportunity to participate in more generalised pelvic and trunk muscle training.

8.1.4.2 Self-Assessment

A female patient may be encouraged to carry out vaginal digital assessment herself. However, it has been shown that only 30% of older women are quite comfortable with the concept of touching their genitalia.[28] If appropriate, self vaginal examination can be explained as a method of proprioception and self-assessment. The method is explained as introducing a clean thumb vaginally, and 'hooking it over' the posterolateral pelvic floor, perhaps when in the bath or shower. If appropriate, it may also be suggested that the individual could get feedback from a sexual partner. One of the side-effects of increased PFM activity is thought to be increased sexual satisfaction, and this in itself may encourage increased effort and compliance to exercise.

A man can palpate his perineal body to feel an upwards movement, and also observe a penile lift during a PFM contraction (see Chapter 16).

8.1.4.3 Frequency and Time of Exercise

Home and work circumstances vary, and any PFME regimen must take this into consideration. Functional activities may act as a reminder, such as the instruction to exercise after voiding. Some may comply with PFME better by practising in clusters of 3 sets of PFME with 2 min rest between each set, to be done 2–3 times daily. Others may benefit from physical reminders. such as stickers placed to catch the eye. The aim is always to have a compliant patient, so time spent in agreeing a 'contract of exercise' is time well spent. Exercising to music may also be useful, but care must be taken regarding tempo, as over-fatigue and an increase in symptoms may result. Asking the patient at each attendance how motivated they feel to continue is not only a good indicator of compliance, but can act as a motivation in itself. Emphasis should always be placed on the 'specific prescription' for the individual and concentration on the PFM whilst exercising.

8.1.4.4 Functional Activity

The need to contract the PFM during any activity which puts the pelvic floor under any additional strain that causes urine loss should be emphasised. The aim is to acquire learned reflex activity. The better the understanding and practise, the more likely someone is to succeed. An exercise diary can be utilised both as a motivator and to provide accurate information as to when the patient has found the best times for exercise (see Appendix 3).

8.1.5 Summary

At present there is no way of predicting who will succeed, so even those patients who may not at first seem like ideal candidates for conservative management should be given the opportunity of PFM re-education, provided that their motivation is high and compliance with treatment is likely. If the patient is prepared to practise assiduously for 3–6 months it can be considered a fair trial of conservative management.[1] It should always be emphasised that maintenance of any strength gain depends on the patient continuing to exercise at their threshold once or twice daily. Lack of exercise will result in the benefit of the exercise regressing in 4–6 weeks.

8.2 Pelvic Floor Stability and Trunk Muscle Co-Activation

R. Jones, M. Comerford and R. Sapsford

8.2.1 Co-activation Synergies

Rehabilitation of the PFM is advocated in the efficient management of urinary or anorectal dysfunction. Until recently, co-activation of any other muscle group during a PFM contraction was considered inappropriate.[29] However, authors in several small studies[30,31] have identified an increase in EMG activity in abdominal muscles during a PFM contraction without visible abdominal movement. Furthermore an increase in PFM EMG activity has been recorded with hip and trunk movements,[32] isometric abdominal e.g. hollowing or bracing[15,31] and other local stabilising muscle activation, i.e. psoas, multifidus, adoption of lumbo-pelvic neutral spine and correct lower limb alignment. It has also been reported that certain abdominal activity can contribute to urethral closure pressure[33] and the time taken to interrupt micturition voluntarily. This was similar whether using isometric abdominal muscles or the PFM and periurethral muscles.[34]

As more is understood about lumbo-pelvic stability, it becomes apparent that for optimal stability function, muscles are required to work not in isolation, but in co-activation synergies.[35–38] These principles should apply to urinary dysfunction and therefore to PFM rehabilitation. Early evidence suggests that activation of the abdominal muscles is a normal response to contraction of the PFM,[31] but further research is aimed at identifying whether the association between abdominal and PFM can be used in clinical practice. Until then, although the efficacy of this approach to rehabilitation has not been proved, rehabilitation strategies have been developed to integrate PFM and trunk muscle function.

Evidence of dysfunction in the local muscle system indicates that the problem is one of motor recruitment or inhibition, not muscle strength or power. For example, in the normal subject, the transversus abdominis (TrA) and the diaphragm have an anticipatory reaction to movement, which is delayed if there is low back pain.[35–40] Results from preliminary investigations indicate that the pubococcygeus has similar anticipatory activity to the diaphragm and TrA.[38] This supports earlier work that demonstrated an anticipatory increase in urethral pressure in healthy women.[41]

Optimal facilitation, recruitment and retraining of pelvic floor dysfunction necessitates rehabilitation of the motor control deficits of the local stabilising muscles, as well as retraining of strength deficits that can be identified. As there is evidence of functional co-activation of the PFM with the other local stability muscle of the trunk, a clinical process of retraining these co-activation synergies can be developed. The other local stability muscles of the trunk are the TrA, segmental fibres of the lumbar multifidus and the posterior fasiculus of psoas, though the latter has not been objectively demonstrated.

8.2.2 Exercises to Facilitate the Local Stability Muscles of the Lumbo-Pelvic Region

The exercises described in this section are examples of some of the many ways of facilitating the local stability muscles of the lumbo-pelvic region. They have all been used clinically to improve the stability function of the spine and to facilitate activation of the PFM.

8.2.2.1 Transversus Abdominis

See Table 8.2 and Figs 8.1 and 8.2.

Clinical Priority A normal breathing pattern should be used independently of a sustained TrA contraction. The most common clinical sign of dys-

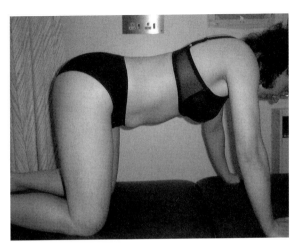

Figure 8.1   Four-point kneeling, abdominals relaxed.

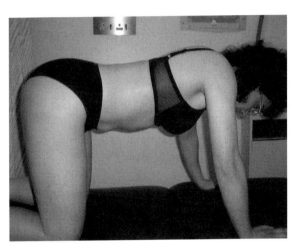

Figure 8.2   Four-point kneeling, activation of transversus abdominis.

function is that the contraction can only be sustained if the subject holds their breath, or that the contraction varies with breathing. During active retraining of TrA it is essential to identify and eliminate substitution strategies. However, O'Sullivan[36,39] has demonstrated that it is not necessary to eliminate the oblique abdominal muscles completely for effective rehabilitation.

Just as each of the abdominal muscles has been seen to function independently, preliminary research suggests that TrA activation facilitates a pubococcygeal contraction.[15] Association of individual abdominal muscles with different muscles of the pelvic floor has been suggested, but has not been verified. However, identification of various abdominal muscle substitution strategies may be an indication that PFM other than pubococcygeus are

Table 8.2.   Activation of transversus abdominus (TrA)

Action to facilitate	Palpation	Observation (Figs 8.1, 8.2)
● A 'drawing in' or hollowing action isolated to the lower abdominal wall with minimal upper abdominal wall involvement ● This action should attempt to minimise spinal rib cage movement and should not cause lateral flaring or bracing of the waist.[38,42] It should be sustained independently of normal breathing[38,43]	● 2 cm down and 1 cm medial to the anterior superior iliac spine (ASIS) ● Palpate for slow TrA tensioning of the low abdominal wall fascia without anterior displacement. The bulge is due to expansion of the internal obliques or intra-abdominal pressure	● Lower abdominal wall should lead the contraction ● Movement should be minimal ● No spinal, pelvic or rib cage movement

predominantly activated. A suggestion to assist this is: 'try to pull your tailbone up towards your pubic bone'. Train the co-activation pattern with 10s sustained contractions repeated 10 times whilst breathing normally in a variety of functional postures.

8.2.2.2 Lumbar Multifidus

It is thought that the lumbar multifidus (LM) may work as a force couple with the PFM to stabilise the sacrum.[44] Conversely, assymetrical contraction of the PFM or LM may contribute to pelvic instability (Table 8.3).

Table 8.3. Activation of lumbar multifidus

Action to facilitate	Palpation	Observation (Figs 8.3, 8.5)
• A specific isometric contraction of lumbar multifidus, involves palpable radial expansion or 'swelling' of the muscle as it generates tension • The 'swelling' action should be localised and should minimise spinal or pelvic movement[38,45]	• Sit with the spine in neutral alignment. • Place fingers/thumbs on LM immediately besides the spine • Lean slightly forward from the hips (spine neutral) and feel the muscles tension • Lean slightly back from the hips until the muscles relax • Try to tension the muscle. Feel the muscle harden and hold this tension (Fig. 8.4) • The lateral abdominals and pelvic floor should co-activate automatically	• A slight muscle contraction • No bracing, holding the breath, spinal or pelvic movement

Clinical Priority If the muscles cannot be relaxed, try the prone position to relax the muscles prior to specific activation. If the multifidus cannot be activated, end expiration can be used to facilitate the contraction, but the contraction should be maintained during breathing. The most common clinical sign of dysfunction is that the contraction can only be sustained if the subject holds their breath. If the multifidus can be efficiently recruited, add in PFM co-contraction. Train the co-activation pattern with 10s contractions repeated 10 times whilst breathing normally in a variety of functional positions.

8.2.2.3 Psoas

The psoas has direct fascial links to the diaphragm superiorly and to the coccygeal PFM inferiorly. It is frequently observed clinically that there is asymmetry of contraction of PFM, psoas, TrA and LM. Psoas retraining is effective in correction of asymmetrical recruitment (Table 8.4).

Table 8.4. Activation of psoas

Action to facilitate	Palpation	Observation (Figs 8.4, 8.5)
• Distract one leg and instruct the patient to pull the leg back into the socket. This involves minimal movement of the leg	• Palpate the ASIS and the anterior thigh	• No pelvic motion • No strong bulge of the anterior thigh muscles • No co-contraction rigidity due to dominance of the limb muscles (check that it is possible to passively rotate the leg with minimal resistance)

8.2.2.4 Specific Psoas Recruitment

The stability role of the psoas is to longitudinally pull the head of the femur into the acetabulum with the spine in neutral alignment, producing axial compression along its line of pull. This 'pulling in' or 'shortening the leg' action should be localised to the hip and pelvis and should attempt to minimise any

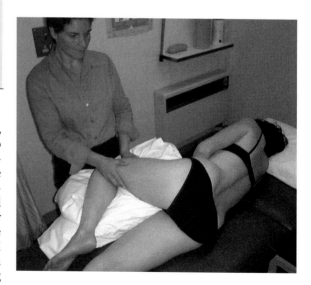

Figure 8.3 Activation of psoas in side lying.

lateral tilt, anterior or posterior tilt or rotation of the pelvis. Likewise, any spinal rotation, flexion or extension should be discouraged.

Clinical Priority Initial facilitation can be trained in side lying (Fig. 8.3), supine and incline sitting. Hold the contraction for 10 s and repeat 10 times. If the psoas can be activated efficiently, then co-activation of psoas, PFM and TrA may be trained.

8.2.2.5 PFM, Psoas and TrA Co-Activation

Sit on the ischiums with both feet on the floor. Keep the spine neutral, lean forward (Fig. 8.4) and con-

tract the PFM. The contraction is generally felt in the anterior PFM. Then lean backwards and contract the PFM – this is generally felt in the posterior PFM. Co-activate TrA by hollowing the low abdominal wall.

Co-activate the psoas by placing the heels together and pushing them together with 20% pressure, half expiration and gentle pull of the hips into the sockets.

Clinical Priority It is considered essential to maintain co-activation and breathe in a slow, relaxed manner. Many patients cannot maintain the sustained consistent PFM co-activation as they start to breathe again. The use of isolated breathing patterns i.e. isolated apical, diaphragmatic or basal breathing, is dysfunctional. Progress by taking weight off the feet (slide the feet from side to side), and then add functional positions:

- Standing small knee bend, i.e. with the feet hip width apart, heels remaining on the floor, bend the knees such that the kneecap is over the second toe.
- Standing against a wall with spine neutral, small knee bend as above, bend forwards at the hips.

8.2.2.6 Hand–Knee Diagonal Push (Progression)

Crook lying with the spine supported in neutral, very gently draw in the lower abdominal wall including the periurethral PFM. Hold, then slowly lift one knee towards the opposite hand and push them isometrically against each other on a diagonal line; do not stabilise with the opposite foot or allow a posterior pelvic tilt (Fig. 8.5). Train the co-activation pattern with up to 10s sustained contractions repeated 10 times while breathing normally in a variety of functional postures. Psoas strongly co-activates with the PFM, LM and the oblique abdominals in this procedure.

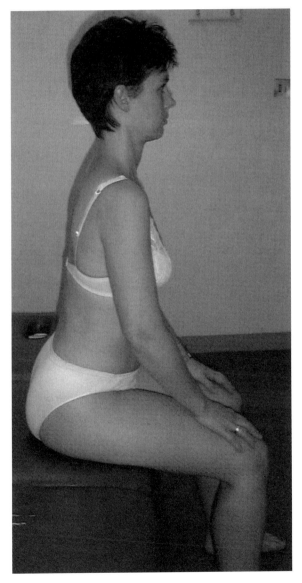

Figure 8.4 Sitting neutral spine forward lean.

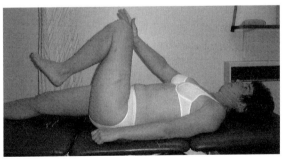

Figure 8.5 Activation of psoas, multifidus, oblique abdominals and pelvic floor muscles in supine.

8.2.3 Integration of Local Stabiliser Recruitment into Normal Function

It is suggested that to integrate an activity or skill into normal, automatic or unconscious function many repetitions must be performed under diverse functional situations.[46] Grimby and Hannerz directly relate proprioceptive dysfunction to dysfunction of tonic or slow motor unit recruitment.[47]

8.2.3.1 Proprioceptive Challenge Training

- Sitting unsupported maintaining a neutral spine: move forwards to backwards at the hip joints; and from side to side holding the PFM synchronised with the other relevant muscle groups (Fig. 8.4).
- Sitting: balance in spine neutral
  - balance boards: progress from a square to a circular balance board.
  - Sit-fit (Sissel UK Ltd): progress from balancing on a single stack to a double stack
  - balance ball training.

8.2.4 Conclusions

O'Sullivan[36,39,40] has demonstrated the clinical effectiveness of integrating the deep stability muscle system into functional movements, activities of daily living and even high loads and provocative positions. This integration is the aim of any rehabilitation programme. TrA or PFM activation must be trained under low load and feel easy before functional integration occurs.

Co-activation of the abdominal, erector spinae, diaphragmatic and PFM is essential to developing the intra-abdominal pressure necessary for spinal stability.[38] These muscles must have efficient tonic recruitment for stability in normal load functions. However, they must also have strength for high load or stressful situations. Any muscle activation that compromises normal function should be avoided.

We still have much to learn about normal muscle function and physiology, and so much more regarding the most effective way to rehabilitate dysfunction. The examples provided here are far from being a fully exhaustive list.

References

1. Agency for Health Care Policy and Research (AHCPR) Urinary Incontinence Guideline Panel (1996) Urinary Incontinence in Adults: Acute and Chronic Management. US Department of Health and Human Services , Rockville, Md.

2. Wilson PD, Samarrai TA, Deakin M, Kolbe E, Brown ADG (1987) An objective assessment of physiotherapy for female genuine stress incontinence. Br J Obstet Gynaecol 94: 575–82.

3. Ferguson KL, McKey PL, Bishop KR et al. (1990) Stress urinary incontinence: Effect of pelvic muscle exercise. Obstet Gynecol 75(4): 671–5.

4. Wells TJ, Brink CA, Diokno AC, Wolfe R, Gillis GL (1991) Pelvic muscle exercise for stress urinary incontinence in elderly women. J Am Geriatr Soc 39: 785–91.

5. Wallace K (1994) Female pelvic floor functions, dysfunctions and behavioural approaches to treatment. Clin Sports Med 13(2): 459–81.

6. Berghmans LCM, Hendriks HJM, Bø K et al (1998) Conservative treatment of stress urinary incontinence in women: a systematic review of randomised clinical trials. Br J Urol 82: 181–91.

7. Theofrastous JP, Wyman JF, Bump RC et al. and the Continence Program for Women Research Group (1997) Relationship between urethral and vaginal pressures during pelvic muscle contractions. Neurourol Urodynamics 16: 553–8.

8. Bø K, Larsen S, Oseid S, Kvarstein B, Hagen R, Jorgenson J (1988) Knowledge about and ability to correct pelvic floor muscle exercises in women with urinary stress incontinence. Neurourol Urodynamics 69: 261–2.

9. Bump RC, Hurt WG, Fantl JA, Wyman JA (1991) Assessment of Kegel pelvic muscle exercise performance after brief verbal instructions. Am J Obstet Gynecol 165: 322–9.

10. Gilpin SA, Gosling JA, Smith ARB, Warrell DW (1989) The pathogenesis of genitourinary prolapse and stress incontinence of urine. A histological and histochemical study. Br J Obstet Gynaecol 96: 15–23.

11. Jones DA, Round JM (1990) Skeletal Muscle in Health And Disease. Manchester University Press, Manchester, UK, pp. 66–8.

12. Bø K (1995) Pelvic floor muscle exercise for the treatment of stress urinary incontinence: An exercise physiology perspective. Int Urogynecol J 6: 282–91.

13. American College of Sports Medicine (1990) The recommended quantity and quality of exercise for developing and maintaining cardiorespiratory and muscular fitness in healthy adults. Med Sci Sports Exerc 22: 265–74.

14. Bø K, Talseth T (1996) Long-term effect of pelvic floor muscle exercise 5 years after cessation of organised training. Obstet Gynecol 87(2): 261–5.

15. Sapsford RR, Hodges PW (2000) Voluntary abdominal exercise and pelvic floor muscle activity. Neurourol Urodynamics 19(4): 510–11.

16. American College of Sports Medicine Position Stand (1990) The recommended quantity and quality of exercises for developing and maintaining cardiovascular and muscular fitness in healthy adults. Med Sci Sports Exerc 22: 265–74.

17. DiNubile NA (1991) Strength training. Clin Sports Med 10(1): 33–62.

18. Shephard RJ, Astrand P-O (1992) Endurance in Sport. The Encyclopaedia of Sports Medicine. An IOC publication, in collaboration with the International Federation of Sports Medicine, Blackwell Scientific, Oxford, pp. 50–61.

19. Astrand P-O, Rodahl K (1988) Textbook of Work Physiology. Chapter 10, Physiological basis of exercise. McGraw-Hill, New York.

20. Miller J, Ashton-Miller J, DeLancey J (1998) A pelvic muscle pre-contraction can reduce cough related urine loss in selected women with mild SUI. J Am Geriatr Soc 46: 870–4.

21. Sampselle CM, Miller JM, Mims BL, DeLancey JOL (1998) Effect of pelvic muscle exercise on transient incontinence during pregnancy and after birth. Obstet Gynecol 91: 406–12.

22. Nielson CA, Sigsgaard I, Olsen M, Tolstrup M et al. (1988) Trainability of the pelvic floor. Acta Obstet Gynecol Scand 67: 437–40.

23. Morkved S, Bø K (1997) The effect of postpartum pelvic floor muscle exercises in the prevention and treatment of urinary incontinence. Int Urogynecol J 8: 217–22.

24. Morkved S, Bø K (2000) Effect of postpartum pelvic floor muscle training in the prevention and treatment of urinary incontinence: a one-year follow up. Br J Obstet Gynaecol 107: 1022–8.

25. Bø K, Larsen S (1992) Pelvic floor muscle exercise for the treatment of female stress urinary incontinence: classification and characterization of responders. Neurourol Urodynamics 11: 497–507.

26. Ramsey I, Thow M (1990) A randomised, double blind placebo controlled trial of pelvic floor exercises in the treatment of genuine stress incontinence. Neurourol Urodynamics 9: 398–9.

27. Bø K (1994) Isolated muscle exercises. In: Schüssler B, Laycock J, Norton P, Stanton S (ed) Pelvic Floor Re-education. Principles and Practice. Springer, Berlin, pp. 134–8.

28. Prashar S, Simons A, Bryant C, Dowell C, Moore KH (2000) Attitudes to vaginal/urethral touching and device placement in women with urinary incontinence. Int Urogynecol J Pelvic Floor Dysfunct 11(1): 4–8.

29. Laycock J (1994) Clinical evaluation of the pelvic floor. In: Schüssler B, Laycock J, Norton P, Stanton S (ed) Pelvic Floor Re-education. Springer, Berlin, pp. 42–8.

30. Bø K, Hagen RH, Kvarstein B et al. (1990) Pelvic floor muscle exercise for the treatment of female stress urinary incontinence: effects of two different degrees of pelvic floor muscle exercises. Neurourol Urodynamics 9(5): 489–502.

31. Sapsford RR, Hodges PW, Richardson CA et al. (2001) Co-activation of the abdominal and pelvic floor muscles during voluntary exercise. Neurourol Urodynamics 20: 31–42.

32. Bø K, Stien R (1994) Needle EMG registration of striated urethral wall and pelvic floor activity patterns. Neurourol Urodynam 13: 35–41.

33. Sapsford RR, Markwell SJ, Clarke B (1998) The relationship between urethral pressure and abdominal muscle activity. Proceedings of the 7th National Conference on Incontinence, 1998, Canberra, p. 37.

34. Sapsford RR, Markwell SJ (1998) Start, now stop the flow. Proceedings of the 7th National Conference on Incontinence, 1998, Canberra, p. 50.

35. Hodges PW, Richardson CA (1999) Altered trunk muscle recruitment in people with low back pain with upper limb movement at different speeds. Arch Phys Med Rehabil 80(9): 1005–12.

36. O'Sullivan PB, Twomey L, Allison G (1997) Evaluation of specific stabilising exercise in the treatment of chronic low back pain with radiological diagnosis of spondylosis or spondylolisthesis. Spine 22(24): 2959–67.

37. Hodges PW, Richardson CA (1996) Inefficient stabilisation of the lumbar spine associated with low back pain. Spine 21: 2640–50.

38. Hodges PW, Richardson CA, Sapsford RR (1996) Therapeutic Exercise for Spinal Segmental Stabilisation in Low Back Pain. Churchill Livingstone, Edinburgh, UK, pp. 53–4.

39. O'Sullivan PB, Twomey L, Allison G (1997) Dysfunction of the neuro-muscular system in the presence of low back pain – implications for physical therapy. J Man Manipulative Ther 5(1): 20–6.

40. O'Sullivan PB, Twomey L, Allison G et al. (1997) Altered patterns of abdominal muscle activation in patients with chronic low back pain. Aust J Physiother 43(2): 91–8.

41. Constantinou CE, Govan DE (1982) Spatial distribution and timing reflex generated urethral pressures in healthy females. J Urol 127(5): 964–9.

42. Richardson CA, Jull GA (1995) Muscle control – pain control. What exercises would you prescribe? Manual Therapy 1: 2–10.

43. Hodges PW, Gandevia SC, Richardson CA (1997) Contractions of specific abdominal muscles in postural tasks are affected by respiratory manoeuvres. J Appl Physiol 83: 753–60.

44. Lee DG (1999) Kinetics of the pelvic girdle. In: Lee DG (ed) The Pelvic Girdle. An approach to the examination and treatment of the lumbo-pelvic-hip region. Churchill Livingstone, Edinburgh, UK, pp. 57–60.

45. Hides JA, Richardson CA, Jull GA (1996) Multifidus muscle recovery is not automatic after resolution of acute, first-episode low back pain. Spine 21(23): 2763–9.

46. Rothstein J, Roy S, Wolf S (1991) The Rehabilitation Specialist's Handbook. F.A. Davis, Philadelphia, Pa.

47. Grimby L, Hannerz J (1976) Disturbances in voluntary recruitment order of low and high frequency motor units on blockades of proprioceptive afferent activity. Acta Physiol Scand 96: 207–16.

9 Improving Patient's Adherence

P.E. Chiarelli

When patients comply with a prescribed medical regimen they are said to be adherent. The problem of the extent to which patients follow the advice given to them by healthcare professionals is a major one.

9.1 How Can Patients Be Encouraged To Adhere To Treatment Protocols?

There is scant evidence specifically relating to patient adherence and programmes developed for the management of bladder control problems. Inference might be drawn from studies relating to behaviour change as well as evidence taken from studies of programmes designed to manage such things as heart disease, asthma and increasing general exercise levels. Demographic characteristics (including age) have not been shown to be associated with patient adherence, but there are a number of factors that should be considered (see below).

9.1.1 Changing Inappropriate Attitudes and Beliefs

A sizeable body of literature has been published showing positive correlation between components of the health belief model (HBM) and patient adherence.[1,2] On the basis of studies of improved adherence, it is suggested that in order to ensure that the patient's beliefs and attitudes are likely to lead to adherence, it is necessary to explore:

- the patient's understanding of the diagnosis and cause of symptoms
- the patients comprehension and recall of the prescribed programme (knowledge)
- the patients beliefs and understanding of the long-term consequences of the condition being suffered
- with the patient, any barriers to treatment
- with the patient, the perceived benefits of adhering to the programme
- ways of increasing the opportunities to act
- providing cues or reminders that might trigger the desired response.

9.1.2 Using Other Principles of Behaviour Change

One of the most frequently identified psychosocial determinants of adherence to physical activity is the individual's perceptions of personal capability or self-efficacy.[3] Self-efficacy relates to an individual's perceptions of their capability to do what is being asked of them. Research in the exercise domain has demonstrated self-efficacy to be implicated in exercise adherence in diseased as well as asymptomatic populations, in large-scale studies and in training studies.[4,5] A study of postnatal women in focus groups has allowed the development of a continence promotion programme based on the HBM which includes principals of behaviour change such as self-efficacy.[6]

9.1.3 Improving Communication with Patients

Research suggests that instead of looking for the source of non-compliance in the patient's uncooperative personality, we should turn to the doctor–patient relationship to see that the patient's needs are being met.[7]

Continence promotion programmes involve varying degrees of patient education and information transfer. Patient adherence to prescribed treatment protocols has been shown to be significantly associated with their satisfaction with communications.[8] Studies dealing with patient recall show that under the best of circumstances patients will only be able to recall two-thirds of the information they are given. Strategies to enhance recall should therefore be incorporated into treatment programmes. Such strategies include:[9]

- primacy (presenting the most important information first)
- stressing and repeating important facts
- using explicit categorization
- using more specific advice
- checking that the patient understands the information given by asking them to repeat it in their own words
- using written instructions and wherever possible, having the patient write the instruction
- the use of reminders.

9.2 Strategies To Increase Patient Motivation

Inherent in the concept of adherence to exercise programmes is the factor of motivation. Studies of adherence with exercise therapy show programmes that include motivational strategies to be more effective.[10,11] Other proven key components of success include:

- goal setting
- negotiating treatment goals and formulating plans that are tailored to the needs of the individual patient's situation and daily routine
- finding specific events in a patient's daily routine to which programme components might be anchored.[12]

Patients find it easier to adhere to programmes that involve fewer lifestyle changes. Although the studies showing associations between higher adherence rates and less complex treatment protocols apply mostly to the prescription of drugs,[9] it seems sensible to assume that the less complex protocols

for the management of bladder and bowel control problems might also have higher adherence rates.

Patients are more likely to comply with treatment programmes that cause the least disruption to their normal daily routine and those that include positive feedback to the patient specifically about their programme adherence.[13] Studies show that when any effective adherence-aiding strategy is withdrawn, adherence levels deteriorate. It is therefore important to check adherence at every consultation.

9.3 Conclusion

Careful attention to the adoption of these strategies at every patient contact might enhance a patient's adherence to their prescribed treatment and, most importantly, their outcomes from treatment.

References

1. Becker MH, Maiman LA (1975) Socio-behavioral determinants of compliance with health and medical care recommendations. Med Care 8: 10–24.
2. Janz NK, Becker MH (1984) The health belief model a decade later. Health Educ Q 11(1): 1–47.
3. Bandura A (1982) Self-efficacy mechanism in human agency. Am Psychol 37(2): 122–47.
4. Knapp D (1988) Behavioural management techniques and exercise promotion. In: Dishman R (ed) Exercise Adherence. Human Kinetics, Champaign, Ill., pp. 203–35.
5. McAuley E, Courneya K, Rudolph D, Lox C (1994) Enhancing exercise compliance in middle-aged males and females. Prev Med 23: 498–506.
6. Chiarelli P, Cockburn J (1999) The development of a physiotherapy continence promotion program using a customer focus. Aust J Physiother 45(2): 111–20.
7. Peck C, King NJ (1986) Medical Compliance. In: King N, Remenyi A (eds) Health Care, A Behavioural Approach. Grune and Stratton, Sydney, pp. 185–91.
8. Ley P, Llewellyn S (1993) Improving patient's understanding, recall, satisfaction and compliance. In: Broome A, Llewellyn S (eds) Health Psychology. Process and applications. Chapman & Hall, Melbourne.
9. Cockburn J, Reid A, Bowman J, Sanson-Fisher R (1987) Effects of intervention on antibiotic compliance in patients in general practice. Med J Aust 147: 324–8.
10. Ice R (1985) Long-term compliance. Phys Ther 65(12): 1832–9.
11. Friedrich M, Gittler G, Halberstadt Y, Cermak T, Heiller I (1998) Combined exercise and motivation program: Effect on the compliance and level of disability of patients with low back pain: A randomized control trial. Arch Phys Med Rehabil 79: 475–87.
12. Hallberg J (1970) Teaching patients self care. Nurs Clin North Am 5: 223–31.
13. Sluijs E, Kok G, Zee J (1993) Correlates of exercise compliance in physical therapy. Phys Ther 73: 771–86.

10 Biofeedback for the Assessment and Re-education of the Pelvic Floor Musculature

J. Haslam

Biofeedback uses an instrument to enable conscious regulation of some body functions by intentional mental control. Different methods can be used in pelvic floor muscle (PFM) re-education, including proprioception and verbal encouragement during digital assessment, vaginal cones, manometric and electromyographic (EMG) feedback. Biofeedback not only helps in PFM awareness, but also provides interest, challenge, reward for effort, a greater feeling of control and progress monitoring.

10.1 Digital Biofeedback

Vaginal or rectal digital PFM assessment of the perineum is a form of biofeedback, by increasing muscle awareness. Verbal feedback of a voluntary contraction can also encourage and assist in enhancing patient effort.

10.2 Use of Biofeedback Equipment

Specific PFM biofeedback equipment uses manometry or surface electromyography (SEMG) as methods of monitoring change. Pressure or SEMG activity can only be considered as a reliable tool of measurement if it is able to yield a reproducible measure of muscle strength, power and duration of contraction prior to fatigue. Informed consent and adequate information must be given and infection control procedures adhered to in the practice of biofeedback.

10.3 Manometric Biofeedback

Manometry is the use of an instrument to detect, assess and record pressure. Kegel used the term "perineometer" for a pressure gauge specific to the PFM.[1] He evolved the instrument for both diagnosis and "non-surgical treatment to women suffering with genital relaxation". Essentially, a pressure perineometer consists of a pressure probe with a connector tube to a manometer. Depending on the sophistication of the equipment, the pressure changes may be shown on a dial, a digital readout, a bar chart or a graphical representation. Different types of probes – air-filled, water-filled, individually made and mass produced – have been reported. Perineometers aim to show changes in pressure caused by the contraction of the perivaginal musculature, to be observable on a manometer gauge. The pressure changes can be measured in centimetres of water (cm H_2O) or millimetres of mercury (mm Hg).

Because the sizes and shapes of perineometer probes are variable, results are not transferable.[2] Anyone using manometry needs to evaluate how any other possible influences are evaluated and eliminated. However, if the same equipment is used following a well-defined protocol, manometry can be most useful both in showing change and in motivating patients.

10.3.1 Research Evidence for the Use of Manometry

Many studies have utilised perineometry both for PFM assessment and as an outcome measure,[3–5] but there is little good-quality research reporting any correlation between manometry and other assessment techniques.

Kegel was a pioneer in PFM therapy but gave only scant information regarding study populations and objective outcomes. In the 1990s Dougherty et al. described a bespoke intravaginal balloon device (IVBD)[6] that was used in further studies.[7–9] However, because of its individual construction the IVBD is considered a research tool and not generally a clinical option.

Other studies have been performed to assess and show the reliability and validity of perineometry;[10,11] reproducibility has also been examined.[12] It has also been shown that the reading for a first PFM contraction is higher than for the next four PFM contractions;[12] this has implications for the clinician determining any changes in PFM contractility. Further investigations have shown the importance of correct placement of the vaginal pressure probe.[13] A six-element sensor for measuring vaginal pressure profiles was devised, allowing measurements to be taken at different vaginal levels. The proximal balloon was shown to correlate with abdominal pressure and the distal balloon sensors responded to contractions of the PFM.[13]

10.3.2 Computerised Manometric Equipment

Before any vaginal biofeedback the patient must be vaginally assessed to ensure the suitability of any probe. Rigorous attention must be paid to patient position and the number and position of any pillows used. If manometry is being used to enhance performance, the patient should be able to observe the screen comfortably during the treatment session.

The pressure probe must be used in accordance with local infection control policies. The probe should be deflated before introduction into the vagina, covered with a suitable condom, located appropriately and then inflated to patient comfort. Over-inflation should be avoided especially if the patient has any sensory impairment. The probe position registering maximally when the patient is at rest determines optimal vaginal positioning. To ensure reproducibility this position must be maintained during any recordings of vaginal pressure during PFM contractions. The inflation should be recorded to ensure the same degree of inflation at any future assessment and treatment sessions. If possible, the distance that the probe is inserted into the vagina needs to be measured and recorded; an adjustable external flange can be useful for this purpose. Any movement of the probe within the vagina during the procedure will invalidate the subsequent readings. If the same patient is to be reassessed at a future date, all conditions must be

Table 10.1. Summary of the essential considerations for reproducibility of perineometry

Each session	Action
Explanation and consent	Must be documented
Reproducible positioning of the patient	Comfort and ease of vision to the screen
Consistent inflation of the probe	Beware under- or overinflation
Consistent probe position	Use a flange if available, otherwise, great care must be taken to ensure a return to baseline between each contraction
Consistency of the PFM warm-up procedure	Always use the same contraction, e.g. the fifth
An equal amount of verbal coaching	Refrain from varying enthusiasm
The same adequate rest periods	Appropriate rest period for the individual
Return to baseline between contractions	If there is no return to baseline it may be the patient is not relaxing or that the probe has slipped

exactly the same for the measurements to be considered valid. For a summary of essential considerations, see Table 10.1.

The clinician has to use their own skills to ensure that once a baseline is fixed, the probe is held accurately to ensure a return to baseline between each PFM contraction (see Fig. 10.1).

A blank screen is used for the initial assessment to determine the most appropriate displays to be used for further assessment, treatment and motivation. Trained PFM should be able to swiftly respond

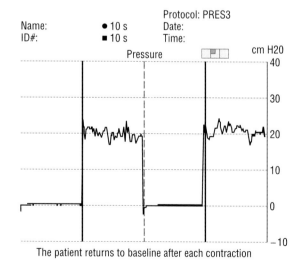

The patient returns to baseline after each contraction

Figure 10.1 The patient returns to baseline after each contraction.

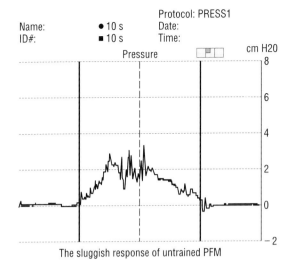

Figure 10.2   The sluggish response of untrained PFM.

to the instruction to both contract and relax (see Fig. 10.1); an untrained pelvic floor will often show a sluggish response to both commands (see Fig. 10.2).

The use of predetermined templates (Fig. 10.3) for either contraction or relaxation (see Section 3 on pelvic pain) can assist in gaining the patient's interest and compliance using either manometry or SEMG.

Other extraneous factors that may affect performance include the time of day, general fatigue and hormonal status. The aim of re-education is not only to have a greater ability to generate force with the PFM but also to have better functional ability to counterbrace whenever there is need. For the patient who has stress leakage during coughing this can be practised during manometry by having them con-

tract their PFM, continue to hold the contraction while coughing and be able to still see the same strength of contraction visible after the cough, until the time of conscious relaxation. This enables an individual to appreciate the activity necessary in a functional manner. Generally, pressure probe design limits the patient positions that can be used for biofeedback.

It has been shown that the abdominal muscles are co-activated with the PFM.[14-16] Monitoring of abdominal activity can take place either by palpation or by the use of EMG surface electrodes judiciously placed on areas of unwanted activity.

10.3.3 Manometric Home Devices

Home devices (Fig.10. 4) can be useful for patients who require additional external proof of their PFM contractility, and can be most useful as a patient motivator. Adequate instructions about infection control and the correct method of use are essential. When an individual probe is used by a single patient there is no need to use a condom to cover the probe; however, normal hygiene procedures should be employed after each use, with adequate storage facilities between uses. It is advisable to provide written instructions regarding the cleansing procedures to be followed. The patient must follow specific instructions to ensure that they do not

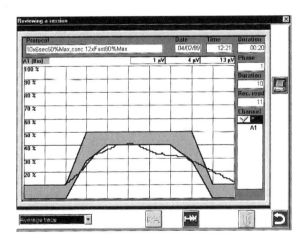

Figure 10.3   Attempting to follow a predetermined shape.

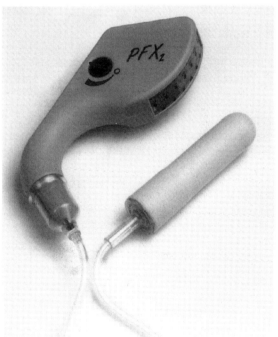

Figure 10.4   The home manometer (Cardio Design Australia).

apparently increase their "score" by gross activity of muscle groups other than the PFM.

10.4 Electromyography Biofeedback

Electromyography (EMG) has recently come into more popular usage as a method of assessment and treatment of pelvic floor dysfunction. EMG is a practical indicator of muscle activity and has been defined as the study of electrical potentials generated by the depolarisation of muscle[17] or, more simply, as the recording of muscle bioelectrical activity.[18] EMG should be considered a monitor of bioelectrical activity correlating to motor unit activity; it does not measure the muscle contractility itself but the electrical correlate of the muscle contraction. It is an electrical and not a kinetic measurement, in other words EMG acts an indicator of the physiological activity. Vaginal, anal or surface electrodes can be used to overview both the rest and contraction phases of PFM activity. The advantage over manometric pressure is that, provided the machinery is of sufficient sophistication with adequate filtering, EMG apparatus can engage the use of the newer types of electrodes that are lightweight and designed to stay in place, hence allowing more functional positions during assessment and treatment.

10.4.1 Neurophysiology Applied to Surface EMG

A motor unit is made up of the anterior horn cell, its myelinated axon and peripheral nerve endings. (Fig. 10.5) The muscle fibres supplied are scattered throughout the muscle. The muscle fibres within the motor unit contract simultaneously through depolarisation of the anterior horn cell, resulting in a nerve action potential along the myelinated motor axon. It is the nerve action potential that causes the

release of acetylcholine and subsequent depolarisation of the motor end plates. The depolarising current along the muscle fibre membrane can be detected by single-needle EMG. Thus, single-needle EMG can detect activity and permit visualization of the individual motor unit action potentials.[17,19] However, surface EMG can only detect an overall pattern of concurrent activity of motor units within the field of the surface electrode. Furthermore, information from surface EMG may be contaminated by crosstalk from other muscles in the area. This lack of selectivity may lead to erroneous conclusions of "co-activation".[20]

There are also inter-patient variables that can affect EMG values, including muscle volume, intervening adipose tissues and motivation of the subjects.[21] Other variables include the EMG equipment, electrodes and the cabling between the two. As surface electrodes measure action potentials from a number of motor units, the smaller the active surface and the closer the electrodes the less the muscle cross-talk and interference from other adjacent striated muscle.

10.4.2 EMG Equipment

The purpose of EMG is to pick up bioelectrical signals from the muscle group under investigation without picking up any of the electrical energy transmitted from elsewhere. The two "active" electrodes detect electrical activity, each with respect to the reference electrode. The two signals are then fed into the differential amplifier which amplifies the difference of the two signals but eliminates any signals common to both. The *common mode rejection ratio* is a measure of how effective the differential amplifier is in eliminating the common mode signal. This is of particular importance to a therapist working in any environment with large amounts of extraneous environmental electromagnetic radiation. It also explains any erroneously high readings that can occur if there is any deterioration of the electrode or poor skin contact. High readings may also be due to battery failure or faults within the cables or the machinery itself. Any unusually high readings should always make the clinician check all possibilities before continuing with the biofeedback. Artefacts of cardiac activity (ECG) may also be picked up, and recognised by regular interference patterns corresponding with cardiac activity. If no fault can be found, the interference may be due to other excessive environmental noise. Equipment that is marketed for therapeutic EMG has the raw EMG signal rectified, smoothed and integrated.

Instruments often have a notch filter to reduce the background noise of the mains frequency (50 Hz in

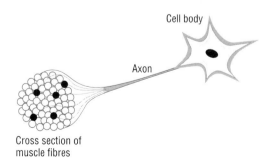

Figure 10.5 A motor unit.

the UK, 60 Hz in the US). The normal frequency distribution of EMG signals resembles that of a bell curve. Lower-frequency signals (0–20 Hz) are often considered unstable, so manufacturers may filter the lower and higher signals by bandpass filters. Clearly any difference in bandwidth filters will lead to different readings, especially at the lower end of the spectrum in examination of very weak PFM.

10.4.3 EMG Biofeedback Practice

The feedback may be in the form of an audio signal or a visual display, or a combination of the two. Simpler equipment for home use may have a series of lights, whereas the more sophisticated equipment has graphical displays that can be used in comparative reports. It must always be remembered that EMG instrumentation varies between manufacturers and models with regard to the sophistication of the amplification and bandpass filters, and different results may be recorded between different machines.

10.4.4 Types of Electrodes

Single fibre and concentric needle electrodes are used to detect activity in single or very few motor units; they may cause discomfort and limit patient mobility. They require good clinical expertise and are used mainly for neurophysiological studies and research purposes.

Therapists can use surface electrodes to assess and treat muscle dysfunction. EMG electrodes must be of good conductivity and be accurately placed on an appropriately cleansed skin surface. The electrodes should be placed closely together on the muscle belly in the direction of the muscle fibres.

Surface Patch Electrodes Surface patch electrodes are usually self-adhesive electrodes for single use. They can be used to detect unwanted activity such as that of the rectus abdominis, or desirable activity such as a PFM contraction. Care must be taken to ensure that the skin conductivity is as good as possible by cleansing the skin appropriately with an alcohol-based cleanser or soap and water to remove dead cells, dirt and natural oils before applying the electrode.[22]

Accurate placement, using anatomical bony points as markers, is recommended. The bipolar arrangement of electrodes detects all muscle activity between them. Close positioning ensures greater accuracy and specificity: wider spacing of electrodes results in a monitoring of bioelectrical activity from a greater area. The reference electrode should ideally be placed an equal distance from each

of the active electrodes. Some makes of equipment require a bony point to be used for the reference electrode, as that is the point of minimal bioelectrical activity. Even when great care is taken regarding accurate electrode placement it is thought unlikely that external surface EMG is totally reproducible and accurate.

Anal Electrodes Anal electrodes record activity from perianal musculature detected through the anal mucosa. The electrodes are generally for single patient use only. The size of the electrode may affect activity. A larger probe may stretch the sphincter and cause a desire to bear down; a smaller one may cause contraction of the anal sphincter even at rest in order to prevent the electrode from slipping out.

Vaginal Electrodes Vaginal electrodes detect PFM activity through the vaginal mucosa. They vary in shape, size and weight, depending on the manufacturer, and these factors can limit the functional positions used in therapy. Vaginal secretions may affect conductivity, and normal hygiene precautions are necessary. Vaginal electrodes are designed for single-patient use unless the manufacturer states that they are autoclavable and this concurs with local infection control policies. Until the mid 1990s vaginal electrodes were limited in their use mainly to the supine position, as their size and design caused discomfort in sitting and their weight made retention in standing very difficult. The development of the Periform intravaginal probe (Neen HealthCare, UK) made the use of vaginal electrodes for biofeedback in positions other than supine more feasible. The Periform is oval in shape to assist in comfortable insertion and to ensure that there is no net downwards force; there is also a central hollow section so that vaginal tissues can form within the hollow, providing a vertical anchor. As the Periform is essentially rectangular in cross-section it resists rotatory movement; moreover, the external flange assists positioning and retention. The design of this probe ensures that it is both lightweight and easy to clean. All of these factors increase the ability of the therapist to treat patients with EMG biofeedback in more functional positions. At present the Periform vaginal electrode is only available in one size (see Fig. 6.8, page 53).

10.4.5 Use of EMG Biofeedback

EMG may be used in assessing resting activity and recruitment activity, for increasing patient awareness and for isolation of activity; however, it has even more variables than manometry. Each type of

EMG equipment may have different parameters for filters, bandwidth and amplification. Each patient is an individual with differing conductivity according to the placement of the electrode. Subcutaneous fatty tissue, skin resistance and the electrode used can all result in different recordings. Electrodes are also variable in conductivity and therefore the same type should be used on each occasion. Any couplant gel used must be specified and also used on further occasions.

10.4.6 Research-Based Evidence for the Use of EMG

There is good evidence for the use of EMG in assessment and rehabilitation of the PFM. It has been shown that there is a good correlation between digital, manometric and vaginal EMG providing that a careful protocol has been followed.[23] It has been shown that EMG compares well with pressure, but that bioelectrical activity of the PFM varies with subject position.[23] There is also a good correlation between perineal EMG and vaginal pressure and also between abdominal EMG and intra-abdominal pressure.[24]

A systematic review[25] concluded that there is a lack of evidence to prove that biofeedback is any more effective than PFM exercises alone in the treatment of stress urinary incontinence. However, this was disputed in a further meta-analysis when it was stated that biofeedback may be an important adjunct to PFM exercise in the treatment of stress urinary incontinence.[26] It has also been shown that home training using EMG-controlled biofeedback is effective[27] in the treatment of female urinary incontinence.

10.5 Other Methods of Biofeedback

Weighted vaginal cones are another method of biofeedback in which the patient harnesses the feeling of vaginal cone slippage to increased proprioception (see Chapter 11).

Another more recently evolved form of biofeedback is that in which a pelvic floor contraction indicator is used in association with the previously mentioned Periform probe (see Fig. 6.8). From this has evolved the Pelvic Floor Educator (Neen Health-Care, UK) (Fig. 10.6). The device is based on the principle of the "Q-tip test" which was developed to demonstrate urethral hypermobility.[28] The Periform or new Pelvic Floor Educator probe is placed vagi-

nally such that the device shows the angle of the vagina at rest and on PFM contraction.[29] When the PFM are contracted the downward deflection of the indicator provides an indication of PFM ability; an upward deflection indicates an inappropriate Valsalva manoeuvre.

Whichever type of biofeedback is used, once the patient has learnt the appropriate activity it should be harnessed functionally. If a patient is using weighted vaginal cones they should be used during increased activity, going up and down stairs, coughing, jumping, etc. If using EMG or manometric pressure feedback, the patient may commence biofeedback in lying but should proceed to treatment in sitting, standing and other functional positions.

10.6 Other Uses of Biofeedback

Biofeedback has also been used in patients suffering with hesitancy and urethral spasm associated with urethral syndrome, aiming to re-educate the patient to have greater awareness of pelvic floor relaxation. It is also useful following ileoanal pouch surgery to ensure that the patient can retain pelvic floor awareness during any period with a temporary stoma, and is extensively used in the treatment of constipation and other bowel dysfunctions (see Chapters 21 and 22).

Biofeedback also has a very important use in assisting the teaching of relaxation to patients

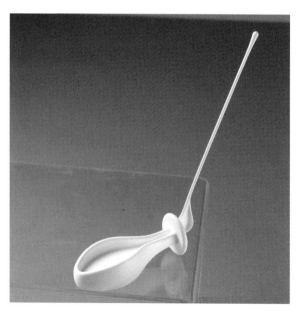

Figure 10.6 The Pelvic Floor Educator (Neen HealthCare UK).

suffering from vaginismus and other sexual disorders (see Chapter 27) and has also been used in the treatment of detrusor instability during cystometry.[30]

Biofeedback is a most exciting modality of treatment that can unfortunately be misused, but with appropriate training and care it provides a formidable weapon in the therapists' armoury.

References

1. Kegel AH (1948) Progressive resistance exercises in the functional restoration of the perineal muscles. Am J Obstet Gynecol 36(2): 238–48.
2. Laycock J, Sherlock R (1995) Perineometers – do we need a gold standard? Proceedings of the ICS Conference, 1995, 169: 144–5.
3. Ferguson KL, McKey PL, Bishop KR et al. (1990) Stress urinary incontinence: effect of pelvic muscle exercise. Obstet Gynecol 75(4): 671–5.
4. Dougherty M, Bishop K, Mooney R, Gimotty P, Williams B (1993) Graded pelvic muscle exercise. Effect on urinary incontinence. J Reprod Med 38(9): 684–91.
5. Griffin C, Dougherty MC, Yarandi H (1994) Pelvic muscles during rest: Responses to pelvic muscle exercise. Nurs Res 43(3): 164–7.
6. Dougherty MC, Abrams R, McKey PL (1986) An instrument to assess the dynamic characteristics of the circumvaginal musculature. Nurs Res 35(4): 202–6.
7. McKey PL, Dougherty MC (1986) The circumvaginal musculature: correlation between pressure and physical assessment. Nurs Res 35(5): 307–9.
8. Samples JT, Dougherty MC, Abrams RM, Batich CD (1988) The dynamic characteristics of the circumvaginal muscles. J Obstet Gynecol Neonatal Nurs (May/June): 194–201.
9. Dougherty M, Bishop KR, Mooney RA, Gimotty PA, Landy LB (1991) Variations in intravaginal pressure measurements. Nurs Res 40(5): 282–5.
10. Bø K, Kvarstein B, Hagen R, Larsen S (1990) Pelvic floor muscle exercise for the treatment of female stress urinary incontinence:– 1 Reliability of vaginal pressure measurements of pelvic floor muscle strength. Neurourol Urodynamics 9: 471–7.
11. Bø K, Kvarstein B, Hagen RR, Larsen S (1990) Pelvic floor muscle exercise for the treatment of female stress incontinence: II. Validity of vaginal pressure measurements of pelvic floor muscle strength and the necessity of supplementary methods for control of correct contraction. Neurourol Urodynamics 9: 479–87.
12. Wilson PD, Herbison GP, Heer K (1991) Reproducibility of perineometry measurements. Neurourol Urodynamics 10(4): 309–10.
13. Whyte TD, McNally DS, James ED (1993) Six-element sensor for measuring vaginal pressure profiles. Med Biol Eng Comput 31: 184–6.
14. Bø K, Stien R (1994) Needle EMG registration of striated urethral wall and pelvic floor muscle activity patterns during cough, valsalva, abdominal, hip adductor and gluteal muscle contractions in nulliparous healthy females. Neurourol Urodynamics 13: 35–41.
15. Sapsford RR, Hodges PW, Richardson CA et al. (1997) Activation of pubococcygeus during a variety of isometric abdominal exercises. Proceedings of the ICS Conference, 1997, pp. 115: 28–9.
16. Sapsford RR, Hodges PW (2000) Voluntary abdominal exercise and pelvic floor muscle activity. Neurourol Urodynamics 19(4): 510–11.
17. Andersen JT, Abrams P, Blaivas JG, Stanton SL (1987) Sixth report on the standardization of terminology of lower urinary tract function. Procedures related to neurophysiological investigations. Electromyography, nerve conduction studies, reflex latencies, evoked potentials and sensory testing. Br J Urol 59(4): 300–4.
18. Vodusek D (1994) Electrophysiology. In: Schussler B, Laycock J, Norton P (eds) Pelvic Floor Re-education. Springer, Berlin, pp. 83–97.
19. Vodusek DB, Bemelmans B, Chancellor K et al. (1999) Clinical neurophysiology. In: Abrams P, Khoury S, Wein A (eds) Incontinence: 1st International Consultation on Incontinence. Health Publication, UK, pp. 157–95.
20. Merletti R, Luca CJ De (1989) Crosstalk in surface electromyography. In: Desmedt J (ed) Computer Aided Electromyography and Expert Systems, Chapter 11. Elsevier, Amsterdam.
21. Basmajian JV, DeLuca CJ (1985) Muscles Alive: Their functions revealed by electromyography (5th ed). Williams & Wilkins, Baltimore, Md.
22. Turker KS (1993) Electromyography: some methodological problems and issues. Phys Ther 73(10): 698–710.
23. Haslam J (1999) Evaluation of pelvic floor muscle assessment, digital, manometric and surface electromyography in females. MPhil Thesis. University of Manchester, Manchester, UK.
24. Workman DE, Cassissi JE, Doherty MC (1993) Validation of surface EMG as a measure of intravaginal and intra abdominal activity: Implications for biofeedback assisted Kegel exercises. Psychophysiology 30: 120–5.
25. Berghmans LCM, Hendriks HJM, Bø K et al. (1998) Conservative treatment of stress urinary incontinence in women: a systematic review of randomised clinical trials. Br J Urol 82: 181–91.
26. Weatherall M (1999) Biofeedback or pelvic floor muscle exercises for female genuine stress incontinence: a meta-analysis of trials identified in a systematic review. BJU Int 83(9): 1015–16.
27. Hirsch A, Weirauch G, Steimer B et al. (1999) Treatment of female urinary incontinence with EMG-controlled biofeedback home training. Int Urogynecol J Pelvic Floor Dysfunct 10(1): 7–10.
28. Crystal D, Charme L, Copeland W (1971) Q-tip test in stress urinary incontinence. Obstet Gynecol 38: 313–15.
29. Laycock J (1998) An update on the management of female urinary incontinence. J Assoc Chart Physiother Women's Health 83: 3–5.
30. Cardozo LD, Abrams PH, Stanton SL, Feneley RCL (1978) Ideopathic bladder instability treated by biofeedback. Br J Urol 50: 521–3.

11 Vaginal Cones

J. Laycock

The pelvic floor muscles work in three ways – tonically, reflexly and voluntarily and it is important to address all three ways in a re-education programme. I believe that cone therapy may achieve this.

11.1 Function and Mode of Action of Cones

Weighted vaginal cones, introduced by Plevnik,[1] are designed to activate the pelvic floor muscles by promoting cone retention. The feeling of losing the cone provides biofeedback to ensure activation of the appropriate pelvic floor muscles; inappropriate muscle contraction, e.g. straining, would reject the cone. Cones are manufactured by several companies, and they come in a variety of shapes, sizes and weights.

Research to assess the mode of action of cones[2] used EMG recordings with intramuscular wire electrodes placed in the left and right pubococcygei. In supine, the insertion of the cone elicited a slight increase in the overall (continuous, tonic) motor unit activity, which increased on standing to a pattern of "waxing and waning", or occasionally, maximum recruitment with no variation. The study concluded that vaginal cones may induce strengthening of pelvic floor muscles as well as a learning effect leading towards a better co-ordinated muscle contraction. Because of the variability in vaginal size, orientation and amount of secretions, cone retention does not give an accurate, reliable measure of pelvic floor muscle strength.

Bø questioned the theoretical framework for cone therapy on pelvic floor muscle training;[3] however, despite this, many studies have demonstrated success rates between 68% and 79%.[4-6] A randomised controlled trial comparing cones with a home pressure biofeedback device (PFX: Cardio Design, Australia) and pelvic floor exercises (the control group) showed significant improvement in all three groups and no statistical difference between the groups.[7]

11.2 Cone Therapy

The following list describes a proposed sequence of events for teaching cone therapy using Aquaflex cones (SSL International, UK), which are available

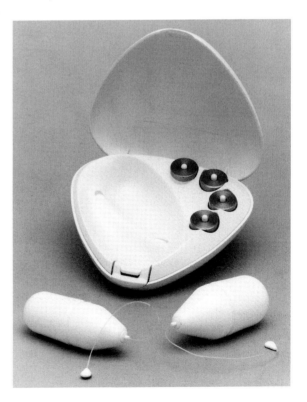

Figure 11.1 Aquaflex cones.

in two sizes of empty shell with weights placed inside (Fig. 11.1).

- The patient introduces an appropriate-sized cone with her index finger to position above pelvic floor (in the position of tampon location). If in doubt about cone size, start with the large cone, empty (no weights).
- Finger withdrawn and underwear replaced.
- Patient instructed to retain the cone in standing. *If successful,*
- Retain in stride standing. *If successful,*
- Retain during walking. *If successful,* record time held and
- Retain going up and down steps. *If successful,*
- Retain while coughing and during activities that cause urine leakage[8]
- Retain cone during activities of daily living
- Perform (patient specific) pelvic floor contractions, i.e. lifting the cone against gravity.

Progression: When cone retained for 5 min:

- Increase weight; when all weights held
- Decrease size of cone
- Increase time – up to 10 min
- Increase duration and repetition of pelvic floor contractions with cone in place.

If the patient cannot retain the cone in standing, cone therapy should be started in supine. The cone is introduced into the vagina and retained against gentle traction on the tail. As muscle contraction awareness increases, more traction is applied. Progression to standing follows the regimen described above. The ability to retain a cone of a certain weight may well depend on the size of the vagina and the amount and type of vaginal secretions; consequently, many women report variable results depending on the stage of their menstrual cycle. Furthermore, many subjects can retain a heavier cone in the morning than in the evening, presumably because of muscle fatigue, and this should be explained beforehand.

Cone therapy can be practised several times each day as part of a pelvic floor re-education programme. However, the results quoted from clinical trials involved one or two cone therapy sessions each day.

Box 11.1

Precautions and contraindications for cone therapy

Vagina too narrow to accept the smaller cone
Pain on insertion
Atrophic vaginitis
Vaginal infection
Moderate to severe prolapse
Menstruation
Within 2 h of intercourse
Seek advice from obstetrician during pregnancy

Some precautions and contra-indications for cone therapy are shown in Box 11.1. Patient compliance also depends on individual attitudes to vaginal devices, and this factor should be considered.

References

1. Plevnik S (1985) New method for testing and strengthening of pelvic floor muscles. Proceedings of ICS, 1985, London, pp. 267–8.
2. Deindl FM, Schussler B, Vodusek DB, Hesse U (1995) Neurophysiologic effect of vaginal cone application in continent and urinary stress incontinent women. Int Urogynecol J 6: 204–8.
3. Bø K (1995) Vaginal weight cones. Theoretical framework, effect on pelvic floor muscle strength and female stress urinary incontinence. Acta Obstet Gynecol Scand 74: 87–92.
4. Pieber D, Zivkovic F Tamussino G et al. (1995) Pelvic floor exercises alone or with vaginal cones for the treatment of mild to moderate stress urinary incontinence in premenopausal women. Int Urogynecol J 6: 14–17.
5. Peattie AB, Plevnik S, Stanton SL (1989) Vaginal cones: a conservative method of treating genuine stress incontinence. Br J Obstet Gynaecol 95: 1049–53.
6. Olah KS, Bridges N, Denning J, Farrar DJ (1990) The conservative management of patients with symptoms of stress incontinence: a randomized prospective study comparing weighted vaginal cones and interferential therapy. Am J Obstet Gynecol 162: 87–92.
7. Laycock J, Brown J, Cusack C et al. (1999) A multi-centre, prospective, randomised, controlled, group comparative study of the efficacy of vaginal cones and PFX. Neurourol Urodynamics 18(4): 301–2.
8. Burton G (1993) Active vaginal cone therapy: a new form of treatment for genuine stress incontinence. ICS suppl., 1993, Rome, pp. 134–5.

12 Electrical Stimulation

J. Laycock and D.B. Vodušek

There are two main types of therapeutic electrical stimulation devices available for physiotherapeutic application: battery-operated units suitable for home and hospital use, and mains-operated units generally used in hospitals. Both are capable of delivering a current intensity sufficient to depolarise sensory and motor nerves. Furthermore, many different names are given to this therapy, which can cause confusion. At high intensity, these devices can be used to strengthen striated muscles in the management of stress incontinence,[1] and normalise micturition reflexes in the treatment of detrusor overactivity and retention.[2-5] The availability of home units has enabled daily or twice daily treatments, resulting in improved health gains.

12.1 Electrodes

Vaginal electrodes are the most commonly used devices for applying electrical currents for lower urinary tract (LUT) problems in women. The vagina offers a route of low impedance, because of the low resistance of the vaginal mucosa and proximity to branches of the pudendal nerves. Anal electrodes are suitable for male patients, and male and female patients with anal sphincter weakness. Anal electrodes can also be used in narrow vaginas, where a vaginal electrode is too big and painful to insert. Electrodes suitable for electrical stimulation may also be used for electromyography (EMG) biofeedback.

To allow ambulatory electrical stimulation and biofeedback, electrodes should be lightweight, and, once in place, remain located within the vagina/anorectum. Such an electrode, the Periform, is described in Chapter 6. In addition to its use as a biofeedback device, the Periform allows clinicians, for the first time, to evaluate the amplitude of current required to produce a motor response, and patients should be encouraged to take sufficient current to produce movement of the indicator.

12.2 Electrical Parameters

Table 12.1 lists some important electrical parameters. More sophisticated equipment allows the clinician to alter these parameters to suit each patient's special requirements.

12.2.1 Frequency

12.2.1.1 Muscle Activation

A biphasic, rectangular pulse is generally recommended, and the number of pulses per second (pps) – the frequency – is selected to mimic the natural firing rate of motoneurons. Eccles et al.[6] described the firing rate of slow motoneurons as 10–20 pulses per second, and the rate for fast motoneurons as 30–60 pulses per second; this represents the discharge rate from the anterior horn cells. To reduce fatigue during electrical stimulation of muscles, the lowest frequency that produces a comfortable tetanic contraction should be selected. The effect of

Table 12.1. Electrical parameters

Parameter	Measurement
Frequency	Hertz (Hz) or pulses per second (pps)
Duty cycle	Time "on" and "off" (in seconds)
Pulse width	Microseconds (μs) or milliseconds (ms)
Pulse shape	Biphasic, symmetrical or asymmetrical
Length of treatment	Minutes

changing the frequency of stimulation on mixed (fast- and slow-twitch) striated muscle fibres of an adequate stimulus is shown in Figs 12.1–12.5.

Figure 12.1 shows the effect of a single pulse on fast- and slow-twitch muscle fibres. Slow-twitch muscle fibres respond with a slow rise in force, followed by a slow decline (long refractory period), whereas fast muscle fibres responding to the same pulse demonstrate a rapid increase and a greater force, followed by a rapid decline (a shorter refractory period).

Figure 12.2 shows that at approximately 8 Hz, the slow-twitch fibres are beginning to relax when the next impulse arrives, and the fast-twitch fibres have time to relax completely between each pulse. There are intermediate fibres that display some fast- and

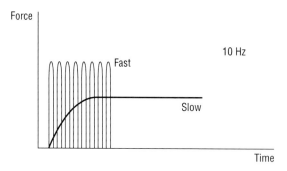

Figure 12.3 Effect of 10 Hz on slow and fast twitch muscle fibres.

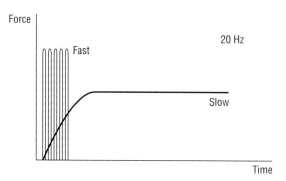

Figure 12.4 Effect of 20 Hz on slow and fast twitch muscle fibres.

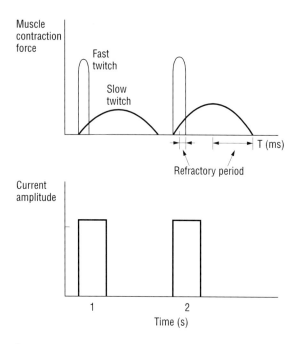

Figure 12.1 Diagrammatic representation of the effect of a single electrical pulse on slow and fast twitch muscle fibres.

some slow-twitch characteristics, but for simplicity, only the slow-twitch and fast-twitch responses are discussed here. At approximately 10 Hz, the slow-twitch fibres do not relax between pulses, but the fast-twitch fibres again have time to relax due to their short refractory period (Fig. 12.3). By increasing the frequency to 20 Hz, the fast fibres may still relax between pulses of electricity (Fig. 12.4). At 50 Hz, a fused tetanic contraction is produced, with the majority of muscle fibres contributing to a strong, forceful contraction, with minimal (if any)

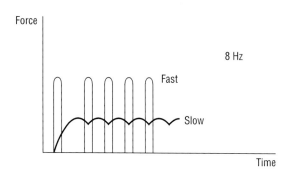

Figure 12.2 Effect of 8 Hz on slow and fast twitch muscle fibres.

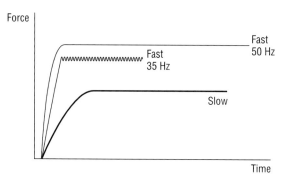

Figure 12.5 Effect of 35 Hz and 50 Hz on slow and fast twitch muscle fibres.

relaxation of the fast-twitch muscle fibres between pulses (Fig. 12.5). This frequency is obviously capable of fatiguing the fast fibres, if the muscle contraction is maintained for several seconds. In view of the propensity of 50 Hz (and higher frequencies) to produce muscle fatigue, a stimulating frequency of 35–40 Hz is proposed; this will produce a forceful contraction, minimising adverse effects due to fatigue (Fig. 12.5). If only a higher frequency, say 50 Hz or 70 Hz, is available, the duty cycle "rest" period (see below) should be increased or the treatment time reduced to minimise fatigue.

12.2.1.2 Detrusor Inhibition

The effect of electrical stimulation on pudendal afferents in the treatment of urge incontinence has been described[2,3] and clinically tested.[7] Optimum electrical parameters have been investigated by Ohlsson.[8] As a result of this comprehensive research, the following conclusions have been reported:

- Maximum vaginal/anal electrical stimulation produces pronounced detrusor inhibition by:
  - reflex activation of sympathetic inhibitory neurones[3,9]
  - reflex central inhibition of parasympathetic excitatory neurones.[3,10]
- Optimal electrical parameters include:
  - maximum current intensity tolerated (up to 80 mA)
  - frequency of 5–10 Hz generally advocated to minimise discomfort
  - pulse width 0.5–1.0 ms
  - duty cycle continuous or short rest periods.

In humans, bladder inhibition has been demonstrated by applying electrical stimulation to non-muscular pudendal afferents, e.g. the dorsal penile nerve.[4] Furthermore, Vodusek et al.[4,11] showed that weaker stimuli, applied in closer proximity to the pudendal nerve, are sufficient to produce bladder inhibition.

12.2.2 Duty Cycle

The duty cycle is the time the current is on and off. Generally speaking, to avoid undue fatigue, when a frequency of 35 Hz or more is selected, the off time should be at least double the on time,[12] and this should be adapted to the strength/weakness and endurance of the voluntary contraction.

The patient always "joins in" with the electrically stimulated contraction, and so the exercise is described as "active assisted" – active contraction, assisted by electrical stimulation. There is debate on the optimum duty cycle at 10 Hz for the treatment of detrusor instability, with many eminent clinicians prescribing continuous stimulation. However, to minimise the likelihood of fatigue, a duty cycle of 10/3 (10 s on, 3 s off) is recommended by the author (JL). During this time the patient is encouraged to contract the pelvic floor muscles submaximally with the stimulating current.

12.2.3 Pulse Width/Phase Duration

The duration of an electrical pulse, measured in microseconds or milliseconds, together with the amplitude, is a measure of the amount of energy transmitted per pulse to the tissues. The recommended pulse width for muscle stimulation is approximately 250 µs, and 500 µs or more recommended for bladder inhibition. When electrical stimulation is used for pain relief smaller pulse widths, in the region of 100 µs, are recommended.[13]

12.2.4 Pulse Shape

There is little, if any, comparative research to indicate which pulse configuration is most effective in producing a comfortable and effective pelvic floor muscle contraction or detrusor inhibition. However, asymmetrical biphasic rectangular pulses have been shown to be effective.

12.2.5 Ramp

The term "ramping" (also known as "surging") refers to the gradual change in current intensity, over 1–2 s, reducing the discomfort felt with a sudden change in amplitude; currents can be "ramped up" and "ramped down".

12.2.6 Length of Treatment

If a muscle-strengthening regimen is too long, fatigue may result, possibly causing an initial worsening of incontinence symptoms. In line with general recommendations for muscle stimulation, the first treatment should be limited to 5 min, and the effects of this treatment monitored. In order to have a training effect, it is necessary to gradually increase the time of treatment over several treatment sessions, and 20–30 min appears to be the optimum time for maximum stimulation reported in research studies. However, many studies have failed to recommend active-assisted therapy, and so patients are only achieving part of the desired effect. Furthermore, one would expect more fatigue with active-assisted therapy and therefore shorter periods of stimulation may be required.

A number of studies have reported using pelvic floor muscle stimulation once a day or twice a day, others alternate days or once per week, for a month, 6 weeks or 3–5 months.[14] A definitive frequency of treatment times and number of sessions has not been established. As with any exercise programme (which is what this is), daily, or twice daily, treatment is advantageous and this is possible if a home unit is available.

Electrical stimulation used for inhibition of an overactive detrusor should be given as often as possible, and may need to be repeated at periodic intervals, as symptoms are prone to recur.

12.3 Transcutaneous Electrical Nerve Stimulation

Surface electrodes over the perineum are thought to be less effective than vaginal electrodes in activating the deep pelvic floor musculature in cases of stress incontinence, because of the high resistance of the skin and the distance to the target nerves. However, good results have been reported with surface electrodes on the dermatomes of S2–4 (see Chapter 6) in the treatment of urge incontinence.[15] Perineal electrodes, clitoral clips and penile electrodes have all demonstrated efficacy. External electrode placement may be preferable to internally located electrodes in some cases.

12.4 Prolonged Effects of Electrical Stimulation

Electrical stimulation of pudendal afferent and efferent nerve fibres may lead to both pelvic floor contraction and inhibition of the overactive detrusor. Both these effects have been demonstrated during actual (ongoing) stimulation; however, there are delayed or "carry-over" effects of such stimulation as well. Short-term carry-over detrusor inhibition has been demonstrated,[4] which might be due to the activation of the spinal opioid system.[16] Carry-over effects of prolonged muscle contraction therapy include hypertrophy of muscle and change of motor unit types. However, apart from "peripheral" effects, we postulate that "central" effects are probably more important.

It seems attractive to analyse the therapeutic effectiveness of electrical stimulation in terms of control theory concepts: the electrically induced afferent input supplements the lost (or limited) physiological neural control. It is important to realise that quite opposite effects can be observed by the same sort of stimulation in different patient groups. Whereas hyperreflexive bladders in patients are inhibited (i.e. to improve storage), the hypo- or areflexive bladders in another group of patients may be activated to improve emptying.[5] It is as if the disrupted neural control is rearranged by electrostimulation by "hitting the switches" and thus turning the control mechanism towards a more functional state.

12.5 Adverse Effects

Abdominal cramps, diarrhoea, anal pain and anal bleeding have been reported with transrectal stimulation, and vaginal stimulation has been reported to cause vaginal irritation, pain and bleeding. The occurrence of adverse effects can be reduced by judicious application of any new modality, starting with a short (5 min) treatment period, and assessing any new symptomology before progressing to the next treatment. Symptoms due to short-term stimulation are generally mild, and disappear within a few days.[14]

12.6 Contraindications and Precautions

Urinary tract infection and atrophic vaginitis should be treated before a course of electrical stimulation.

There is insufficient evidence to support or discourage the use of electrical stimulation in pregnancy or in the presence of malignant tumours, and so most clinicians rightly assume that it is contraindicated. Evidence from a controlled study on pregnant rats[17] concluded that electrical stimulation did not have any adverse effects on the rats or their fetuses. However, this study used a low-frequency current and so these results should not be applied in cases of high-frequency currents, such as interferential therapy or "Russian" stimulation.

Contraindications and precautions are summarised in Boxes 12.1 and 12.2 respectively.

12.7 Conclusions

Electrical stimulation is becoming accepted as a useful therapy for incontinence by an increasing number of clinicians who believe that conservative treatment should be the treatment of choice. Patient

Box 12.1

Contraindications to low-frequency currents to the pelvic region

Patients who do not understand the procedure and instructions

Implanted pacemaker (especially demand type)

Pregnancy

Malignant tumour

Atrophic vaginitis, vaginal infection

Recent or recurrent haemorrhage/haematoma

Box 12.2

Precautions for low-frequency currents to the pelvic region

Selection of appropriate stimulation parameters

Selection of appropriate electrode

Check for allergy to electrode gel

Check for compromised circulation/mucosa

and doctor acceptance of electrical stimulation can be heightened by an appropriate physiologically orientated explanation, i.e. that electrical stimulation supplements and improves the use of available neuromuscular structures. We feel that patients should be encouraged to profit from the increased awareness that electrostimulation provides. Furthermore, electrical stimulation should be logically combined with biofeedback and pelvic floor muscle exercises for muscle strengthening, and with bladder drill and medication for detrusor hyper- and hypoactivity. However, the precise regimens or combinations need to be delineated by further studies.

References

1. Sand P, Richardson DA, Staskin DR et al. (1995) Pelvic floor electrical stimulation in the treatment of genuine stress incontinence: a multicenter, placebo-controlled trial. Am J Obstet Gynecol 173: 72–9.
2. Fall M, Lindstrom S (1991) Electrical stimulation. a physiologic approach to the treatment of urinary incontinence. Urol Clin N Am 18(2): 393–407.
3. Lindstrom S, Fall M (1983) The neurophysiological basis of bladder inhibition in response to intravaginal electrical stimulation. J Urol 129: 405–10.
4. Vodusek DB, Light JK, Libby J (1986) Detrusor inhibition induced by stimulation of pudendal nerve afferents. Neurourol Urodynam 5: 381–9.
5. Plevnik S, Homan G, Vrtacnik P (1984) Short-term maximal electrical stimulation for urinary retention. Urology 24: 521–3.
6. Eccles JC, Eccles RM, Lundberg A (1958) The action potentials of the alpha motoneurones supplying fast and slow muscles. J Physiol 142: 275–91.
7. Eriksen BC, Bergmann S, Mjolnerod OK (1987) Effect of anal electrostimulation with the "Incontan" device in women with urinary incontinence. Br J Obstet Gynaecol 94: 147–56.
8. Ohlsson B, Lindstrom S et al. (1986) Effects of some different pulse parameters on bladder inhibition and urethral closure during intravaginal electrical stimulation: an experimental study in the cat. Med Biol Eng Comput 24: 27–33.
9. Sundin T, Carlsson CA (1972) Reconstruction of several dorsal roots innervating the urinary bladder. An experimental study in cats. 1. Studies on normal afferent pathways in the pelvic and pudendal nerves. Scand J Urol Nephrol 6: 176–84.
10. Sundin T, Carlsson CA, Kock NG (1974) Detrusor inhibition induced from mechanical stimulation of pudendal nerve afferents. Invest Urol 11: 374–8.
11. Vodusek DB, Plevnik S, Vrtacnik P, Janez J (1988) Detrusor inhibition on selective pudendal nerve stimulation in the perineum. Neurourol Urodynamics 6: 389–93.
12. Packman-Braun R (1988) Relationship between functional electrical stimulation duty cycle and fatigue in the wrist extensor muscles of patients with hemiparesis. Phys Ther 68(1): 52–6.
13. Tulgar M, McGlone F, Bowsher D, Miles JB (1991) Comparative effectiveness of different stimulation modes in relieving pain. Part 1. A pilot study. Pain 47: 151–5.
14. Yamanishi T, Yasunda K (1998) Electrical stimulation for stress incontinence. Int Urogynecol J 9: 281–90.
15. Webb R, Powell H (1992) Transcutaneous electrical nerve stimulation in patients with idiopathic detrusor instability. Neurourol Urodynamics 11(4): 327–8.
16. Dray A, Metsch R (1984) Opioid receptors and inhibition of urinary bladder motility in vivo. Neurosci Lett 47: 81–4.
17. Wang Y, Hassouna MH (1999) Electrical stimulation has no adverse effect on pregnant rats and fetuses. J Urol 162: 1785–7.

13 Prosthetic Devices, Inserts and Plugs for the Management of Stress Incontinence

D. Tincello

Genuine stress incontinence accounts for two-thirds of hospital referrals for incontinence. Physiotherapy produces significant improvement in up to 90% of patients, with minimal side effects.[1] However, some patients will have no significant benefit from physiotherapy and eventually require surgery. Retropubic suspension procedures are generally considered the best operations in terms of cure rate, but side-effects include voiding dysfunction, detrusor instability and enterocele formation.[2]

13.1 Prosthetic Devices

Over recent years, prosthetic devices have developed in an attempt to provide an alternative to physiotherapy or surgery. Several vaginal devices and urethral inserts have become available and they have been assessed in studies of varying design and quality. Each device is considered separately, with a discussion of its design and mode of action, and the available data are examined critically.

13.2 Intraurethral Plugs

Neilsen et al.[3,4] described the concept of an intraurethral plug with a balloon tip to ensure correct positioning within the urethra. The original device was tested on 22 patients of whom 75% were either continent or improved on pad testing.[3] The device appeared to be less effective in patients with larger volumes of leakage. A modified device was assessed in a 3-month study involving 40 patients:[4] 22 patients withdrew from the study, and 16 of those who continued the study were continent or rarely wet. The changes in individual leakage were highly variable, and some patients became worse. Only 9 patients opted to continue using the device after the study was completed. Six patients developed urinary tract infections and 2 of these were found to have the device within the bladder.

The Reliance urinary control insert was the natural descendant of the Neilsen device, and this has been available since the mid-1990s (Fig. 13.1).

Two published studies have examined the device.[5,6] A multicentre study with 4-month follow-up showed

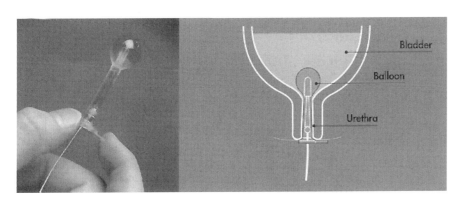

Figure 13.1 The Reliance urinary control insert (left panel) with a schematic representation of the device in situ (right panel). Courtesy of Astra Ltd.

the Reliance insert to be highly effective, with 80% continence rates and overall 95% improvement.[5] The most common reason cited by patients for withdrawing from the study was discomfort. A global measure of quality of life (the Short Form 36) showed significant improvement in results from patients who completed the study.[5] A 12-month follow-up study of 63 women with stress or mixed incontinence on cystometry testing found that 56 patients (89%) completed the study and 82% of these were continent with the device in situ. After 12 months, 79% were continent and 16% were improved. The device had a high level of side-effects, with up to 84% of patients having microscopic haematuria and 24% gross haematuria.[6] Some clinicians still express doubt about the long-term safety of the device, in view of the incidence of haematuria and migration into the bladder.[7]

13.3 Intravaginal Tampons and Pessaries

Intravaginal devices have been developed which produce upward pressure around the bladder neck. The earliest attempts to achieve continence were carried out using contraceptive and Hodge pessaries,[8,9] and produced rates of improvement of around 60%.

The Introl bladder neck support prosthesis is a polythene ring with two blunt prongs pointing superiorly (Fig. 13.2).

In a prospective study of 32 women with 4-week follow-up, 2 patients withdrew and 83% of women were dry with the device in place.[10] Urodynamic evaluation showed that the device mimicked the effects of colposuspension. Twenty-two of these patients (73%) were enrolled in a longer-term study of the device and the majority (68%) continued with

the device for 1 year.[11] These data have been confirmed by two other studies. Of 57 patients 29% were dry and another 51% had a reduction in leakage of at least 50% after 3 months.[12] There were 16 dropouts from the study. Foote et al.[13] found a success rate of 88% in 26 women using this device. Two studies in patients with both stress incontinence and mixed incontinence (GSI and detrusor instability) confirm these findings.[14,15] The results are similar to those of the other papers.

The Conveen continence guard is a shaped foam tampon with a plastic applicator (Fig. 13.3). The springiness of the foam ensures a good fit within the vagina with support of the bladder neck. Twenty-six women with symptoms of stress incontinence were studied with continence in 41% and significant improvement in a further 45%.[16] Nineteen women wished to continue with the device and were followed up for a further 12 months:[17] 68% were sub-

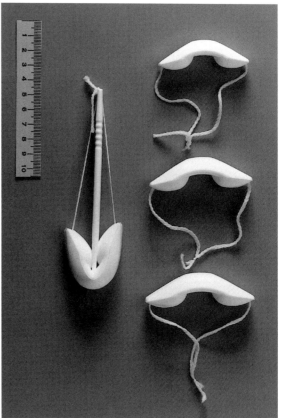

Figure 13.3 Conveen continence guard (in three different sizes) with applicator. [From Kozman EL, Frazer MI, Holland N. The use of mechanical devices in the management of stress incontinence. In Studd J (ed) Progress and Obstetrics and Gynaecology 13. Churchill Livingstone, Edinburgh, 1998, with permission].

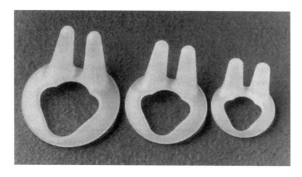

Figure 13.2 The available sizes of the Introl bladder neck prosthesis. From Davila et al.[15]

jectively dry and 26% significantly improved, 86% were objectively improved on repeat pad testing and there were no significant or serious complications. These data have been confirmed in a larger study of 126 women with 75% continent or improved.[18]

13.4 Extraurethral Devices

Whereas the intraurethral devices attempt to reproduce intrinsic sphincter function and the vaginal devices provide support to the bladder neck to reduce mobility, the extraurethral devices act by occluding the external urethral meatus. Two devices are available: the FemAssist personal urinary control device and the Continence control pad.

The FemAssist is a 30mm silicone rubber cup, which is held over the external urethral meatus by a weak vacuum generated by the central teat. We first studied this device in a short-term study involving 27 women with proven stress incontinence.[19] Six patients were continent with the device and 50% had reduced leakage, but 25% of the patients had a worse pad test result with the device in place. However, the reduction in median pad test loss across the whole group was statistically significant. Only 56% expressed an interest in using the device.

An American study over a 1-month period involved 155 women,[20] of whom 62% completed the study and 45% were continent while wearing the device; 39% wished to continue with the device. A second study of 100 women with a 4-week follow-up[21] found that 41% of the study group dropped out, but the other patients reported significant reductions in pad test losses, leakage frequency and pad use and 93% wished to continue with the device.

We have recently conducted a prospective 3-month study of the FemAssist device.[22] The majority of patients withdrew from the study or failed to attend for review appointments. Only 2 of 41 completed the 3-month study protocol. The data that we collected confirmed our suspicions about the variable benefit obtained with this device, and the dropout rate clearly indicated that the device was unacceptable to our patient population. It is difficult to explain the difference in results between our data and those of others, except to assume that the women recruited in other studies were more highly motivated to persevere with the device and therefore achieved a better result. Nevertheless, there was a high dropout rate in both these studies (38% and 41% respectively). This discrepancy in data may reflect underlying bias in the studies published to date.

The Continence Control pad (a soft adhesive rubber pad which fits over the urethral meatus) has been assessed in two studies.[23,24] Over a 2-week period the pad produced significant improvement in 58% of patients and continence in 17%.[23] In this study 411 women used the device for 12 weeks;[24] 85% of women completed the study and significant reductions in pad loss, reported leakage and leakage severity were found. Few of the subjects reported achieving continence with the device.

13.5 General Considerations

All the published studies described above suffer from several problems. The first is obviously that they cannot be blinded. More importantly, each study was a case series with the patients acting as their own controls. There are no randomised controlled studies of these devices. There is a high likelihood of selection bias in the studies reported, and publication bias is almost certain to be present. The use of variable length follow-up and different outcome data between studies renders comparison difficult. For these reasons, the quality of the data leaves serious doubts about the utility of these devices. It is therefore a cause for some concern that these devices have become increasingly prevalent and that two of them have been licensed by the US Food and Drug Administration (FDA) for the treatment of incontinence.

13.6 Areas for Future Research

There is a pressing need for a large randomised controlled trial with a well-defined set of outcome measures with long-term follow up. Long-term results (5–10 years) are particularly important. A randomised comparison of the two most effective devices, the Introl and Reliance, would also be valuable. It is vital that good quality, methodologically sound research is conducted in this area in the interests of evidence-based practice and clinical governance.

References

1. Bø K, Talseth T, Holme I (1999) Single blind, randomised controlled trial of pelvic floor exercises, electrical stimulation, vaginal cones, and no treatment in management of genuine stress incontinence in women. BMJ 318: 487–93.
2. Jarvis GJ (1994) Surgery for genuine stress incontinence. Br J Obstet Gynaecol 101: 371–4.
3. Nielsen KK, Kromann-Andersen B, Jacobsen H et al. (1990) The urethral plug: a new treatment modality for genuine urinary stress incontinence in women. J Urol 144: 1199–202.
4. Nielsen KK, Walter S, Maegaard E, Kromann-Andersen B (1993) The urethral plug II: an alternative treatment in

women with genuine urinary stress incontinence. Br J Urol 72: 428–32.

5. Staskin D, Bavendam T, Miller J et al. (1996) Effectiveness of a urinary control insert in the management of stress urinary incontinence: early results from a multicenter study. Urology 47: 629–36.

6. Miller JL, Bavendam T (1996) Treatment with the Reliance urinary control insert: one-year experience. J Endourol 10: 287–92.

7. Vierhout ME, Lose G (1997) Preventive vaginal and intra-urethral devices in the treatment of female urinary stress incontinence. Curr Opin Obstet Gynecol 9: 325–8.

8. Suarez GM, Baum NH, Jacobs J (1991) Use of standard contraceptive diaphragm in management of stress urinary incontinence. Urology 37: 119–22.

9. Nygaard I (1995) Prevention of exercise incontinence with mechanical devices. J Reprod Med 40: 89–94.

10. Davila GW, Ostermann KV (1994) The bladder neck support prosthesis: a nonsurgical approach to stress incontinence in adult women. Am J Obstet Gynecol 171: 206–11.

11. Davila GW (1996) Introl bladder neck support prosthesis: a nonsurgical urethropexy. J Endourol 10: 293–6.

12. Kondo A, Yokoyama E, Koshiba K et al. (1997) Bladder neck support prosthesis: a nonoperative treatment for stress or mixed urinary incontinence. J Urol 157: 824–7.

13. Foote A, Moore KH, King J (1996) A prospective study of the long term use of the bladder neck support prosthesis. Neurourol Urodynamics 15: 404–6.

14. Moore KH, Foote A, Siva S, King J, Burton G (1997) The use of the bladder neck support prosthesis in combined genuine stress incontinence and detrusor instability. Aust N Z J Obstet Gynaecol 37: 440–5.

15. Davila GW, Neal D, Horbach N et al. (1999) A bladder-neck support prosthesis for women with stress and mixed incontinence. Obstet Gynecol 93: 938–42.

16. Thyssen H, Lose G (1996) New disposable vaginal device (continence guard) in the treatment of female stress incontinence. Design, efficacy and short term safety. Acta Obstet Gynecol Scand 75: 170–3.

17. Thyssen HH, Lose G (1997) Long-term efficacy and safety of a disposable vaginal device (continence guard) in the treatment of female stress incontinence. Int Urogynecol J 8(133): 130–2.

18. Hahn I, Milsom I (1996) Treatment of female stress urinary incontinence with a new anatomically shaped vaginal device (Conveen Continence Guard). Br J Urol 77: 711–15.

19. Tincello DG, Richmond DH (1997) Preliminary experience with a urinary control device in the management of women with genuine stress incontinence. Br J Urol 8: 752–6.

20. Versi E, Griffiths DJ, Harvey M (1998) A new external urethral occlusive device for female urinary incontinence. Obstet Gynecol 92: 286–91.

21. Moore KH, Simons A, Dowell C, Bryant C, Prashar S (1999) Efficacy and user acceptability of the urethral occlusive device in women with urinary incontinence. J Urol 162: 464–8.

22. Tincello DG, Adams EJ, Bolderson J, Richmond DH (2000) A urinary control device for management of female stress incontinence. Obstet Gynecol 95: 417–20.

23. Eckford SD, Jackson SR, Lewis PA, Abrams P (1996) The continence control pad–a new external urethral occlusion device in the management of stress incontinence. Br J Urol 77: 538–40.

24. Brubaker L, Harris T, Gleason D, Newman D, North B and The Miniguard Investigators Group (1999) The external urethral barrier for stress incontinence: a multicenter trial of safety and efficacy. Obstet Gynecol 93: 932–7.

14 Surgery for Genuine Stress Incontinence

V. Khullar, L. Cardozo and K. Boos

Over 150 different surgical techniques have been described for the treatment of genuine stress incontinence. The number of procedures indicates that the mechanism of continence and the pathophysiology of genuine stress incontinence are uncertain, and each method has complications associated with it. The majority of operations can be by the system shown in Table 14.1. This chapter covers only the procedures most likely to be encountered.

Table 14.1. Surgical techniques for treatment of stress incontinence

Vaginal approach	
Anterior colporrhaphy	
Urethrocleisis	
Periurethral bulking agents	GAX collagen
	Macroplastique
	Autologous fat
Abdominal approach	
Marshall–Marchetti–Krantz procedure	
Burch colposuspension	
Vagino-obturator shelf	
Needle suspension	
Stamey	
Pererya	
Gittes	
Combined abdomino-vaginal approaches	
Sling procedures	Organic slings (rectus sheath, fascia lata)
	Synthetic slings (Mesilene, silastic, vicryl, Gore-tex)
Laparoscopic procedures	
Laparoscopic colposuspension	
Salvage operations	
Artificial urinary sphincter	
Neourethra	
Urinary diversion (ileal conduit)	
Mitroffanoff procedure	

14.1 Anterior Colporrhaphy

Anterior colporrhaphy (anterior repair) has a contentious place as a continence operation. The operation, first described by Kelly,[1] involves a midline incision in the anterior vaginal wall; the urethra and bladder are dissected free and two silk mattress sutures are used to plicate the paraurethral tissues. Redundant vaginal skin is excised and the incision is closed. This procedure has been used to treat primary genuine stress incontinence in the presence of a cystocele, the operation being a better treatment for prolapse than for incontinence. Subjective cure rates vary between 48%[2] and 90%.[3] The objective cure rates have varied between 30% and 70%.[4] In most randomised comparative studies the objective cure rate after 5 years for this procedure has been poor.

14.2 Burch Colposuspension

This procedure is performed abdominally through a low transverse incision. The bladder neck is mobilised and sutures are placed into the ipsilateral paravaginal tissue and into the ileopectineal ligament on both sides. The procedure corrects co-existent anterior vaginal wall prolapse.

The subjective success rates of this procedure range between 89% and 100%,[5-7] and the objective cure rates are between 73% and 90%.[4]

14.3 Slings

The operation is generally performed through a combined vaginal and abdominal procedure, though either approach may be used independently. An

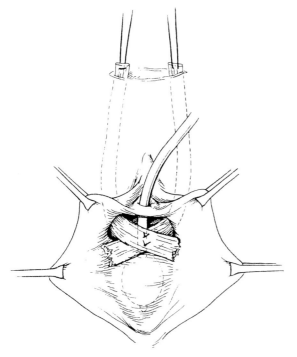

Figure 14.1 Suburethral sling in which autologous fascia or synthetic material is passed into the retropubic space and tied above the fascia of the rectus abdominis muscle. [From Cardozo L (ed) Urogynecology, Churchill Livingstone, Edinburgh, 1997, with permission].

organic or synthetic material is placed under the urethra at the level of the bladder neck (Fig. 14.1); the synthetic materials have a higher rate of erosion and infection. The ends of the sling can be attached to the

rectus sheath or the ileopectineal ligament. Cure rates are very similar to the Burch colposuspension.[4]

14.4 Bladder Neck Suspension

This group of procedures involve passing sutures mounted on a long needle on either side of the bladder neck from the rectus sheath to the paravaginal fascia, or vice versa. The main modifications involve the attachment of the suture to the paravaginal tissue. These procedures are more commonly used in frail or elderly people because they can generally be carried out under local anaesthetic. The initial cure rates are good but the long-term cure rates are poor, being as low as 2% after 10 years, mainly because the suture tears through the paravaginal tissue.

14.5 Injectables

Many different substances have been injected around the bladder neck either paraurethrally (Fig. 14.2) or transurethrally. The advantage of this operation is that it can be performed under local anaesthetic and the procedure may be performed as a day case.[4] The main injectables in use at present are macroplastique, which is a silicone-based compound, and collagen. The main problem with this technique is that the cure rate is lower than for other procedures.[8,9]

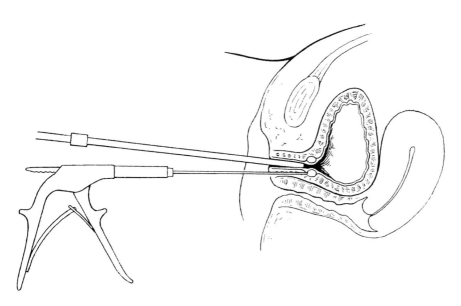

Figure 14.2 Periurethral bulk-enhancing agents. This diagram demonstrates the paraurethral technique under cystoscopic control. [From Cardozo L (ed) Urogynecology, Churchill Livingstone, Edinburgh, 1997, with permission].

Table 14.2. Postoperative complications of major urogynaecological surgery

Immediate complications
  Haemorrhage and shock
  Bladder injury during surgery

Early complications
  Dysfunction to other systems, e.g. paralytic ileus, respiratory
    infection, urinary tract infection
  Secondary haemorrhage
  Deep vein thrombosis
  Pain
  Nausea and vomiting
  Dehydration

Late complications
  Constipation
  Urinary tract infection
  Voiding difficulties
  Urinary urgency and de-novo detrusor instability

14.6 Laparoscopic Colposuspension

The Burch colposuspension may be carried out using laparoscopic techniques and there appear to be initial advantages, including reduced hospital stay and the absence of a large abdominal incision. Unfortunately the cure rates at 2 years do not appear to be as good as for an open procedure.[4]

All women undergoing continence surgery must have an adequate explanation of the procedure, its cure rate and its associated complications. After a continence procedure, most women will be catheterised and often this will involve a suprapubic catheter because voiding without a postmicturition residual may take time to occur.

All major urogynaecological surgery has associated postoperative complications (Table 14.2). Some women develop detrusor instability following surgery for genuine stress incontinence. These women may need to be treated with bladder drill and anticholinergic therapy.

14.7 Conclusion

Surgery for genuine stress incontinence requires careful counselling of the patient and correct patient selection. All procedures have benefits as well as complications, and these should be taken into account when deciding on whom to operate and which operation.

References

1. Kelly HA (1913) Incontinence of urine in women. Urol Cutan Rev 17: 291–3.
2. Low JA (1967) The management of severe anatomic urinary incontinence by vaginal repair. Am J Obstet Gynecol 97: 308–15.
3. Green T (1975) Urinary stress incontinence; differential diagnosis, pathophysiology and management. Am J Obstet Gynecol 122: 368–400.
4. Hill S (1997) Genuine stress incontinence. In: Cardozo L (ed) Urogynecology. Churchill Livingstone, Edinburgh, UK, pp. 240–85.
5. Burch JC (1961) Urethrovesical fixation to Cooper's ligament for correction of stress incontinence, cystocele and prolapse. Am J Obstet Gynecol 81: 281–90.
6. Glesen JE (1962) A review of 60 Marshall–Marchetti operations. J Obstet Gynecol Br Emp 69: 397–402.
7. Jarvis GJ (1994) Surgery for stress incontinence. Br J Obstet Gynaecol 101: 371–4.
8. Monga AK, Robinson D, Stanton SL (1995) Periurethral collagen injections for genuine stress incontinence: a 2-year follow-up. Br J Urol 76: 156–60.
9. Buckley JF, Lingam K, Lloyd SN et al. (1993) Injectable silicone macroparticles for female urinary incontinence (abstract). J Urol 149: 402A.

15 The Importance of Fluids

R. Addison

15.1 The Amount to Drink

Burns,[1] in a review of nine studies, identified a daily range for adult fluid intake between 1000 ml and 2500 ml, with an average of 1500 ml. Fluid intake requirements alter according to the health status of the patient and vary according to temperature and activity. It is generally recommended that adults should aim to excrete approximately 1.5 l (3 pints) of urine per 24 h, and this entails drinking 6 – 8 cups of fluid. Clearly there are complications and dangers of dehydration, including increased plasma concentrations of drugs and risk of thrombus formation.

15.2 Fluid Restriction

Patients with some lower urinary tract symptoms (LUTS) logically restrict fluid intake as a coping strategy. A study (n = 847) of incontinent patients categorised as "pad users"[2] found that 91% restricted evening fluids, 100% restricted fluids if going out, those on diuretics were likely to restrict intake, and many patients were constipated; furthermore, there was no attempt to replace fluids, and these practices could happen several times per week. Norton[3] suggests that fluid restriction may be counter-productive, decreasing bladder capacity, increasing urinary tract infection in "at risk" groups, increasing constipation, causing dysuria and worsening some LUTS. In contrast, Griffiths[4] showed that selective fluid restriction may be therapeutic. This study of 128 elderly Canadian nursing home residents showed that in severe urge incontinence, night voiding programmes combined with evening fluid restriction could be of value.

15.3 Types of Fluid

Some drinks are therapeutic and some are considered harmful, especially when combined with medication. In simple terms, water is probably the best drink.

15.3.1 Caffeine

Caffeine, a xanthine, is one of the most widely consumed drugs in the world and is found in coffee, tea, cocoa, cola and other soft drinks and many over-the-counter medications. When absorbed, the highest concentration of caffeine is found in muscle tissue and significant improvement in aerobic exercise following caffeine ingestion has been reported.[5] However, as well as skeletal muscle stimulation, caffeine is known to have a diuretic effect and may produce symptoms of urgency and frequency.

The effect of caffeine on women with detrusor instability (n = 20) and normal women (n = 10) has been investigated by means of repeated cystometry.[6] This study showed a significant increase in the detrusor pressure rise on bladder filling after caffeine administration compared with no caffeine in the unstable group, and no abnormality in the normal group. These results suggest that the increased pressure rise is due to decreased bladder compliance, possibly as a result of an excitatory effect on detrusor smooth muscle comparable to that described for skeletal muscle. A trial of caffeine withdrawal is worthwhile, especially for patients with detrusor instability, those reporting bypassing of a Foley catheter, and those who report urgency and frequency after drinking caffeinated beverages. A word of caution: the amount of caffeine should be reduced gradually over 7–10 days to prevent withdrawal symptoms.

A study on the effect of caffeine on the urethral pressure in female dogs[7] showed a decrease in pressure following more than 125 mg of caffeine and this supported earlier work demonstrating an inhibitory effect of caffeine on urethral smooth muscle. This suggests that patients with stress incontinence or low urethral pressures should eliminate caffeine for a trial period and evaluate any changes in their symptomology.

15.3.2 Tea

There is some evidence for the therapeutic effect of drinking tea due to its antioxidant properties; this is thought to reduce the likelihood of high blood pressure, some cancers, high cholesterol levels and strokes.

15.3.3 Herbal Teas

Herbal teas and infusions have become very fashionable and they are often considered healthy drinks; however, this may not always be the case.[8] Newall[9] expressed concern regarding some herbal teas and pregnancy, reporting potential risk of abortion. Furthermore, breast-feeding may incur some hazards as babies take longer to excrete certain substances, as do some subjects with heart, kidney and liver diseases. A Canadian study of the digoxin-like factors found in 46 packaged and 78 herbal teas showed that Breathe Easy, Blackcurrant, Pleurisy Root, Chaparral and Peppermint had the highest amount and Raspberry Patch, Red Zinger, Boneset and Cracked Rosehips produced the lowest amount of digoxin-like effects.[10]

15.3.4 Grapefruit Juice

Grapefruit juice may be harmful to some subjects; a study on the effect of grapefruit juice on patients taking calcium antagonist antianginal preparations containing felodipine and nifedipine demonstrated an enhanced effect of these drugs resulting in hypotension, vasodilation and an increased heart rate.[11] Furthermore, grapefruit juice was shown to increase plasma concentrations of cimetidine (prescribed to reduce gastric acid secretion) and inhibit stereoselective metabolism of nitrendipine.[12]

15.3.5 Cranberry Juice

Research into the effect of cranberry juice on the lower urinary tract has shown that, if taken in sufficient quantity (300 ml per day), it may be of value for patients who suffer from repeated urinary tract infections where *E. coli* is the predominant affecting organism. Cranberry juice does not work by making urine more acidic[13] but by the bacteriostatic effect produced by the condensed tannins, which reduces the adherence of organisms and thereby minimises colonisation.[14-16] Because of the naturally bitter and highly acidic nature of cranberries, cranberry juice has added sugar and water, and so may not be suitable for diabetics.

15.3.6 Alcohol

Some alcohol drinks have therapeutic properties. Red wine or grape juice equivalent is said to regulate cholesterol levels, prevent blood clots and reduce the risk of heart disease. However, there are many anecdotal references to the merits and perils of some drinks and more research is needed to guide our practice in all aspects of fluid manipulation.

References

1. Burns D (1992) Working up a thirst. Nurs Times 88(26): 44–5.
2. McKeever MP (1990) An investigation of recognised incontinence within a health authority. J Adv Nurs 15: 1197–207.
3. Norton C (1986) In: Norton C (ed) Nursing for Continence. Beaconsfield Publishers, Beaconsfield, UK, pp. 98–9.
4. Griffiths DJ, McCracken PN, Harrison GM, Gormey EA (1993) Relationship of fluid intake to voluntary micturition and urinary incontinence in geriatric patients. Neurourol Urodynamics 12(1): 1–7.
5. Williams JH, Barnes WS, Gadberry WL (1987) Influence of caffeine on force and EMG in rested and fatigued muscle. Am J Phys Med 66(4): 169–85.
6. Creighton SM, Stanton SL (1990) Caffeine: does it affect your bladder? Br J Urol 66: 613–14.
7. Palermo LM, Zimskind PD (1977) Effect of caffeine on urethral pressure. Urology X(4): 320–4.
8. McKay DW, Seviour JP, Comerford RT et al. (1995) Herbal tea: an alternative to regular tea for those who form calcium oxalate stones. J Am Diet Assoc 95(3): 360–1.
9. Newall CA, Anderson LA, Phillipson JD (1996) Herbal Medicines. A guide for healthcare professionals. Pharmaceutical Press, London.
10. Longerich L, Johnson E, Gault MH (1993) Digoxin-like factors in herbal teas. Clin Invest Med 16: 210–18.
11. Bailey DG, Spence JD, Munoz C et al. (1991) Interaction of citrus juices with felodipine and nifedipine. Lancet 337: 268–9.
12. Soons PA, Vogels BAPM, Roosemalo MCM et al. (1991) Pharmacokinetics and drug disposition. Grapefruit juice and cimetidine inhibit stereoselective metabolism of nitrendipine in humans. Clin Pharmacol 50(4): 394–403.
13. Fellors CR, Redman BC, Parrott EM (1933) The effect of cranberries on urinary acidity and blood alkali reserve. J Nutrition 6(5): 455–63.
14. Avorn J, Monmaem M, Gurwitz JH et al. (1994) Cranberry juice ingestion reduces bacteriuria and pyuria in older women. JAMA 271(10): 751–4.
15. Sobota AE (1984) Inhibition of bacterial adherence activity of cranberry juice. Potential use for treatment of urinary tract infection. J Urol 131: 1013–16.
16. Zafiri D, Ofek I, Adar R et al. (1989) Inhibitory activity of cranberry juice on adherence of Type 1 and Type P fimbriated escherichia coli to eucaryotic cells. Antimicrob Agents Chemother 33(1): 92–8.

16 The Male Patient

R. Addison

16.1 Assessment of the Male Pelvic Floor

The pelvic floor musculature in men consists of three layers. The levator ani forms the pelvic diaphragm, supporting the bladder and the proximal urethra. The medial portion of this deep layer, the puborectalis muscle, also helps the faecal continence mechanism by maintaining the anorectal angle. The most superficial layer consists of several muscles including the ischiocavernosus and the bulbocavernosus (BC), which play a role in penile erection and ejaculation. The urogenital diaphragm, situated between the two layers described above, contains the external urethral sphincter, which is the main structure responsible for urinary continence. Pathology of the pelvic floor may be responsible for a wide range of disorders, including urinary and faecal incontinence, constipation, impotence and ejaculation problems[1].

Wyndaele et al. (1996) examined male volunteers in the supine position with legs relaxed. The BC muscle was examined by placing two fingers underneath the scrotum, on the mid-line, ventral to the perineal body. The external anal sphincter (EAS) was examined by placing the distal phalanx of the index finger in the anal meatus; the puborectalis muscle was examined by the index finger in the anal canal, directed laterally and dorsally.[1]

Contraction of the individual muscles was described as follows: for the BC muscle, a thickening of the muscle under the skin, together with a slight downward movement of the penis; for the EAS, a squeezing of the examining finger, and for the puborectalis, a displacement of the rectal wall and examining finger ventrally and inwards. The right and left puborectalis muscle can be evaluated separately.[1] The tone of the anal canal may be reduced if the rectum is distended and this should be documented.

As with the female pelvic floor muscle assessment (Chapter 6), information is gleaned from observation and palpation, and different techniques and positions have been described. Peterson[2] describes an inward movement (retraction) of the penis during a contraction, others describe a lifting of the penis, and others a downward movement of the penis. Clearly, it is important to identify which muscles are producing the movement. All studies agree that anal retraction can be observed during a pelvic floor contraction and a reflex pelvic floor contraction on coughing should be noted. Many clinicians prefer to assess the pelvic floor muscles with the patient in the left-lateral position (for a right-handed examiner) with hips and knees flexed.

Approximately 80% of the resting tone in the anal canal is due to the tone of the internal anal sphincter, and this can be evaluated by resistance to insertion of the index finger. However, reflex relaxation of the internal anal sphincter may occur as a result of insertion of the examining finger. In the left-lateral position, the strength of the puborectalis is determined by hooking the distal phalanx of the examining index finger around the muscle, directed posteriorly.

The PERFECT muscle assessment (see Chapter 6) can be applied to the assessment of EAS and puborectalis.

Other methods of assessing pelvic floor muscle contractility include EMG using external surface or anal electrodes, and manometry, using an anal pressure probe (see Chapter 21).

16.2 Voiding Techniques

The first and most important factor in relation to voiding problems is the environment. Is it conducive to micturition and acceptable to the patient? Several voiding techniques have been found to be successful for men who have no physical obstruction to their urinary flow such as an enlarged prostate, a urethral stricture or lesion. Patients with mild sphincter spasm may be helped by these voiding techniques, either singly or combined. Using a Valsalva (gentle straining) and Credé manoeuvre (pressing on the lower abdomen, over the bladder) has been shown to increase the intraabdominal pressure, thus increasing the intravesical pressure and promoting micturition. However, the danger of possible reflux of urine up the ureters to the kidneys has been highlighted, and caution with these techniques is advised.[3,4] Furthermore, urethral obstruction may result from manual expression.

16.2.1 Double Voiding

This may help men with residual urine and voiding problems. After micturition ceases, the patient contracts the pelvic floor; this helps to 'milk' any drops of urine in the prostatic urethra into the bladder and also inhibits further detrusor contraction (see micturition reflexes, Chapter 2) allowing a hypotonic detrusor to rest. The patient can then walk around for a minute, return to the toilet and complete micturition.

Some patients will respond to sensory stimulation – turning taps on so they can hear running water, or putting their hands in water. Various other methods have also been described. Abdominal wall tapping (percussion) over the bladder, sustained and repeated, may stimulate a detrusor contraction.[3,4] However, in patients with a neurogenic bladder, this may cause detrusor-sphincter dyssynergia. Patients with multiple sclerosis have been shown to respond to mechanical vibration over the bladder.[5] Johnson[6] describes stroking of the abdomen or thigh to stimulate micturition. Other techniques include anal digital stimulation, pulling pubic hairs, pouring cold or warm water over the abdomen or genitalia, and stroking the cleft between the top of the buttocks.[3,6]

It is helpful if a number of techniques are taught so that the patient can experiment and find the most useful. Ultrasound is invaluable in evaluating the effectiveness of these voiding techniques. If none of the measures suggested here is effective, the patient may have to perform intermittent self-catheterisation.[7]

16.3 Post-Micturition Dribble

At the end of micturition, a few drops of urine may be left in the male urethra; movement may cause this urine to leak out, and this is termed post-micturition dribble (PMD). This is a normal occurrence in all men and is not classed as true incontinence, although to some men it is problematic. Some self-help measures can minimise the problem, but PMD may still happen to some degree from time to time.

Patients are advised to wait a few moments for the last drops of urine to be passed. Then they should lean slightly forward, and pull the penis downwards, shaking gently to allow any further drops of urine to pass. Still leaning slightly forward, they should try to pass more urine; they may pass a few more drops. This is the double voiding technique described above. Next, using two or three fingers, upward and forward pressure is applied to the perineal area posterior to the scrotum, to expel any remaining drops of urine. This may need to be done two or three times and is referred to as urethral milking.[8–10]

A further method of treating PMD is by a course of pelvic floor exercises. A randomised controlled study[2] showed that pelvic floor muscle exercises were more effective in treating PMD than urethral milking.

References

1. Wyndaele JJ, Eetvelde B Van (1996) Reproducibility of digital testing of the pelvic floor muscles in men. Arch Phys Med Rehabil 77: 1179–81.
2. Paterson J, Pinnock CB, Marshall VR (1997) Pelvic floor exercises as a treatment for post micturition dribble. Br J Urol 79: 892–7.
3. Colburn D (1994) The Promotion of Continence in Adult Nursing. Chapman & Hall, London, pp. 95–7.
4. O'Hagan M (1996) Neurogenic bladder dysfunction. In: Norton C (ed) Nursing for Continence. Beaconsfield Publishers, Beaconsfield, UK, pp. 170–91.
5. Dasgupta P, Haslam C, Goodwin R, Fowler CJ (1996) The use of vibration to empty the bladder. Neurourology Urodynam 15(4): 266–7.
6. Johnson JH (1980) Rehabilitative aspects of neurogenic bladder dysfunction. Nurs Clin North Am 15(2): 293–307.
7. Wyndaele JJ, Maes D (1990) Clean intermittent self-catheterisation: a 12 year follow-up. J Urol 143: 906–8.
8. Colburn D (1994) The Promotion of Continence in Adult Nursing. Chapman & Hall, London, pp. 86–7.
9. Denning J (1996) Male urinary incontinence. In: Norton C (ed) Nursing for Continence. Beaconsfield Publishers, Beaconsfield, UK, pp. 163–4.
10. Millard RJ (1996) Bladder Control, A Simple Self-Help Guide. Maclennan Petty, Sydney, pp. 107–8.

17 Bladder Training and Behavioural Therapy

J. Haslam

At birth a baby has no bladder or bowel control. As the central nervous system develops, the child becomes aware of the sensations of a full bladder and an impending bowel movement. When their higher centres are sufficiently well developed and the culture in which they live determines they should be "trained", they become continent. Children respond to parents and others expressing pleasure at them delivering their urine and faeces in the correct place at an appropriate time; they have undergone behavioural training. The components to achieve success are a neurologically intact system, normal anatomy, comprehension of what is needed, an appropriate environment and a reason to succeed.

17.1 Detrusor Instability and the Overactive Bladder

Those with detrusor instability have lost their previous cortical domination of bladder activity. A therapeutic intervention aims to teach an individual how to inhibit any unwanted detrusor contractions and control any sensations causing frequency and urgency. The newer term "overactive bladder" refers to the symptoms of frequency and urgency with or without urge incontinence in the absence of any local pathologic or metabolic factors that would account for the symptoms.[1] Bladder training and behavioural therapy can be useful both for the overactive bladder and for those with acquired disorders.

17.2 Normal Bladder Behaviour

Normal bladder capacity is usually stated as 400–600 ml, but micturition patterns are based on common beliefs and individuals tend to use their own voiding pattern as a standard.[2] The largest voided volume is often considered as a measure of the bladder's physiological capacity, but this does not allow for the possibility of a post-micturition residual. In a study of 151 normal women over 2 days, the range of largest volume voided was 200–1250 ml[2] and the mean was 460 ml. It was also shown that the individuals' mean voided volume was 90–610 ml, with the mean between the individuals being 250 ml.

Normal frequency of micturition is usually stated as 4–6 times per day; this was confirmed when it was found that the symptom-free women voided between 3 and 6 times per day with a mean of 5.8 voids.[2] It was also shown that there was a variation in total volumes voided: the range was 600–3100 ml per day, with a mean of 1430 ml.

A further study[3] of 33 symptom-free women showed similar total voided volumes per 24 h and voiding frequency as in the previous study.[2] It was also found[3] that functional bladder capacity was significantly higher during the night in the normal female (daytime 237 ml, night-time 379 ml). It seems that symptom-free "normal" women vary in frequency, bladder capacity and total volumes voided, but the usual suggested parameters concur with the mean in a normal population.[2,3]

17.3 Assessment

An appropriate assessment must be carried out before any intervention. If there are any symptoms of frequency and urgency, urinalysis must be performed to ensure that the patient is not suffering from a urinary tract infection (UTI) and appropriate action taken. Urodynamic assessment is considered by many to be important for a definitive diagnosis, and should be considered before any surgery is undertaken.[4] A pretreatment positive cystometrogram also gives a poorer prognosis for effective therapy than a negative cystometrogram.[5] However, often no urodynamic changes are seen after bladder training and behavioural therapy, despite significant changes in symptoms.

17.3.1 History Taking

The patient needs to be questioned regarding the history of their problem and how it has evolved over time, including nocturnal enuresis as a child, recurrent UTI and any recent life events that may have affected their condition. Full information regarding their medical, surgical, obstetric and gynaecological history should also be obtained. The possibility of any neurological condition also needs to be eliminated, first by questioning, followed by physical examination as appropriate. The effect of the condition on the patient's life can also be evaluated by the use of a validated quality of life instrument. Further evaluation and actions may need to be taken if there are any problems of mobility or the home environment. Assumptions should not be made regarding voiding habits; specific questions regarding toileting behaviour need to be asked. It has been shown[6] that 85% of women crouch over the seats of public toilets, and of those with detrusor instability 51% crouched over the toilet even at a friend's house. This behaviour may result in a reduction of flow rate and increase in post-micturition residual volumes.

17.3.2 Frequency/Volume Chart

The self-completed frequency/volume chart has been recommended for many years.[7-10] However the number of days necessary for completion has been debated. It has been shown[11] that a 7-day diary is a reproducible measure in women with stress urinary incontinence, but also the first 3 days correlate well with the last 4 days, suggesting that a 3-day trial is sufficient. Further consideration has been given to whether the chart should be sent out before the first attendance or after individualised instruction when first attending.[12,13] The essential concern is that the instructions should be clear, taking literacy and linguistic skills into consideration, in order to ensure that the patient is fully aware of what is required.

The chart should state the need to measure urine output (by the use of a jug or other appropriate container, in a fully sitting position) indicating the times of voiding over the required number of days. Patients should also be asked to indicate the times

and amounts of urine loss, times of urgency, pad changes, and the types, volumes and times of drinks taken (see Appendices 1 and 4). This can elicit useful information such as details of inappropriate fluids and patterns of drinking.

17.3.3 Physical Examination

Any concern about a patient's neurological status requires further testing of motor and sensory function (see Chapters 4 and 6). Part of behavioural therapy is empowering the individual to harness the effect of the perineo-detrusor inhibitory reflex,[14] so it is essential to determine the contractility of the pelvic floor musculature and to ascertain the appropriate level of exercise.[15]

17.4 Behavioural Therapy

Behavioural therapy involves learning new patterns of response or re-establishing previously learnt behaviour to concur with what is considered to be "normal". Its chief advantage is that it has little or no side-effects, and leaves open the possibility of more invasive options. The difficulty with the treatment is that it requires patient determination and compliance, and may take some time to succeed. Determination is necessary to achieve success: an individual has to be encouraged and supported throughout their therapy, initially by providing information on how the bladder works, then by how the therapy is aimed at learning to consciously re-dominate their bladder.

17.4.1 Bladder Training and Re-education

Jeffcoate and Francis first described "bladder discipline" as a method in which someone can gain awareness, correct bad habits and gain voluntary control of their bladder.[16] These ideas were developed and further investigated[17,18] and methods of bladder training reviewed,[19] including methods of bladder training in older people.[19]

Bladder training has been carried out as an inpatient treatment, to ensure rigour and strict adherence to the bladder training protocol.[20,21] However, later protocols have evolved using outpatient treatment over varying periods.[22,23] Success rates have varied between 12% and 90%,[21-23] with 42–80% of those successful patients remaining symptom free.

17.4.2 Practical Advice

The completed bladder chart needs to be reviewed by the clinician and the patient together. There has to be an agreement as to what is feasible and practical, and confirmation that the patient is fully aware that it is his or her own will-power and compliance with advice that will result in success. Written instructions with charts for the patient to complete with times of void should be provided, to monitor compliance with the therapy. Patients should also be advised that the desirable maximum of appropriate fluids is partly determined by their activity. The aim is to have a throughput of no more than 1500 ml per day; this is usually achieved by drinking 1.5–2 l of fluid per day, depending on activity and temperature. Strategies for decreasing the feeling of urgency should also be discussed with the patient; these are summarised in Box 17.1.

A patient who is following a mandatory scheme (see Table 17.1) must realise that they have to use their skills and determination to reach the next time of voiding. Once they have managed the schedule successfully for two successive days, the time between voids is then increased by 15–30 min. The aim is eventually to be able to have 3–4 h between voids.

Box 17.1

Methods of assisting in the reduction of urgency

Remove any causative stimuli, e.g. turn off any running taps

Stopping still and crossing legs may be helpful

Apply perineal pressure by sitting on something hard, e.g. the arm of a chair, a rolled towel

Apply manual pressure to the perineum – clitoral stimulation or penile squeezing if possible

Contract the PFM, aiming to hold for 20 s

Distract your mind by thinking of some complex but possible task, e.g. the alphabet backwards or a mathematical problem, until the sensation subsides.

Standing on your toes may be helpful

Changing position can be useful for some people

17.5 Bladder Training in Association with Drug Therapy

Behavioural therapy, including biofeedback, was compared with anticholinergic medication in a group suffering urge and mixed incontinence.[24] After four sessions of behavioural therapy over 8 weeks, there was an 80.7% reduction in episodes of urinary incontinence in the behavioural group compared with 68.5% in the drug group and 39.4% in the placebo group. At the end of therapy only 14% of the behavioural group wished to try other treatment as opposed to 75% of people in the other two groups.

In a further study a telephone-based bladder retraining programme was offered to 123 women.[25] Of these women 55% either never started or were non-compliant to treatment without any clear explanation being ascertained. There was, however, an increased compliance rate to bladder retraining in those women who were also taking concurrent anticholinergic medication. It may be that a face-to-face contact with a concerned health professional is necessary.

Other studies have shown that bladder retraining is better than[26] or similar to anticholinergic therapy.[27] It is believed that drug therapy should always be associated with instructions for timed voiding in order to improve the patients' warning time.[28]

17.6 Bladder Training Versus Pelvic Floor Muscle Training

It has been found in a group of older women that bladder training had very similar results to a similar group undergoing pelvic floor muscle training.[29] It would seem clinically sensible to advocate pelvic floor muscle exercise (PFME) as part of the therapeutic intervention. Many women with stress incontinence also suffer with the symptoms of urgency and frequency, and should improve their musculature with PFME therapy in association with bladder training.

17.7 Other Therapies

Biofeedback has been used during cystometry for patients to observe bladder activity. Auditory and visual biofeedback was used for patients to learn to inhibit bladder contractions over 4–8 1h sessions at

Table 17.1. Methods of bladder training

Type of bladder training	Voiding times	Type of patient
Mandatory scheduled voiding	A set frequency of voiding is determined. The person is not allowed to use the toilet under any circumstances until the next scheduled time of void	Those people whose lifestyle permits such a intervention. This method has been pursued in in-patient therapy
Self-scheduled voiding	Aiming to increase their voiding times, the person is "allowed" to use the toilet if the sensation of urgency becomes intolerable	Useful for the individual who is very anxious about their ability to succeed, and who needs to be convinced of their ability
Habit retraining	The times are varied according to patient needs and requirements, therefore, the periods between voids are not consistent throughout the day	Most helpful in those people whose work dictates possible times of voiding, e.g. teachers
Regular timed voiding	Set times of voiding are used to ensure that there is no further damage caused to the upper and lower urinary tract	Those with neurogenic bladders associated with spinal lesions that require intermittent self-catheterisation
Prompted voiding	The person is regularly asked if they would like to go to the toilet and taken if they say yes	Institutionalised patients with severe cognitive and mobility problems

weekly intervals.[30] Using subjective and objective methods of assessment, 81% of the patients improved. Five years later, of the 11 women who were initially cured or improved, 4 remained completely cured, 2 had undergone surgery and 5 had relapsed. Those who had relapsed had tried drug therapy without much success.[31] The usefulness of more traditional biofeedback assisted behavioural training for elderly men and women has also been investigated.[23,32,33] It appears from the evidence that biofeedback is a technique that may enhance other treatments, but has yet to be proved effective for all patients.

Hypnotherapy has also been shown to be of value for the treatment of detrusor instability,[34,35] as has psychotherapy in association with bladder drill.[36] Acupuncture[37,38] is yet another complementary therapy that has been tried and found to decrease symptoms in bladder instability (see Chapter 32). Electrostimulation has been used for many years to inhibit detrusor contractions.[39,40] The frequency, pulse width, duty cycle and intensity parameters are all of importance for an effective treatment (see Chapter 12).

17.8 Conclusions and Recommendations

Behavioural therapy should always be considered as the initial treatment in most of those with an overactive bladder.[28] The therapy includes education, bladder training, functional training and PFM rehabilitation. Other complementary therapies seem to have some efficacy, although there is a lack of evidence from randomised controlled trials.

Patients should always have a choice in their treatment when there is a variety of effective research-based alternatives. Behavioural therapies benefit from a lack of side-effects, but do require great motivation and compliance from the patient. As a greater understanding of the physiology and pathophysiology of the overactive bladder is gained, it may become possible to match the therapeutic interventions more closely with the disorder. Methods of bladder training are summarised in Table 17.1.

When the Department of Health (2000) reported on good practice in continence services, an integrated service offering an assessment and management treatment plan followed by treatment and audit in the community was recommended.[41] It is by both randomised controlled trials and local audit that best practice will become more apparent. Behavioural therapy seems to be an ideal non-invasive therapy to be used in the community setting.

References

1. Abrams P, Wein AJ (2000) Overactive bladder and its treatments. Urology 55(4A): 1–2.
2. Larsson G, Victor A (1988) Micturition patterns in a healthy female population, studied with a frequency volume chart. Scand J Urol Nephrol Suppl 114: 53–7.
3. Kassis A, Schick E (1993) Frequency-volume chart pattern in a healthy female population. Br J Urol 72: 708–10.
4. Homma Y, Batista JE, Bauer SB (1999) Urodynamics. In: Abrams P, Khoury S, Wein A (eds) Incontinence. 1st International Consultation on Incontinence. Health Publication Ltd, UK, pp. 353–99.

5. Payne CK, Bø K, Mattiasson A (2000) Overactive bladder and its treatments – questions and answers. BJU Int 85(3): 14–16.

6. Moore KH, Richmond DH, Sutherst JR, Imrie AH, Hutton JL (1991) Crouching over the toilet seat: prevalence among British gynaecological outpatients and its effect upon micturition. Br J Obstet Gynaecol 98: 569–72.

7. Frewen WK (1970) Urge and stress incontinence. Fact and fiction. J Obstet Gynaecol Br Commonw 77: 932–4.

8. Turner Warwick R, Milroy E (1979) A reappraisal of the value of routine urological procedures in the assessment of urodynamic function. Urol Clin North Am 6: 63–70.

9. Mundy A (1988) Detrusor instability. Br J Urol 62: 393–7.

10. Lose G, Fantl JA, Victor A et al. (1998) Outcome measures for research in adult women with symptoms of lower urinary tract dysfunction. Neurourol Urodynamics 17: 255–62.

11. Nygaard I, Holcomb R (2000) Reproducibility of the seven-day voiding diary in women with stress urinary incontinence. Int Urogynecol J 11: 15–17.

12. Abrams P, Klevmark B (1996) Frequency volume charts: an indispensable part of lower urinary tract assessment. Scand J Urol Nephrol (Suppl) 179: 47–53.

13. Robinson D, McClish DK, Wyman JF et al. (1996) Comparison between urinary diaries completed with and without intensive patient instructions. Neurourol Urodynamics 15: 143–8.

14. Mahoney DT, Laferte RO, Blais DJ (1980) Integral storage and voiding reflexes. Urology IX(1): 95–106.

15. DiNubile NA (1991) Strength training. Clin Sports Med 10(1): 33–62.

16. Jeffcoate TNA, Francis WJA (1966) Urgency incontinence in the female. Am J Obstet Gynecol 94(5): 604–18.

17. Frewen WK (1980) The management of urgency and frequency of micturition. Br J Urol 52: 367–9.

18. Frewen WK (1982) A reassessment of bladder training in detrusor dysfunction in the female. Br J Urol 54: 372–3.

19. Hadley EC (1986) Bladder training and related therapies for urinary incontinence in older people. JAMA 256(3): 372–9.

20. Frewen WK (1978) An objective assessment of the unstable bladder of psychosomatic origin. Br J Urol 50: 246–9.

21. Jarvis JG, Millar DR (1980) Controlled trial of bladder drill for detrusor instability. Br Med J 281: 1322–3.

22. Fantl JA, Wyman JF, McClish DK et al. (1991) Efficacy of bladder training in older women with urinary incontinence. JAMA 265: 609–13.

23. Wyman JF, Fantl JA, McClish DK et al. (1998) Comparative efficacy of behavioural interventions in the management of female urinary incontinence. Am J Obstet Gynecol 179: 999–1007.

24. Burgio KL, Locher JL, Goode PS et al. (1998) Behavioural vs drug treatment for urge urinary incontinence in older women: a randomized control trial. JAMA 280: 1995–2000.

25. Visco AG, Weidner AC, Cundiff GW, Bump C (1999) Observed patient compliance with a structured outpatient bladder retraining program. Am J Obstet Gynecol 181: 1392–4.

26. Jarvis JG (1981) Controlled trial of bladder drill and drug therapy in the management of detrusor instability. Br J Urol 53: 565–6.

27. Columbo M, Zanetta G, Scalambrino S et al. (1995) Oxybutinin and bladder training in the management of female urinary urge incontinence: A randomized study. Int Urogynecol J 6: 63–7.

28. Payne CK (2000) Behavioral therapy for overactive bladder. Urology 55(4A): 3–6.

29. Wyman JF, Fantl JA, McClish DK et al. (1991) Bladder training in older women with urinary incontinence: Relationship between outcome and changes in urodynamic observations. Obstet Gynecol 77: 281–6.

30. Cardozo LD, Abrams PD, Stanton SL, Feneley RCL (1978) Ideopathic bladder instability treated by biofeedback. Br J Urol 50: 521–3.

31. Cardozo LD, Stanton SL (1984) Biofeedback: a 5 year review. Br J Urol 56(2): 220.

32. Burgio KL, Engel BT (1990) Biofeedback-assisted behavioural training for elderly men and women. J Am Geriatr Soc 38: 338–40.

33. Burns PA, Pranikoff K, Nochajksi TH et al. (1993) A comparison of effectiveness of biofeedback and pelvic muscle exercise treatment of stress incontinence in older community dwelling women. J Gerontol 48: M167–74.

34. Freeman RM, Baxby K (1982) Hypnotherapy for incontinence caused by the unstable detrusor. Br Med J 284: 1831–4.

35. Freeman RM, Guthrie KA, Baxby K (1985) Hypnotherapy for idiopathic detrusor instability: a two year review. Br Med J 290: 286.

36. Macaulay AJ, Stern RS, Holmes DM et al. (1987) Micturition and the mind: psychological factors in the etiology and treatment of urinary symptoms in women. Br Med J 294: 540–3.

37. Chang PL (1988) Urodynamic studies in acupuncture for women with frequency, urgency and dysuria. J Urol 140: 563–6.

38. Philp T, Shah PRJ, Worth PHL (1988) Acupuncture in the treatment of bladder instability. Br J Urol 61: 490–3.

39. Fall M, Ahlstrom K, Carlsson CA et al. (1986) Contelle: pelvic floor stimulator for stress–urge incontinence. A multicenter study. Urology 27: 282–7.

40. Vodusek DB, Light JK, Libby JM (1986) Detrusor inhibition induced by stimulation of pudendal nerve afferents. Neurourol Urodynamics 5: 381–9.

41. DoH (2000) Good Practice in Continence Services. Department of Health, London.

18 Voiding Problems in Women

J. Haslam

Urinary retention can be defined as the inability to void.[1] Bladder emptying difficulties can result from a myogenic, psychogenic or neurogenic problem, or a bladder outlet obstruction. Any of these can result in difficulty in the initiation to void, a low flow rate or a post-void residual of urine. The elderly in particular may suffer with detrusor hyperactivity with impaired contractility (DHIC).[2]

18.1 Dangers of Incomplete Emptying

An over-distended bladder during or after labour, perineal pain, gynaecological surgery or painful herpetic lesions may all inhibit bladder activity.[1] Bad bladder habits can also be self-imposed: it has been shown that many women crouch over, rather than sit down on a toilet seat to void,[3] and this may contribute to disordered voiding. Volume and types of fluids and some medication may also affect bladder function. Furthermore, those with neurological disease sometimes first manifest as having a problem with incomplete bladder emptying, due to detrusor sphincter dyssynergia or detrusor hypocontractility.[4]

If left untreated, incomplete emptying or a high-pressure bladder may lead to damage of the upper urinary tract.[5] If there is any suspicion of an incomplete void, the patient should have an ultrasound bladder scan or in–out catheter (if no scanner is available) to assess any post-void residual. If there is significant residual urine (100 ml over) it should be considered in the context of the amount voided, any current known pathology and any other possible causes of the symptoms.

Chronic residual urine can lead to an ever-increasing likelihood of recurrent urinary infections requiring an escalating provision of medication.

This is a cost both to the individual and to the health service. Any women with high post-void residuals should have a full assessment and ultimately may require the teaching of clean intermittent self catheterisation (CISC) and continue to be monitored. The teaching of this technique is described in some detail in Chapter 4.

A chronic obstruction can ultimately lead to high intravesical pressures resulting in hydronephrosis and kidney damage,[5] so an obstruction of any kind should be investigated and medical referral made as appropriate.

This chapter considers the techniques that a therapist may teach a patient to assist voiding, after determining that the use of the techniques will not compromise their health.

18.2 Detrusor Hypoactivity and Inappropriate Relaxation of the Pelvic Floor Muscles and Urethral Sphincter

It is believed that one-third of women void by relaxation of the urethra with an accompanying contraction of the detrusor, one-third by urethral relaxation alone and one-third by a combination of straining and detrusor contraction[5]. Hesitancy may be apparent when there is a need to void in a public toilet, at the first large void of the day, immediately after delivery or after gynaecological surgery. A slow stream can be the result of an obstruction, a low detrusor pressure, a neuropathy of the pelvic nerves or a combination; an interrupted stream can result from the lack of a sustained detrusor contraction, a lack of co-ordination between the detrusor and sphincters (detrusor sphincter dyssynergia often seen in neurological patients), obstruction or the use of unsustained straining.

Any patient with post-void residuals without obvious cause should be given a full neurological assessment.

18.3 Neurogenic Bladder

In patients with a neurogenic bladder the aims must be to keep low pressure within the bladder, to empty the bladder regularly to completion and to avoid reflux at all times. Triggered voiding, CISC, medication, electrostimulation, the use of appliances, surgery or an indwelling catheter may all be considered if appropriate. However, the neurogenic patient with post-void residuals has to be treated with extreme caution to avoid any possible complications. Video-urodynamics are considered essential before instructing a patient to use any trigger mechanisms. Any sign of reflux or inadequate detrusor contraction means that triggered voiding is inappropriate. Autonomic dysreflexia with symptoms of paroxysmal hypertension, anxiety, sweating, headache and bradycardia[6] may be triggered by reflex voiding. If triggered voiding is deemed appropriate, the triggers for an individual may vary: these include suprapubic pressure or percussion (at least 7–8 percussions with intervals of a few seconds[6]), thigh scratching or anorectal manipulation.[7] Suprapubic tapping can result in a gross reflex of both the detrusor and urethral sphincter, but ceasing tapping at the initiation of the void should result in relaxation of the sphincter while the slower-reacting detrusor continues to contract.[6] Tapping can then be repeated if necessary. If there is any doubt that the manoeuvre is possibly causing further problems, it must be ceased immediately.

18.4 Outflow Obstruction in Women

Constipation accompanied by a rectocele, cystocele or urethrocele may all contribute to outflow obstruction. The obstruction may also be caused by urethral stricture or by bladder neck suspension surgery. Those undergoing such surgery should be assessed before surgery to determine if they are at risk of postoperative voiding dysfunction. If this is likely they should be appropriately counselled and taught CISC prior to surgery.

18.5 Prevention of Post-Void Residual Urine

Children should be taught good habits during their early toilet training experiences, sitting with their feet supported.[8] Women should be told always to sit down comfortably to void, and to allow time to void fully without hurrying. Voluntary stopping and starting of urine flow should be discouraged, as this goes against normal voiding reflexes.[9,10] Anyone with abnormal detrusor or urethral function should completely desist from midstream stopping. Constipation should be avoided, and a healthy diet encouraged. Any pregnant women wishing to undergo epidural anaesthesia for childbirth should be counselled regarding appropriate bladder care both during labour and after delivery. If a woman is having epidural anaesthesia, she should be catheterised during labour. If the catheterisation is not continued after delivery, the woman should be advised to attempt voiding once voluntary control of the lower limbs has returned, regardless of whether she feels the need to void or not, as bladder sensation returns only many hours after limb sensation has returned.[11] It is essential to check for post-micturition residuals in women who have had traumatic deliveries, those with a long period without bladder emptying after epidural anaesthesia, or those who relate any urinary symptoms. This is best done by ultrasound bladder scanning.

Urinalysis can be used to initially discover the likelihood of a urinary tract infection or abnormal blood sugar levels indicative of diabetes. Diabetes can be a cause of pelvic nerve neuropathy which in turn can cause post-void residuals. Further appropriate referral should be made if any abnormalities are detected.

18.6 Investigations and Treatment of Post-Void Residual Urine

- Uroflowmetry can be useful in determining flow rates; further urodynamic investigations may be warranted in investigating the problem.
- Appropriate catheterisation protocols and procedures should be in place for patients after gynaecological surgery and those with voiding problems after delivery.
- Neuromuscular stimulation may be indicated to assist in normalising normal reflex activity using

Table 18.1. Possible advice to promote full voiding

Privacy	Comfort and privacy are necessary to void easily. Particular attention should be paid to this, especially in long-stay accommodation
Sitting	Women should always sit down properly on the toilet with the feet supported, relaxing the pelvic floor muscles and allowing sufficient time to void to completion
Double voiding	After the initial void, stand up, move around then sit down and attempt to void again
Credé manoevre	The hand gives gentle downward pressure supra-pubically. This is a potentially hazardous manoevre and should only be used in those with an underactive detrusor and underactive/ incompetent sphincter mechanism causing low urethral resistance.[1] This may also assist in stimulating the detruso-detrusor reflex[9]
Leaning forwards	Leaning forwards may promote micturition[12]
Tapping	Tapping over the bladder may assist in triggering a reflex detrusor contraction, especially in those patients with an autonomic neurological dysfunction[5]
Stroking/tickling	Stroking or tickling the lower back to stimulate the micturition reflexes has also been reported as helpful in some patients[5]
Whistling	Whistling provides a sustained outward breath with a gentle increase in intra-abdominal pressure
Pubic hair	Some people can initiate a detrusor contraction by pulling pubic hair; this is thought to have a reflex action on the bladder
Valsalva manoeuvre	This is the act of holding the breath with a closed glottis while increasing abdominal pressure. As this action has the potential to increase genital prolapse, rectal prolapse and haemorrhoids,[5] it should only be used with great caution. The same precautions must be taken as when using a Credé manoeuvre
Running water	The sound of running water can promote a detrusor contraction,[13] but care must be taken not to promote detrusor instability by over use of this technique
Warm water	In those with a traumatised perineum and pelvic floor the action of pouring warm water over the perineum can aid in promoting relaxation and therefore assist in voiding
Relaxation	General relaxation techniques should be taught to patients who are generally tense and anxious about their condition. The method chosen should be one that is most appropriate for the individual
Prolapse	A women with a large cystocele may need to be taught to reduce the prolapse before voiding while awaiting surgery
Queen Square bladder stimulator	This suprapubic vibration device has also been found useful in neurogenic patients with detrusor hyper-reflexia who are not severely disabled[3]

correct parameters (see Chapter 12). Some centres have used intravesical stimulation to promote detrusor contraction, but this is not widely available.

- Drugs including cholinergic agonists, alpha blockers, prostaglandins and diazepam have all been suggested as being potentially useful.[5]
- Those people with an inability to relax their pelvic floor muscle (PFM) may respond to biofeedback.
- CISC should only be taught by a suitably trained professional.
- Urethral dilatation may be used in the case of urethral stricture causing difficulty in voiding. Stricture therapy using CISC may then need to be continued.

18.7 Conclusions

There are many possible causes of difficulty in voiding to completion. Each patient needs to be assessed and treated individually, and the simple measures described in Table 18.1 may be of help. However, triggered voiding may be considered dangerous in the patient with a neurogenic bladder. Care should always be taken to monitor all patients, even if they do not have a neurogenic bladder. Appropriate investigations and referrals should always be made if the use of these simple measures to empty the bladder does not lead to an improvement.

References

1. Faerber GJ (1994) Urinary retention and urethral obstruction. In: Kursch ED, McGuire EJ (ed) Female Urology. JB Lippincott, Philadelphia, pp. 517–32.
2. Resnick N, Yalla S, Laurino E (1986) An algorithmic approach to urinary incontinence in the elderly. Clin Res 34: 832–7.
3. Moore KH, Richmond DH, Sutherst JR, Imrie AH, Hutton JL (1991) Crouching over the toilet seat: prevalence among British gynaecological outpatients and its effect upon micturition. Br J Obstet Gynaecol 98: 569–72.
4. Dasgupta P, Haslam C, Goodwin R, Fowler CJ (1997) The 'Queen Square bladder stimulator': a device for assisting emptying of the neurogenic bladder. Br J Urol 80: 234–7.

5. Wall LL, Norton PA, DeLancey JOL (1993) Bladder emptying problems. In: Practical Urogynaecology. Williams & Wilkins, Baltimore, Md, pp. 274–92.

6. Madersbacher H, Wyndaele JJ, Igawa Y et al. (1999) Conservative management in the neuropathic patient. In: Abrams P, Khoury S, Wein A (eds) Incontinence. Health Publication Ltd, UK, pp. 777–82.

7. Rossier A, Bors E (1964) Detrusor responses to perineal and rectal stimulation in patients with spinal cord injuries. Urol Int 10: 181–90.

8. Wennergren HM, Ogerg BE, Sandstedt P (1991) The importance of leg support for relaxation of the pelvic floor muscles. Scand J Urol Nephrol 25: 205–21.

9. Mahoney DT, Laferte RO, Blais DJ (1980) Integral storage and voiding reflexes. Urology IX(1): 95–106.

10. Bump RC, Hurt WG, Fantl A, Wyman JF (1991) Assessment of Kegel pelvic muscle exercise performance after brief verbal instruction. Am J Obstet Gynecol 165: 322–9.

11. Khullar V, Cardozo LD (1993) Bladder sensation after epidural analgesia. Neurourol Urodynamics 12(4): 424.

12. Devreese AM, Nuyens G, Staes F, Vereeken RL, De Weerdt W, Stappaerts K (2000) Do posture and straining influence urinary-flow parameters in normal women? Neurourol Urodynamics 19(1): 3–8.

13. Skehan M, Moore KH, Richmond DH (1990) The auditory stimulus of running water: Its effect on urethral pressure. Neurourol Urodynamics 9(4): 351–3.

19 Drugs Acting on the Lower Urinary Tract

D. Tincello

In this chapter the drugs available for the treatment of lower urinary tract (LUT) disorders are described, with the exception of antibiotics for urinary tract infections. The discussion is limited to prescribed medications, which are grouped according to diagnoses.

19.1 Detrusor Instability: Anticholinergic Drugs

Detrusor instability is a condition characterised by uninhibited detrusor muscle activity. Several drugs are available which suppress the muscle activity by acting at the neuromuscular junction of the detrusor muscle (a muscarinic cholinergic receptor). The drugs have characteristic side-effects: dry mouth, dry eyes, headaches, blurred vision and constipation. The balance between side-effects and the effect on the bladder determines the clinical utility of each drug.

Oxybutynin (Ditropan, Lorex Synthélabo; Cystrin, Pharmacia & Upjohn)[1,2] is a tertiary amine with anticholinergic, antispasmodic and local anaesthetic properties.[3] It provides excellent symptom relief in terms of urgency and frequency, but the efficacy of the drug is hampered by severe side-effects.[4-7] Data from randomised controlled trials have shown that side-effects occur in over 80% of patients and that up to 25% discontinue the medication.[3,5] Keheller et al.[8] reported that only 18% of patients continue oxybutynin for more than 6 weeks. Measures such as salivary stimulants do not increase compliance in the medium term.[9] Oxybutynin has been administered intravesically. The circulating levels of active drug are much lower[2] and the incidence of side-effects is reduced while symptomatic improvement is maintained.[10-12]

Tolterodine (Detrusitol, Pharmacia & Upjohn)[13] has less marked effects on the salivary glands than on the bladder.[14] The incidence of side-effects (10%) is less than with oxybutynin,[13] but the efficacy is comparable to that of the maximum dose of oxybutynin.[15,16] In a pooled analysis of randomised controlled trials, only 8% of patients discontinued medication.[17] A randomised controlled trial involving 293 patients confirmed these findings.[18] Quality of life data improves after treatment, suggesting that the theoretical advantage of tolterodine is translated into real benefit.[19] Long term data (i.e. 5 years or more) are yet to be published, but it is likely that this drug will allow patients to have significant long-term relief from the symptoms of detrusor instability.

Flavoxate (Urispas, Shire Pharmaceuticals Ltd) is an antispasmodic agent with direct action on the smooth muscle of the urinary tract.[20] It is a useful second line drug because of the absence of significant anticholinergic side-effects[21] and because it does not impair voiding function.[20]

Propantheline (Pro-Banthine, Baker Norton Pharmaceuticals) tends not be used often in modern practice because it has less efficacy than oxybutynin[22] without any appreciable benefit in terms of side-effect profile. It is now used primarily for the treatment of enuresis in adults.

19.2 Detrusor Instability: Antidepressant Drugs

Antidepressant drugs have been used for detrusor instability and are particularly useful when nocturia is a significant problem.

- *Imipramine* (Tofranil, Novartis) significantly improves incontinence in an elderly population.[23]
- *Doxepin* (Sinequan, Pfizer Ltd) is a tricyclic antidepressant with significant anticholinergic properties, which reduced nocturia, urinary leakage and nocturnal enuresis in a randomised trial of patients who failed to respond to conventional drug regimes.[24]

19.3 Genuine Stress Incontinence: Oestrogens

Genuine stress incontinence is caused by a weakness of the urethral sphincter mechanism. Sphincter tone is maintained by the sympathetic autonomic nervous system with voluntary tone added by the somatic nerves.

Oestrogen has been used in postmenopausal women to improve the mucosal oedema and periurethral tissue "tone". A review of published studies[25] and a meta-analysis by the Urogenital Therapy Committee of the Cochrane Collaboration[26] both show no effect of oestrogen treatment on either subjective or objective criteria of incontinence.

However, oestrogen treatment does prevent recurrent urinary tract infections in postmenopausal women and alleviates the symptoms of sensory urgency with an associated increase in quality of life.[27] It is therefore worth considering oestrogen replacement on this basis alone.

19.4 Genuine Stress Incontinence: Sympathomimetic Drugs

Several drugs which have sympathetic adrenergic effects have been used to treat stress incontinence. Fourteen days of treatment with norephedrine produced an increase in functional urethral length associated with subjective symptomatic improvement.[28] A randomised trial of 2 weeks treatment with *phenylpropanolamine* demonstrated increased mean urethral closure pressure and subjective improvement in 71% of patients compared to 36% of controls.[29] A controlled trial of 6 weeks of norephinephrine in 44 women with objective measurement of leakage (pad testing) found no difference in outcome.[30]

Thirty-six women were included in a 4-week period with *phenylpropanolamine and oestriol* in combination.[31] Both treatments reduced reported leakage episodes, but only the phenylpropanolamine (alone or in combination) produced any objective reduction in pad test loss. A similar study with 6 weeks follow-up found that phenylpropanolamine produced a significant continence rate (48% vs. 28%) and a significant reduction in leakage (30%) on pad testing.[32] It appears that phenylpropanolamine, either alone or in combination with oestriol, is an effective agent for the management of stress incontinence, but no long-term data are available. Pharmacological treatment for stress incontinence is rarely used in practice in the UK, probably because of concerns regarding the long-term risks of cardiovascular disease, in addition to the significant success rates associated with physiotherapy and surgery.

19.5 Sensory Disorders

Oestrogen administration has been shown to improve the symptoms of sensory urgency in postmenopausal women.[27] Simple measures such as alkalinisation of the urine with *potassium citrate* can help to alleviate the symptoms in women of all ages. Care must be taken to exclude urinary tract infection, although avoiding unnecessary antibiotic use. Interstitial cystitis can cause sensory urgency and should always be considered in patients with refractory symptoms. The treatment of interstitial cystitis lies outside the scope of this chapter, but Erickson and Davies have recently reviewed the disease.[33]

19.6 Summary

Drug therapy has been the mainstay of treatment of detrusor instability for many years, and recent advances in the tolerability and specificity of anticholinergic medication is likely to improve the management of patients with unstable bladders still further. The available evidence suggests that pharmacological treatment of genuine stress incontinence is effective and may avoid surgery in up to a third of patients.[30] This option does not appear to have established itself in modern practice owing to a combination of moderate efficacy and concerns about long-term safety.

References

1. Diokno AC, Lapides J (1972) Oxybutynin: a new drug with analgesic and anticholinergic properties. J Urol 108: 307–9.

2. Massad CA, Kogan BA, Trigo-Rocha FE (1992) The pharmacokinetics of intravesical and oral oxybutynin chloride. J Urol 148: 595–7.

3. Yarker YE, Goa KL, Fitton A (1995) Oxybutynin. A review of its pharmacodynamic and pharmacokinetic properties, and its therapeutic use in detrusor instability. Drugs Aging 6: 243–62.

4. Kirkali Z, Whitaker RH (1987) The use of oxybutynin in urological practice. Int Urol Nephrol 19: 385–91.

5. Tapp AJ, Cardozo LD, Versi E, Cooper D (1990) The treatment of detrusor instability in post-menopausal women with oxybutynin chloride: a double blind placebo controlled study [see comments]. Brit J Obstet Gynaecol 97: 521–6.

6. Riva D, Casolati E (1984) Oxybutynin chloride in the treatment of female idiopathic bladder instability. Results from double blind treatment. Clin Exp Obstet Gynecol 11: 37–42.

7. Moisey CU, Stephenson TP, Brendler CB (1980) The urodynamic and subjective results of treatment of detrusor instability with oxybutynin chloride. Br J Urol 52: 472–5.

8. Kelleher CJ, Cardozo LD, Khullar V, Salvatore S (1997) A medium-term analysis of the subjective efficacy of treatment for women with detrusor instability and low bladder compliance. Br J Obstet Gynaecol 104: 988–93.

9. Tincello DG, Adams EJ, Sutherst JR, Richmond DH (2000) Oxybutynin for detrusor instability with adjuvant salivary stimulant pastilles to improve compliance: results of a multicentre, randomised controlled trial. BJU Int 85: 416–20.

10. Brendler CB, Radebaugh LC, Mohler JL (1989) Topical oxybutynin chloride for relaxation of dysfunctional bladders. J Urol 141: 1350–2.

11. Enzelsberger H, Helmer H, Kurz C (1995) Intravesical instillation of oxybutynin in women with idiopathic detrusor instability: a randomised trial. Br J Obstet Gynaecol 102: 929–30.

12. Greenfield SP, Fera M (1991) The use of intravesical oxybutynin chloride in children with neurogenic bladder. J Urol 146: 532–4.

13. Jonas U, Hofner K, Madersbacher H, Holmdahl TH (1997) Efficacy and safety of two doses of tolterodine versus placebo in patients with detrusor overactivity and symptoms of frequency, urge incontinence, and urgency: urodynamic evaluation. Int Study Group World J Urol 15: 144–51.

14. Nilvebrant L, Andersson KE, Gillberg PG, Stahl M, Sparf B (1997) Tolterodine – a new bladder-selective antimuscarinic agent. Eur J Pharm 327: 195–207.

15. Abrams P, Freeman RM, Anderstrom C, Mattiason A (1996) Efficacy and tolerability of tolterodine vs oxybutynin and placebo in patients with detrusor instability. J Urol 157 (Suppl): 103.

16. Drutz HP, Appell RA (1997) Enhanced tolerability of tolterodine compared to oxybutynin in an controlled clinical study. Int Urogynecol J 8 (Suppl): S14.

17. Appell RA (1997) Clinical efficacy and safety of tolterodine in the treatment of overactive bladder: a pooled analysis. Urology 50: 90–6.

18. Abrams P, Freeman R, Anderström C, Mattiasson A (1998) Tolterodine, a new antimuscarinic agent: as effective but better tolerated than oxybutynin in patients with an overactive bladder. Br J Urol 81: 801–10.

19. Kobelt G, Kirchberger I, Malone-Lee J (1999) Quality of life aspects of the overactive bladder and the effect of treatment with tolterodine. BJU Int 83: 583–90.

20. Guarneri L, Robinson E, Testa R (1994) A review of flavoxate: pharmacology and mechanism of action. Drugs Today 30: 91–8.

21. Delaere KP, Michiels HG, Debruyne FM, Moonen WA (1977) Flavoxate hydrochloride in the treatment of detrusor instability. Urol Int 32: 377–81.

22. Thuroff JW, Bunke B, Ebner A et al. (1991) Randomized, double-blind, multicenter trial on treatment of frequency, urgency and incontinence related to detrusor hyperactivity: oxybutynin versus propantheline versus placebo. J Urol 145: 813–16.

23. Castleden CM, Duffin HM, Gulati RS (1986) Double-blind study of imipramine and placebo for incontinence due to bladder instability. Age Ageing 15: 299–303.

24. Lose G, Jorgensen L, Thunedborg P (1989) Doxepin in the treatment of female detrusor overactivity: a randomized double-blind crossover study. J Urol 142: 1024–6.

25. Sultana CJ, Walters MD (1995) Estrogen and urinary incontinence in women. Maturitas 20: 129–38.

26. Fantl JA, Cardozo LD, McClish DK (1994) Estrogen therapy in the management of urinary incontinence in postmenopausal women: a meta-analysis: first report of the Hormones and Urogenital Therapy Committee. Obstet Gynecol 83: 12–18.

27. Cardozo LD, Kelleher CJ (1995) Sex hormones, the menopause and urinary problems. Gynaecol Endocrinol 9: 75–84.

28. Ek A, Andersson KE, Gullberg B, Ulmsten U (1978) The effects of long-term treatment with norephedrine on stress incontinence and urethral closure pressure profile. Scand J Urol Nephrol 12: 105–10.

29. Lehtonen T, Rannikko S, Lindell O et al. (1986) The effect of phenylpropanolamine on female stress urinary incontinence. Ann Chir Gynaecol 75: 236–41.

30. Lose G, Rix P, Diernaes E, Alexander N (1988) Norfenefrine in the treatment of female stress incontinence. A double-blind controlled trial. Urol Int 43: 11–15.

31. Kinn A, Lindskog M (1988) Estrogens and phenylpropanolamine in combination for stress urinary incontinence in postmenopausal women. Urology 32: 273–80.

32. Ahlstrom K, Sandahl B, Sjoberg B et al. (1990) Effect of combined treatment with phenylpropanolamine and estriol, compared with estriol treatment alone in postmenopausal women with stress urinary incontinence. Gynecol Obstet Invest 30: 37–43.

33 Erickson DR, Davies MF (1998) Interstitial cystitis. Int Urogynecol J 9: 174–83

III Colorectal Disorders

20 An Anatomical Overview

D. Kumar

20.1 Anatomy of the Anorectum

20.1.1 Anal Canal

The anal canal is approximately 3–4 cm in length; it extends from the anal skin margin to the level of the pelvic diaphragm (the pelvic floor). The anal canal is surrounded by the two sphincter muscles (Fig. 20.1). The inner circular smooth muscle area of the rectum becomes thickened and forms the internal anal sphincter, which is easily palpated on digital examination. The internal sphincter is involuntary but provides a resting tone that helps to keep the anal canal closed at all times. The external anal sphincter consists of striated muscle and has three distinctive parts: the subcutaneous, superficial and deep. The deep part of the external anal sphincter fuses with the puborectalis muscle at the top of the anal canal and helps to maintain continence.

The puborectalis muscle maintains the anorectal angle by pulling the rectum forward at the anorectal junction. The puborectalis forms part of the levator ani muscle and is its most medial component.

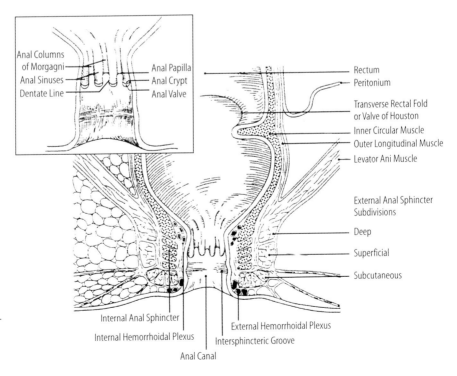

Figure 20.1 Section of the rectum and anal canal, demonstrating the internal and external anal sphincters and the valves of Houston.

Lateral to the puborectalis lies the pubococcygeus, then the iliococcygeus and the most lateral is the ischiococcygeus. Together these muscles form the pelvic diaphragm or the pelvic floor, and support the pelvic viscera.

The anal canal is very richly supplied by nerves; the upper half is supplied by both sympathetic and parasympathetic nerve fibres. The preganglionic sympathetic nerve fibres originate from the second to the fourth lumbar splanchnic nerves and the post ganglionic fibres to the sigmoid colon, rectum and upper anal canal via the pelvic plexus. The preganglionic parasympathetic nerves originate in the sacral cord (S2–4). These emerge as the nervi errigentes and become the pelvic sphanchnic nerves. The lower half of the anal canal is supplied by branches of the pudendal nerve called the inferior rectal nerves. The external anal sphincter is also supplied by branches of the pudendal nerves.

20.1.2 Rectum

The rectum is approximately 15 cm long and lies in the sacral hollow. The beginning of the rectum is identified by the disappearance of tenia coli and appendices epiploicae which are present in the colon. The rectum has a complete coat of longitudinal muscle.

The anterior and posterior muscles are slightly shorter than the lateral muscle and this configuration produces three lateral shelves called the superior, middle and inferior rectal valves or valves of Houston. The rectum is supplied by both sympathetic and parasympathetic nerve fibres similar to those of the upper anal canal. The sensory fibres of the rectum are derived from the autonomic nervous system and enter the chord at the L1, L2, S2, S3 and S4 levels. The rectum is relatively insensitive to painful stimuli but does respond to distension and stretch.

20.1.3 Mechanism of Continence

A number of theories have been put forward to explain anorectal continence. The flutter valve theory argues that intra-abdominal pressure forces applied to a high-pressure zone in the lower rectum produces occlusion of this area of the rectum, thus preventing passage of rectal contents into the anal canal. However, Duthie observed a high-pressure zone within the anal canal and therefore argued against the flutter valve theory.[1] He proposed that for a flutter valve to produce a high-pressure segment the intra-abdominal forces would have to be applied below the levator muscles. Parks put

forward the flap valve theory and stressed the importance of an acute anorectal angle which helped in the application of intra-abdominal forces to the anterior rectal wall.[2] During a rise in intra-abdominal pressure, the top of the anal canal is occluded by anterior rectal mucosa which plugs it and prevents rectal contents reaching the anus. According to Parks, incontinence occurs when there is excessive perineal descent and the anorectal angle becomes obtuse. He developed the postanal repair operation to recreate the anorectal angle.

Rectal filling results in lowering of resting anal canal pressures which is due to inhibition of internal anal sphincter activity. This reflex activity is called the recto-anal inhibitory reflex. Local intrinsic nerve pathways then lead to an increase in internal sphincter pressure thus maintaining continence. The recto-anal inhibitory reflex allows the rectal contents to come into contact with the specialised anal sensory epithelium which then initiates the anal sampling reflex.

Two other factors, rectal compliance and gastrointestinal transit, also help in maintaining continence. Rectal filling is appreciated from volumes of 10 ml or more and the rectum can tolerate 300 ml before a feeling of fullness is noticed. This is achieved by the accommodation reflex, and once the maximum tolerable volume is achieved, there is an urgent desire to defecate. Similarly, rapid colonic or gastrointestinal transit results in rapid filling of the rectum, resulting in urgency or urge incontinence. This can occur in the presence of a normal and competent sphincter complex.

20.1.4 Mechanism of Defecation

Defecation is a complex act which is under the influence of the central nervous system. Rectal filling, distension and stimulation of the anorectal mechano receptors provide the stimulus for the initiation of the act of defecation. It has two main components:

- the rise in intra-abdominal pressure which is achieved by the contraction of the abdominal wall muscles and contraction of the pelvic floor muscles
- the evacuation of the rectum achieved by relaxation of the anal canal and contraction of the rectal wall.

Defecation can occur without abdominal wall contraction, however, especially in circumstances when the stools are loose. In addition to the central cortical control, there is a spinal centre in the lumbo-sacral region which can maintain reflex defecation following transection of the spinal cord at this level. The onset of defecation in this case is marked by descent of the pelvic floor, followed by propulsive contractile activity in the sigmoid colon which propels faeces to the rectum. Rectal filling induces the conscious urge to defecate and causes relaxation of the internal sphincter muscle. This sequence is completed by the decision to defecate. The external anal sphincter relaxes, and faeces are expelled by alternating contraction and relaxation of the levator muscles. This is aided by a rise in intra-abdominal pressure transmitted through the relaxed pelvic floor. Defecation is not possible when the pelvic floor is raised, presumably because intra-abdominal pressure cannot then be transmitted to the recto-anal contents. The colon also contributes to the mechanism of defecation by producing high-amplitude contraction waves in the proximal colon immediately prior to defecation.

20.2 Aetiology and Pathophysiology of Anorectal Disorders

20.2.1 Aetiology and Pathophysiology of Faecal Incontinence

Continence is maintained by an interaction of several factors including normal transit of a normal-consistency stool, normal capacity rectum to provide an adequate reservoir, and a normal voluntary control and reflex function provided by the anal sphincter complex. The most common cause of faecal incontinence in adult healthy women is obstetric trauma. Other causes include pudendal nerve neuropathy and iatrogenic causes such as damage to the sphincter muscles during surgical operations. Neurological causes of faecal incontinence include upper motor neurone lesions and lower motor neurone lesion or peripheral nerve lesions from the sacral outflow or the pudendal nerve. In patients with diabetes, mixed motor and sensory loss may result in faecal incontinence. Direct trauma to the sphincters can also cause faecal incontinence. It may also be the presenting symptom in patients with faecal impaction and idiopathic constipation. Similarly, patients with rectal prolapse and those with proctitis may also have associated incontinence. In children Hirschsprung's disease and anorectal malformation can also result in faecal incontinence.

20.2.1.1 Obstetric Trauma

It is now well established that in healthy adult women the most common cause of faecal incontinence is sphincter damage during childbirth. Often there is a history of a difficult vaginal delivery, forceps-assisted delivery or a perineal tear.[3]

Sultan et al in a study of 128 women found that pudendal nerve latencies were significantly prolonged after vaginal deliveries.[4] Only a third of those who had a prolonged pudendal nerve latency were still affected after 6 months, suggesting that most women who sustained sphincter trauma during childbirth appeared to recover normal nerve function. With the availability of better imaging technology we now know that sphincter disruption is the most common form of obstetric damage.[5] Approximately a third of all primiparous women develop a sphincter defect involving one or both muscles following a vaginal delivery.[6] Patients who sustain external sphincter damage also have impaired sensation which appears to persist in the upper anal canal at 6 months.[7]

20.2.1.2 Iatrogenic Sphincter Trauma

This is usually the result of operation on the anal canal for fissures, fistula-in-ano and haemorrhoids. It is now well established that anal manual dilatation also results in damage to the anal sphincter complex.

20.2.1.3 Faecal Impaction

Faecal impaction is common in geriatric patients, and is easily seen as a cause of faecal incontinence.[8] In younger patients it is often associated with a megarectum or congenital anorectal malformation.

20.2.1.4 Internal Anal Sphincter Dysfunction

Swash et al. found ultrastructural changes in internal anal sphincter biopsies in patients with neurogenic anorectal incontinence.[9] Pharmacological studies have demonstrated a poor response to adrenaline stimulation and lack of response to electrical field stimulation of internal anal sphincter biopsies from patients with neurogenic incontinence.[10,11]

20.2.2 Aetiology and Pathophysiology of Constipation (see also Chapter 22.2)

Constipation is a symptom, and its causes can be organic or functional. Before making a diagnosis of chronic idiopathic constipation, specific causes such as metabolic and endocrine abnormalities, neurological lesions, drugs and muscular lesions, as well as gastrointestinal tract disorders, need to be excluded.

An anatomical and morphological variation in the size of the colon and rectum and consistency and size of the stool can have a significant impact on the mechanism and the frequency of defecation. Small hard stools are more difficult to expel than soft stools of the same shape and volume. Stool form and consistency also correlate with transit time; hard stools are passed when the transit time is long and a soft mushy stool is associated with rapid transit through the colon. The consistency of stool depends on its water content; longer residue time in the colon results in a harder stool. In some patients with constipation the length of the colon is abnormal (this is often referred to as a redundant colon on contrast radiology). Using a continuous colonic profusion and a dye dilution technique, colonic volumes were found to be about 50% greater in constipated patients than in control subjects.

In patients with a megarectum and a megacolon there is thickening of the muscle layers in the rectum and the colon; this may be in response to a zone of functional obstruction. The megabowel most commonly involves the rectum and the rectosigmoid. In children there is often a history of faecal soiling. Some patients have normal and others delayed transit times.[13]

20.2.2.1 Idiopathic Constipation: Motility Disorder

Perfused tube manometry over a period of 24 h has shown that colonic motility consists of low-amplitude contractions most of the time but high-amplitude propagating contractions were noted early in the morning, after waking and before defecation.

During defecation, the peristaltic wave progresses to the distal bowel and causes internal sphincter relaxation. In patients with constipation the frequency and duration of the high-amplitude pressure waves is reduced.

20.2.2.2 Abnormalities of Sensation

Rectal volume sensation can be recorded by distending a balloon in the rectum and noting the volumes at which first sensation, urgency and pain are experienced. Patients with constipation require a greater volume to produce their initial sensation and urgency but have a normal maximum tolerated volume when compared with controls.[13] Rectal sensation can also be tested by applying a slowly increasing current to the rectal mucosa.

Constipated patients demonstrate an elevated mean sensory threshold compared with a control group. However, there is considerable overlap between constipated patients and the control population.

20.2.2.3 Abnormality of the Pelvic Floor

Some patients with chronic idiopathic constipation exhibit abnormalities of pelvic floor function and may be unable to expel a water-filled balloon from the rectum. Rectal function may be abnormal in patients with slow colonic transit, but also in patients who have a normal colonic transit time. The latter abnormality is more commonly seen in patients with increased pelvic floor descent and those who have a history of chronic straining resulting in pelvic nerve damage.

Electromyography (EMG) studies of the striated external anal sphincter muscles have shown that many patients with severe constipation have paradoxical contraction of the muscle during straining.[14] It has been suggested that inappropriate contraction of the puborectalis and external sphincter muscles is responsible for blocking rectal emptying. This phenomenon has been termed "anismus". However not all patients with constipation exhibit this EMG abnormality, and moreover some normal subjects and patients with other anorectal conditions may have this abnormality as well. It is conceivable that the phenomenon of paradoxical pelvic floor contraction may be an abnormal learned response rather than an inherent abnormality of the neuromuscular mechanisms.

20.3 Assessment and Investigations

20.3.1 Evaluation of a Patient with Faecal Incontinence

All patients presenting with faecal incontinence should have a careful history taken. Special attention should be paid to the stool consistency, history of straining and a previous history of difficult vaginal delivery with or without the use of forceps.

A physical examination of the abdomen and anorectum should be carried out (see Chapters 21 and 22). Neurological symptoms should also be recorded. Attention should be paid to symptoms suggestive of colonic or rectal disease such as the presence of diarrhoea and the leakage of mucus or blood in patients with inflammatory bowel disease. Any history of previous pelvic or anal surgery, especially anal dilatation, fistula surgery and prolapse repairs, should be documented.

20.3.2 Anorectal Investigations

20.3.2.1 Anal Manometry

A variety of pressure measurement equipment is commercially available. Using these devices, the function of both internal and external anal sphincters is assessed by measuring anal canal pressures. The manometry assembly is inserted into the rectum and then gradually withdrawn. When the high-pressure zone is reached, the distance from the anal verge is recorded and the pressure in the anal canal measured at 1 cm intervals as the catheter is withdrawn further. This records the resting pressure produced by the internal anal sphincter as well as the resting sphincter length. Manometry is the only method of measuring resting tone in the anal canal.

The internal anal sphincter is responsible for approximately 70–80% of the resting tone in the anal canal. Measurement of the resting tone therefore provides an assessment of the internal anal sphincter function. The procedure is repeated but this time the patient is asked to voluntarily squeeze the external anal sphincter so that the maximum squeeze pressure produced by the external sphincter can be recorded. Voluntary squeeze pressure is the greatest pressure achieved above resting pressure during a maximal voluntary contraction. It is mainly an expression of the external anal sphincter function. The patient should be instructed not to use the gluteal muscles during voluntary squeeze as this will result in an erroneous recording of the squeeze pressure. In the majority of patients with incontinence the resting and squeeze pressures are significantly lower than in normal subjects. Patients who are incontinent to liquid and solid stool have lower squeeze pressures than those who are incontinent to liquid stool alone, and the length of the high-pressure zone is shorter in patients with incontinence than in normal subjects.

20.3.2.2 Rectal Volume Sensation

This can be measured by using a latex balloon tied to a rubber tube, which is attached to a three-way

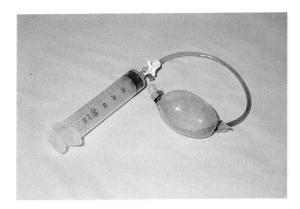

Figure 20.2   Latex balloon for rectal sensitivity evaluation.

tap and a syringe (Fig. 20.2). The balloon assembly is inserted into the rectum and known aliquots of air are injected into the balloon. The volume of air at first perception is the threshold volume. The volume at which the patient can perceive the presence of an inflated balloon inside the rectum determines the volume at constant sensation and volume at which the patient has an uncontrollable desire to defecate is the maximum tolerated volume.

In patients with faecal incontinence due to rectal factors, the volume at constant sensation is often below normal. The maximum tolerable volume may also be impaired in patients with faecal incontinence. In some patients constant sensation or maximum tolerability at a low volume may be the only abnormality. These patients often have symptoms of severe urgency associated with faecal incontinence.

20.3.3 Neurophysiological Studies

20.3.3.1 Electromyography

Electromyography is used to assess denervation or reinnervation in patients with faecal incontinence. It is commonly performed by using a concentric or single fibre needle electrode (See Chapter 7.10). The concentric needle electrode has a relatively large uptake area and records the activity of several motor units; the EMG activity will be reduced where the number of functioning fibres is reduced. Patients with neuropathic faecal incontinence have reduced activity in both puborectalis and external anal sphincter muscles. By contrast, the single fibre EMG allows analysis of changes in single muscle fibres. It demonstrates reinnervation of previously denervated muscle fibres by surrounding neurons and is expressed as fibre density. It is increased in patients with neurogenic faecal incontinence and is said to be a sensitive and specific marker of neuropathy.[15]

20.3.3.2 Pudendal Nerve Terminal Motor Latency

Pudendal nerve terminal motor latency measures conduction in the terminal part of the pudendal nerve. The pudendal nerve is stimulated as it crosses the ischial spine whilst recording the evoked potential in the external anal sphincter. This is studied using a specifically designed device mounted on a glove.[10] Recordings are made from both sides of the pelvis, as pudendal nerve damage may be asymmetrical in some patients. Pudendal nerve terminal motor latency is prolonged in patients with idiopathic faecal incontinence. However, it must be remembered that pudendal nerve terminal motor latency and fibre density increase with age and this should be considered when interpreting the data.

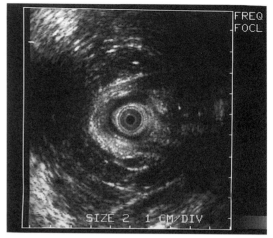

Figure 20.5   Internal and external anal sphincter defect.

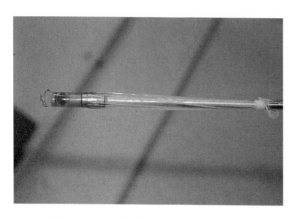

Figure 20.3   Anal ultrasonography equipment.

20.3.4 Endoanal Ultrasound

Endoanal ultrasound provides high-resolution images of both the internal and external anal sphincter and the puborectalis muscles. The examination is performed with the patient in the left lateral position and serial images are obtained at rest and during squeeze in the lower, mid and upper anal canal. The equipment used to perform endoanal ultrasonography is shown in Fig. 20.3. The normal ultrasound (Fig. 20.4) consists of a compete ring of internal sphincter muscle surrounded by the mixed echogenic uninterrupted external sphincter. In patients with a direct sphincter injury or obstetric trauma, a sphincter defect is seen in the internal and/or external anal sphincter (Fig. 20.5). It also provides a dynamic assessment of the sphincter muscles on voluntary contraction.

20.3.5 Evaluation of a Patient with Constipation (see also Chapter 22.3)

The patient should have a thorough general physical and systemic examination to elicit signs of hypothyroidism and other associated medical conditions. Haematological and biochemical abnormalities should be excluded by a full blood count, urea and electrolyte estimation, thyroid function tests and liver function tests. Serum calcium should also be checked in all patients. A barium enema examination should be performed to exclude a mechanical reason for constipation. After all possibilities of an organic cause for constipation have been excluded, a complete functional evaluation of the patient with chronic idiopathic constipation should be made.

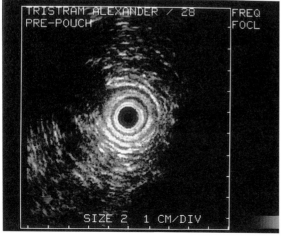

Figure 20.4   Normal ultrasound of the anal canal.

This should include an assessment of colonic transit, rectal transit and pelvic floor function. In some cases additional assessment with colonic motility or small bowel motility measurement may be necessary.

20.3.5.1 Colonic Transit

Radiological techniques involving ingestion of radio-opaque markers of different shapes and sizes on different days followed by several abdominal radiographs over the subsequent 5–7 days are commonly used but are time consuming and subject the patients to excessive radiation.

Colonic scintigraphy is the method of choice in the author's unit for the assessment of colonic transit. It is performed in outpatients without bowel preparation. The subject ingests a capsule which is methacrylate coated and contains 2 MBq of indium-111 as the radionuclide. Imaging starts within 4 h. Radioactive (cobalt-57) markers are applied to bony landmarks to permit correct alignment of images. Imaging is continued hourly between 9 a.m. and 5 p.m. on the first day, and the subject returns home overnight. Imaging is continued for 2 further days between 9 a.m. and 5 p.m. On days 2 and 3 images are acquired at 4-hourly intervals. Subjects are encouraged to maintain as normal a lifestyle as possible. They are asked to collect faecal samples and record the time of evacuation. These activities permit subsequent measurement of evacuated radioactivity.

From the computerised data, dynamic images are generated and the position of the colon determined. To evaluate segmental colonic transit, regions of interest (ROI) are defined on scans and transit through each region is separately determined. Four regions of interest are used:

- ROI 1 is the caecum, ascending colon and hepatic flexure
- ROI 2 is the transverse colon
- ROI 3 is the splenic flexure
- ROI 4 is the descending colon, sigmoid colon and rectum.

The proportion of the scintographic counts in each region on each image is calculated and the distribution of scintigraphic activity throughout the colon with time is determined. Scintigraphy has advantages over other methods of measuring colonic transit in that a repeated or continuous observations can be obtained without additional radiation hazards. The estimated dose equivalent is less than one abdominal radiograph. The measurement of radiation counts in stool samples within closed containers makes the process of faecal examination convenient and aesthetically acceptable. Scintigraphic transit measurement also has the advantage over other methods in that segmental colonic transit can be quantified. The main problem with scintographic transit measurement is poor image resolution which can sometimes lead to difficulty in differentiating the colon from overlapping small bowel.

20.3.5.2 Rectal Transit

Chronic idiopathic constipation may be due to impaired rectal evacuation, slow colonic transit or a combination of both functional abnormalities.

Assessment of rectal evacuation is therefore an important component of the evaluation of the constipated patient. The variety of different methods of assessing rectal evacuation testify to the difficulties and the lack of consensus about the optimum method.

20.3.5.3 Barium Proctography

Conventional assessment of anorectal function with barium proctography involves evacuation of a barium-labelled artificial stool. Barium proctography is widely used for assessment of anorectal angle, pelvic floor descent, rectoceles and mucosal prolapse. However, it is debatable how important it is to evaluate these parameters. The anorectal angles in constipated patients and in controls are similar and there is no relationship between symptoms and the anorectal angle. Pelvic floor descent, rectoceles and mucosal prolapses are probably the result rather than the cause of impaired rectal evacuation. Another drawback with barium proctography is safety. A typical investigation involves 1–2 min of fluoroscopy and 2–3 radiographs

20.3.5.4 Isotope Defecography

The drawback of conventional proctography led to the development of a quantitative scintigraphic method of assessing defecation. Scintigraphic defecography involves evacuation of a radiolabelled artificial stool.

Radioactive markers, each containing 1 MBq activity are placed over the subjects pubis, lumbosacral junction and coccyx to promote alignment of images. With the subject in the left lateral position, 200 ml of an oat porridge and water mixture containing 100 MBq technetium is introduced intrarectally. The subject is imaged whilst seated on a commode with a gamma camera head against the left hip. Dynamic digital images are acquired during evacuation for up to 10 min and stored on computer.

The images are replayed and a rectal region of interest is drawn around the bolus of scintigraphic activity in the rectum. Rectal emptying curves are obtained. Rectal percentage of evacuation time and evacuation rate are easily calculated. Ano-rectal angle, pelvic floor descent and rectocele can all be measured with reference to the markers and the anal canal. The advantage of scintigraphic defecography is that it provides quantitative and dynamic information on rectal evacuation. The other main advantage is the minimal radiation dose administered to the patient.

20.4 Conservative and Medical Management of Faecal Incontinence

The principles governing conservative management of faecal incontinence are:

- keep the stool formed
- keep the rectum empty.

See also Chapter 21. The roles of dietary measures and pelvic floor exercises and re-education are also discussed in subsequent chapters.

20.4.1 Keep the Stool Formed

Keeping the stool formed is extremely important, as a compromised anal sphincter finds it difficult to control liquid stool and maintain continence. Stool consistency also influences rectal function in that liquid stool makes urge incontinence worse than does solid stool.

Stool consistency can be altered either by dietary manipulation or by use of constipation agents or both. It is important to recognise that the introduction of a high-fibre diet or fibre supplements in the diet can be used to soften the stool as well as to make it formed. This can be achieved by regulating the amount of oral fluids. If the stool is already liquid, then the introduction of fibre supplements with limited oral fluids makes the stool firm as the fibre draws fluid from the stool itself.

Constipating agents that work by slowing intestinal and colonic motility are also beneficial. The agents most commonly used are codeine phosphate

and loperamide. These agents increase the residue time for the stool in the colon and therefore provide a better opportunity for absorption of water from the stool. Loperamide has an added beneficial effect in that it also increases the resting tone in the internal sphincter function, which may be beneficial in patients who have internal sphincter weakness.

Occasionally, a combination of fibre supplements and constipating agents can work better than either of these used in isolation. This also has the advantage that a very small dose of the motility reducing agent is required.

20.4.2 Keep the Rectum Empty

Keeping the rectum empty is an important aspect of the management of faecal incontinence. It is particularly important in the elderly patient who often has faecal loading or impaction. In these patients faecal incontinence is secondary to the faecal impaction, and often the treatment of faecal impaction results in complete resolution of the symptom of faecal incontinence.

The simplest way of keeping the rectum empty is by regular use of glycerine suppositories, which can be brought over the counter. Two suppositories a day will give an adequate and satisfactory bowel action. In some patients suppositories do not provide a satisfactory answer and in those circumstances daily enemas or washouts may be necessary.

In a small number of patients, particularly young children, antegrade continence enemas may be necessary. This procedure involves bringing the appendix to the surface as a small opening providing access to the colon. The patient irrigates the colon with half a litre of water and this clears the colon completely, leaving an empty bowel.

20.5 Conservative and Medical Management of Constipation

Most patients with constipation can be managed successfully by conservative means. Less than 10% will require surgical intervention. The conservative measures include dietary manipulation, judicious use of laxatives and specific drug therapy. Once a mechanical cause for constipation has been excluded, all patients should be given advice regarding a high-fibre diet, fibre supplementation and increased oral fluid intake prior to rectal and colonic transit studies. Any electrolyte abnormalities or impairment of thyroid function should be corrected. More than half of all patients presenting with the symptom of constipation will respond to such measures. Dietary manipulation is discussed in more detail in Chapter 22.

A precise definition of the extent of the problem and the segments of the colon or rectum involved helps in deciding whether the treatment should consist of oral laxatives, rectal suppositories or enemas, or a combination of both. Approximately 20% of patients will have only rectal problems, a third will have a combination of rectal and colonic problems, another third will have colonic problems alone and the remainder will have normal transit constipation. In patients with colonic inertia only, judicious use of laxatives provides the most satisfactory results. This may be combined with dietary measures or fibre supplementation. Such patients will not respond to treatment with rectal suppositories or enemas. In contrast, patients with delayed rectal transit will respond extremely satisfactorily to regular use of suppositories or enemas. Oral laxatives are of no benefit to such patients. Patients who have a combination of rectal and colonic transit abnormality need a combination of oral laxatives and suppositories or enemas.

There is a resurgence of interest in the development of more targeted drug therapy for chronic idiopathic constipation, but at present no satisfactory targeted treatment is available.

References

1. Duthie HL (1971) Anal continence. Gut 12: 844–52.
2. Parks AG (1975) Anorectal incontinence. Proc R Soc Med 68: 681–90.
3. MacArthur C, Lewis M, Knox EG (1991) Health and childbirth. Br J Obstet Gynaecol 98: 1193–204.
4. Sultan AH, Kamm MA, Hudson CN (1994) Pudendal nerve damage during labour: prospective study before and after childbirth. Br J Obstet Gynaecol 101: 22–8.
5. Deen KI, Kumar D, Williams JG, Oliff J, Keighley MRB (1993) The prevalence of anal sphincter defects in faecal incontinence: a prospective endosonic study. Gut 34: 685–8.
6. Sultan AH, Kamm MA, Hudson CN, Bartram CI (1993) Anal sphincter disruption during vaginal delivery. N Engl J Med 329: 1905–11.
7. Cornes H, Bartolo DCC, Stirrat GM (1991) Changes in anal canal sensation after childbirth. Br J Surg 78: 74–7.
8. Barratt JA (1992) Colorectal disorders in elderly people. Br Med J 305: 764–6.
9. Swash M, Gray A, Lubowski DZ, Nicholls RJ (1988) Ultrastructural changes in internal anal sphincter in neurogenic faecal incontinence. Gut 29: 1692–8.
10. Lubowski DZ, Nicholls RJ, Burleigh DE, Swash M (1988) Internal anal sphincter in neurogenic faecal incontinence. Gastroenterology 95: 997–1002.
11. Speakman CTM, Hoyle CHV, Kamm MA, Nicholls RJ, Burnstock G (1990) Adrenergic control of the internal anal sphincter is abnormal in patients with idiopathic faecal incontinence. Br J Surg 77: 1342–4.
12. Verduron A, Devroede G, Bouchoucha M (1988) Megarectum. Dig Dis Sci 33: 1164–74.
13. Kamm MA, Lennard-Jones JE, Thompson DG et al. (1988) Dynamic scanning defines a colonic defect in severe idiopathic constipation. Gut 29: 1085–92.
14. Preston DM, Lennard-Jones JE (1985) Anismus in chronic constipation. Dig Dis Sci 30(5): 413–18.
15. Neill ME, Swash M (1980) Increased motor unit fibre density in the external anal sphincter in ano-rectal incontinence: a single fibre EMG study. J Neurol Neurosurg Psychiatry 43: 343–7.

21 Faecal Incontinence

C. Norton

21.1 Prevalence

Faecal incontinence has been variously defined. For the purposes of this chapter, it will be taken to mean "the involuntary or inappropriate passage of faeces".[1] The term "anal incontinence" is usually used to denote any involuntary leakage, whether of solid, liquid or gas. Although the problem does increase with advancing age and disability, there are also large numbers of young otherwise healthy adults with this distressing symptom. The most recent community study in the western world surveyed 2570 households comprising 6959 people in the USA by telephone interview and found that 2.2% of the population reported some anal incontinence (0.8% were incontinent of solid stool, 1.2% of liquid stool and 1.3% of flatus). Two-thirds of those reported as anally incontinent were under 65 years old, and 63% were female. These results are in response to the question "in the last year, have you or anyone in your household experienced unwanted or unexpected or embarrassing loss of control of bowels or gas?"[2] Ten per cent of those reporting incontinence had more than one episode per week, one-third had restricted their activities as a result of their incontinence and only 36% had consulted a doctor about it.[2]

Except in the under-30 age group, more men than women were incontinent in all age groups. Of those with incontinence, only 20% of those attending the GP had mentioned their incontinence, and under half had told their gastroenterologist; 10% avoided leaving their home for fear of an accident. Drossman[3] similarly found more men than women with some symptoms (7.9% vs. 7.7%), but the men were more likely to have minor soiling, whereas more women were grossly incontinent (0.9% women vs. 0.5% of men).

In people over 65 years living at home 3.7% report faecal incontinence at least once a week and 6.1% needed to wear pads in case of bowel leakage.[4] Twenty-one per cent of elderly people living in a home or hospital are faecally incontinent at least weekly,[5] and for most people in institutional care faecal incontinence is compounded by urinary incontinence. Among frail elderly people in nursing homes prevalence of over 20% is common, but rates of over 90% are also reported,[6] suggesting that variation may be due to factors other than the ageing bowel (such as institutional regimes and policies).

People with neurological disease or injury are especially vulnerable to loss of bowel control. It should be noted that in the colorectal literature "neurogenic incontinence" usually refers to incontinence caused by damage to the pudendal nerve, rather than to patients with neurological problems. This can cause confusion. Over one-third of people who have a stroke have faecal incontinence on admission to hospital. This falls to 10% at 6 months, with older patients, women, and those with the most severe strokes, diabetes or another disabling disease being most at risk.[7] It seems that this faecal incontinence may be a product more of immobility and dependency than of neurological damage.[8]

Spinal cord injury (SCI) commonly causes major bowel dysfunction, with 11% reporting faecal incontinence weekly or more, and only 39% having reliable bowel continence.[9] Many people with neurological problems are dependent on others for toileting needs. Half of SCI patients need help to manage their bowels, 53% used digital anal stimulation and two-thirds used manual removal of faeces. Half take over 30 min for a bowel routine; one in five need over 1 h.[9] Multiple sclerosis is associated with constipation in over 40% and faecal incontinence in over 50%; those with greatest disability being most affected by both.[10] However, people with neurological conditions are not exempt from bowel problems due to other aetiologies.[11]

21.2 Assessment

Incontinence of faeces is a devastating symptom in our hygiene- and odour-conscious society. As with any problem, investigation starts with talking to the patient. It is essential that, whichever member of the multidisciplinary team the incontinent or constipated person presents to, she or he is met by an empathetic and positive response. It is important to build a relationship of trust with the patient if the whole picture is to be openly and frankly discussed,

and to establish a vocabulary of words that are mutually understood and acceptable.

Investigation must include a detailed history of bowel function, symptoms and the effect on life-style. Various formats have been suggested for assessment.[12] The following areas should be considered.

21.2.1 Usual Bowel Pattern

• *How often do you open your bowels?*

"Normal" bowel function varies between 1–3 times a day and once in 3 days.[13] It is probably a minority of the total population (40% of men and 33% of women) who have their bowels open once each

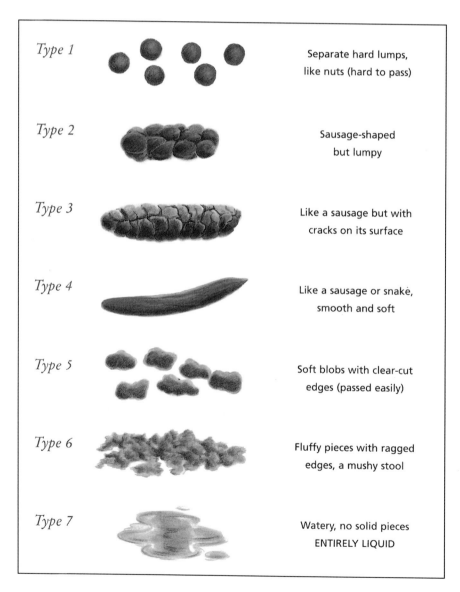

Type 1		Separate hard lumps, like nuts (hard to pass)
Type 2		Sausage-shaped but lumpy
Type 3		Like a sausage but with cracks on its surface
Type 4		Like a sausage or snake, smooth and soft
Type 5		Soft blobs with clear-cut edges (passed easily)
Type 6		Fluffy pieces with ragged edges, a mushy stool
Type 7		Watery, no solid pieces ENTIRELY LIQUID

Figure 21.1 Bristol Stool Form Scale. With permission from Dr K. Heaton.

day.[14] Most are irregular in bowel habit, with young women being the most irregular.

"Constipation" means different things to different people. Infrequent bowel motions, if the stool is easy to pass and not hard, are not a cause for concern or intervention. Conversely, some very constipated people can produce a stool several times per day, but only at the expense of long hours of straining on the toilet. It is important to record if the patient reports a recent change in the frequency of bowel motions, as this may indicate underlying disease or malignancy. Any recent unexplained change in bowel habit in a patient over 40 years should be investigated by barium enema radiography or by colonoscopy. Asking the patient to keep a diary or chart of bowel actions for a week often provides useful baseline information.

21.2.2 Usual Stool Consistency

- *What is your stool (bowel motion) like; is it loose, soft but formed, hard or hard pellets?*
- *Does this vary?*

Record if stool consistency has altered and if the patient reports a change in stool colour. Patients with irritable bowel syndrome are particularly prone to a very variable stool consistency. Where the patient has difficulty in describing the stool, a visual prompt may be helpful (Fig. 21.1).[14] Type 3 or 4 is the most usual consistency, but in women only 56% of stools are these "normal" types; in men 61% of stool are these types.[14] If the stool is loose, this makes both passive and urge faecal incontinence far more likely. Pellet stool is common in slow transit constipation.

21.2.3 Faecal Incontinence

It is quite difficult to gauge severity, as many people restrict their lifestyle to limit the possibility of urge incontinence, so it may actually happen very infrequently, yet still be a major problem, and many find it difficult to estimate the amount lost (minor stain, teaspoonful, tablespoonful, whole bowel motion). It is helpful to question separately about the two major symptom types of urge or passive incontinence.

21.2.4 Urgency and Ability to Defer Defecation

- *When you need to open your bowels, do you need to rush to get to the toilet?*
- *How long can you hold on for?*

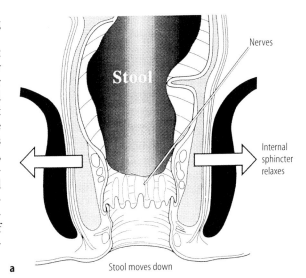

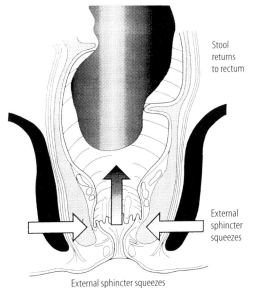

Figure 21.2 Section of the rectum and anal canal: **a** Stool moves down. **b** External sphincter squeezes.

Normally defecation can be deferred for long periods of time, as the urge to defecate is opposed by voluntary contraction of the external sphincter,[15] which should generate sufficient pressure to prevent immediate stool expulsion and to return the stool to the rectum (Fig. 21.2).

If the external sphincter is not functioning well, the squeeze may be insufficient to suppress the urge to defecate, even when the stool is of a normal consistency. A reduced squeeze pressure and an inability to sustain a submaximal contraction have been found to correlate with the symptom of urgency.[16,17] Patients generating high bowel pressures seen in inflammatory bowel disease or irritable bowel syndrome may report severe urgency. In instances where a patient is suffering from diarrhoea this is especially difficult, due both to increased bowel pressures opposing sphincter function and to loose stools.

21.2.5 Urge Incontinence

- *Do you ever not get to the toilet in time and have a bowel accident?*

This often highlights a weakness or defect in the external anal sphincter, which is unable to oppose rectal contractions and so allow delay in defecation. It is possible that a vicious circle develops – any bowel sensation is interpreted as urgent and likely to lead to incontinence – this causes great anxiety, even panic, which in turn exacerbates the sense of urgency. Some people have very infrequent episodes, but self-impose major lifestyle restrictions and never venture far from a toilet "just in case".

21.2.6 Passive Soiling

- *Do you have any leakage from your back passage, of which you are unaware?*
- *Is this liquid or solid?*
- *Does this occur at any time or only after you have opened your bowels?*

The internal anal sphincter is comprised of smooth muscle and is responsible for resting tone in the anal canal. A weak or disrupted sphincter will not close the anal canal completely, and therefore if the stool is loose or soft, some will remain in the anal canal and will ooze out after defecation. Passive soiling is associated with internal anal sphincter damage on ultrasound.[18] These patients complain of great difficulty in cleaning the anus after defecation and subsequent soiling, possibly for several hours. Others experience passive soiling at any time without being aware of it, or loss of stool exacerbated by physical exertion such as walking or playing sport. Passive loss of pellet stool or loss of copious amounts of mucus may result from a rectal prolapse (see below).

21.2.7 Flatus

- *Can you control wind?*
- *Are you able to tell the difference between wind and the need to empty your bowels?*

This also examines the function of the sphincters and whether they are able to maintain an airtight seal. Some patients report incontinence of liquid or solid stool occurring on passing flatus because they are unable to distinguish between flatus and stool.

21.2.8 Presence of Blood and Mucus

- *Do you pass any blood or mucus when you have your bowels open?*

Fresh blood may be passed if a patient has haemorrhoids or an anal fissure. Darker blood may indicate underlying disease or malignancy. The presence of blood and mucus in an individual with a history of straining may indicate the presence of a solitary rectal ulcer. Copious mucus with normal bowel function may indicate a villous adenoma; with disturbed bowel function, mucus is a frequent accompaniment to the irritable bowel syndrome. When a patient reports passing blood or mucus further investigation is warranted.

21.2.9 Pain

- *Do you have pain associated with opening your bowels?*
- *Is this before opening your bowels and relieved by opening your bowels, or is it a pain as you actually pass a stool?*

Pain with an urge to defecate may be reported by patients with inflammatory bowel disease or irritable bowel syndrome, making it difficult to defer defecation. They may refer to a colicky or spasmodic "stabbing" pain. Pain with defecation is often caused by haemorrhoids or an anal fissure. Chronically constipated people often report abdominal discomfort, especially accompanied by bloating.

21.2.10 Evacuation Difficulties

- *Do you have difficulty opening your bowels?*
- *Do you need to strain? If so, how long for?*
- *Do you ever need to insert a finger into your back passage or vagina to help the stool out?*
- *Do you need to push on the area by your back passage?*
- *Does it feel as if you have not completely emptied your bowels?*

These questions examine whether the patient suffers from an evacuation difficulty. People with chronic constipation often just describe defecation as "unsatisfying", that it is always difficult to go and they never feel as if the bowel is properly emptied. Many repeatedly return to the toilet and some spend long periods, even hours, straining without result. Those with a very weak pelvic floor often feel unable to propel the stool out of the anal canal as this moves down every time they strain. The front wall of the rectum may bulge into the vagina with attempted defecation and sometimes, gentle backward pressure with a finger in the vagina may aid complete evacuation of any stool "trapped" in a rectocele. Constipation is often associated with bloating of the abdomen: some women even report needing two sets of clothes, their normal wardrobe and clothes a size or two larger for the end of the day or for when the bowels have not been opened for several days.

21.2.11 Sensation of Prolapse

Some people may report a dragging feeling, or even that the rectum protrudes from the anus, particularly during or after straining. Most prolapses will reduce spontaneously after defecation, but occasionally the patient may find it necessary to manually replace the rectum when it has prolapsed.

21.2.12 Pads or Pants

- *Do you need to wear a pad due to problems with leakage from your bowels?*
- *If so, what type of pad?*
- *Do you need to change your underwear during the day due to leakage?*
- *If yes, how often?*

Patients may wear pads due to urinary incontinence and so it is important to identify if pads or underwear are changed due to faecal incontinence. Also, patients who describe urgency may always wear a pad due to fear of incontinence rather than actual accidents.

21.2.13 Medication

Many preparations can influence bowel function, either to constipate or to loosen the stool.

21.2.14 Past Medical History

The history may give important clues about causation. Major neurological disease, abdominal surgery, diabetes, thyroid disease, psychological disturbances and many other disorders may have an influence on bowel function. Any anal trauma may be relevant, as

may unwanted anal intercourse, which has been found to be associated with internal anal sphincter damage.[19] Many women date the onset of bowel symptoms to gynaecological surgery, especially hysterectomy.[20]

21.2.15 Obstetric History

- *How many babies have you had?*
- *Were forceps used for any of these deliveries?*
- *Did you tear, or did you have stitches?*
- *How heavy were the babies?*
- *Were there any problems with bowel control following the deliveries?*

Women who have had difficult deliveries, particularly assisted by forceps or involving a third-degree tear, are especially likely to report faecal incontinence.[21] Prolonged labour (particularly the second stage) and heavy babies can cause trauma and damage to the anal sphincters. Women with pre-existing irritable bowel syndrome are known to be more likely than others to develop faecal urgency postpartum (64% vs. 10%) and poor control of flatus (35% vs. 13%), at least in the short-term.[22]

21.2.16 Diet, Smoking, Weight and Fluid Intake

Many people find that what they eat influences their bowel function. Nicotine is thought to slow upper gut motility and increase total transit time,[23] but it seems that it can speed rectosigmoid transit,[24] and this fits with many people reporting clinically that smoking a cigarette facilitates initiation of defecation. It is not known whether obesity has an adverse effect on bowel control. Some people with anorexia become very constipated; others abuse laxatives; a few seem to experience pelvic floor problems, possibly secondary to excessive exercise regimes or muscle wasting.

Caffeine is a known gut stimulant[25] and will exacerbate urgency in many patients (personal observations).

21.2.17 Skin Problems

Some patients with faecal incontinence seem to have few problems with skin excoriation. Others suffer greatly from soreness and itching. Certainly, if there is diarrhoea, there is the possibility of small-bowel digestive enzymes in contact with the skin. If there is both urinary and faecal leakage, this seems to make things worse. Some postmenopausal women may have skin problems due to hormone deficiency and oestrogens have been suggested to have some beneficial effect on symptoms of faecal incontinence.[26] Where skin problems prove resistant to simple skin care and barrier creams it is worth seeking a dermatological opinion, as there may be secondary infection or a treatable skin condition.

21.2.18 Bladder Control

- *Do you have any problems with leakage from your bladder?*
- *Does urine leakage occur if you cough, sneeze or laugh?*
- *Do you need to rush to the toilet to pass water?*

These questions help to identify any other continence symptoms. Referral for further investigations may be indicated. Up to a quarter of women attending a urodynamic clinic for investigation of urinary incontinence will admit to faecal incontinence on a postal questionnaire, but only 15% do so on direct questioning, emphasising the difficulty many women have in admitting this symptom.[27] Possibly surprisingly, faecal incontinence seems to be more often associated with detrusor instability than with genuine stress incontinence, possibly reflecting the overlap of irritable bowel syndrome with an unstable bladder.[28]

21.2.19 Effect on Lifestyle, Relationships and Psychological Factors

Some patients report feeling very restricted, planning their journeys around toilet facilities; others may become housebound. Obviously such behaviour will have a profound effect on the individual, and any partner and family. Patients often report avoiding a sexual relationship because of feeling dirty, or a fear that an episode of incontinence will occur. It is known that children born with congenital anorectal abnormalities and with persistant faecal incontinence have an increased risk of behavioural and social problems than their peers.

21.2.20 Examination

It has been suggested that a good history and physical examination can predict findings of anorectal physiology studies in many cases. A low resting tone in the anal canal on digital examination is associated with passive leakage, and there is often gaping of a "funnel-shaped" anal introitus if gentle traction

is applied away from the anal verge.[18] Reduced strength and duration of voluntary contraction has been found to correlate with the symptom of urgency.[16,18] Urge incontinence is also associated with reduced puborectalis squeeze and an increased anorectal angle; many patients also report urge and stress urinary incontinence.

In men, digital examination has been found to be reliable except for assessment of fatigue.[29] It is increasingly recognised that fatigue of voluntary squeeze is an important parameter of assessment, and it is possible to work out a fatigue rate index using manometry.[30] It is not known whether digital examination can accurately assess the rate of fatigue of an anal squeeze. It has been found that digital examination is especially poor at estimating resting tone.

Aspects of physical examination other than the resting and squeeze tone of the anal canal should include:

- Inspection of the perianal skin for excoriation, presence of soiling, any congenital abnormalities, and any haemorrhoids or skin tags.
- Inspection of the perineum for scarring from episiotomy or tears. However, perineal inspection has been shown not to correlate well with the presence or absence of occult anal sphincter damage as seen on anal ultrasound, and an apparently intact perineum does not preclude underlying sphincter damage.[31]
- Inspection of the posterior wall of the vagina for any rectocele at rest and on straining.
- Where there is any suspicion from the history of rectal prolapse, this will seldom be apparent if the patient is examined lying down. The best way to check for prolapse is to sit the patient on a commode or toilet, sitting forward on the toilet seat and leaning forward, and ask her to strain as hard as she can. A prolapsing rectum will be visible or can be felt at the anal verge or below.
- Perineal descent of greater than 2 cm on straining is considered abnormal.
- The contours of the lower back may reveal previously unsuspected spina bifida occulta.
- The presence of a loaded rectum may suggest constipation or faecal impaction, particularly in a frail or immobile person; however, digital rectal examination provides an unreliable indicator of colonic loading, particularly where stools are soft and putty-like rather than hard.[32] Plain abdominal radiograph may be helpful.
- A general assessment of physical abilities and any disabilities that might impair the individual's coping with independent toileting.

Table 21.1. Assessment of faecal incontinence – checklist

Main complaint	Evacuation difficulties?
Duration of symptoms/trigger for onset	Straining?
Usual bowel pattern	Incomplete evacuation?
Usual stool consistency (Bristol Chart)	Need to digitate anally or vaginally, or support the perineum?
Type: Colour:	
Faecal incontinence:	Painful defecation?
How often? How much?	
Urgency? Time can defer	Bloating?
Urge incontinence	Sensation of prolapse?
Difficulty in wiping	Pads/pants
Post-defecation soiling	Bowel medication
Passive soiling	Current medication
Events causing:	
Flatus? Flatus control	Past medical history (including psychological)
Ability to distinguish stool/flatus?	History of depression?
Abdominal pain relieved by defecation	Previous bowel treatments and results
Abdominal bloating?	Obstetric history: parity, difficult deliveries
Rectal bleeding?	Dietary influences
Mucus?	Smoker?
Nocturnal bowel problems?	Height/weight
	Fluids – caffeine
	Skin problems
	Bladder problems
	Effect on lifestyle, relationships etc.

A checklist of points is provided in Table 21.1. Jorge and Wexner [12] have proposed a format for recording the findings from a physical examination (Table 21.2).

21.2.21 Rating the Severity of Incontinence

Several rating scales for faecal incontinence have been proposed. The scale found to have the highest validity is given in Table 21.3.[50]

21.3 Dietary Management of Faecal Incontinence and Faecal Urgency

It is worth experimenting a little to see if each individual can find anything that upsets bowel control. Food rich in fibre is the most common contributor to poor bowel control. Fibre supplements have been found to contribute to faecal incontinence in frail immobile people.[32] There are no trials on the effect of fibre reduction on faecal continence, but clinically a lot of patients derive benefit from moderating their fibre intake.

Table 21.2. Physical examination results

Inspection	Palpation	Endoscopy
Perineal soiling	Resting tone	Intussusception
Scars	Squeeze tone	Solitary rectal ulcer
Anal closure	Sphincter defects	Scarring
Muscular defects	Anal canal length	Mucosal defects
Loss of perineal body	Anorectal angle	Neoplasm
Rectal prolapse	Rectal content	Inflammation
Muscular contraction	Soft tissue scarring	Inflammatory bowel disease
Perineal descent	Rectocele	Infectious colitis
Anal skin reflex to pin prick	Intussusception	Others
Anatomic anorectal pathology	Rectovaginal fistula	Fistula
Haemorrhoids		
Skin tags		
Fistula		
Mucosal ectropion		
Fissure		
Others		

From Jorge and Wexner[12].

Table 21.3. St Mark's faecal continence score

	Never	Rarely (<1 mth)	Sometimes (<1 week)	Usually (<1 day)	Always (Daily)
Solid	0	1	2	3	4
Liquid	0	1	2	3	4
Gas	0	1	2	3	4
Lifestyle	0	1	2	3	4

	No	Yes
Need to wear a pad/plug/ change underwear for soiling	0	2
Taking constipating medicines	0	2
Lack of ability to defer defecation for 15 min	0	4

Total score:

Very spicy or hot food can upset some people. Other foods to consider include milk products and chocolate, which some people find make their stools looser. A few people find that artificial sweeteners (in many low-calorie foods, drinks and chewing gum) have a tendency to make their stools looser. If the patient thinks that there may be a link with what they eats, keeping a diary may reveal if there is a pattern. A course of antibiotics can upset the bowel, and live natural yoghurt or lactobaccilus drink (e.g. "Yakult") can help to restore a more regular habit.

Conversely, some foods may help to make stools firmer and therefore easier to control: arrowroot biscuits, marshmallow sweets or very ripe bananas help some people.

Incontinence of flatus is difficult to treat. Dietary changes, such as reduction in bran products, vegetables and caffeine can reduce the amount of flatus produced for some people. Some patients report that products such as live natural yoghurt and aloe vera are helpful in reducing flatus.

21.3.1 Drinks

Types of drink can make a difference to some people; again this is individual and it is worth experimenting. Alcohol seems to cause the bowels to be loose and urgent for some people, but less so for others. Different types of alcoholic drink can affect people in different ways.

Some people have a bowel that seems to be very sensitive to caffeine (found in coffee, tea, cola drinks and expensive chocolate). Caffeine seems to stimulate the bowel and so makes the stools move through faster. This means that less fluid is taken from the stools, which are then looser, and may produce urgency. For the patient with urgency, frequency or loose stool it is worth trying to spend at least a week without any caffeine (decaffeinated tea, coffee and cola are available at most supermarkets), to see if this helps. If things are better without caffeine, then the patient has a choice of whether or not to drink it. Someone who drinks a lot of caffeine should not stop it all suddenly, as headaches may result: advise people to cut down gradually.

Everyone needs to drink approximately 1–1.5 l (2–3 pints) of fluid a day. Beyond this, the amount you drink probably has little effect on the bowels, as any excess fluid intake that your body does not need is processed by the kidneys and passed out as urine, not from the bowel. Increasing fluid intake has been found not to increase stool output or weight in healthy volunteers.[33] Significant fluid deprivation does decrease stool frequency and weight, but only if fluid intake is severely restricted.[34] There does not seem to be a difference between normal and constipated people in either their fluid or fibre intake, and seems that there is a threshold of fluid intake beyond which there is no further increase in stool output for increasing intake. This means that the common advice to constipated people to drink more may in fact not be of any benefit.

21.3.2 Environmental Factors

People who are unwell or generally weak may be unable to generate enough abdominal effort to stimulate a defecation reflex. Poor toilet facilities or lack of privacy may exacerbate this. Confused people may fail to realise what social behaviour is required for toileting, and ignore the call to stool.

21.4 Treatment

J. Laycock

The physiotherapy treatment of faecal incontinence will clearly depend on the results of assessment and investigations. If the patient is incontinent of liquid or soft stool, every attempt should be made to firm the stool and keep the rectum empty (see Chapter 20). Where weakness of the external anal sphincter (EAS) or puborectalis is demonstrated, specific muscle re-education and training should be introduced. The principles and practice of the various modalities are well described in Chapters 8–12 and apply just as well to anal incontinence as to urinary incontinence, and so only a brief resume is included in this chapter; however, there is a more detailed section on the different types of biofeedback for anal incontinence (below).

21.4.1 Pelvic Floor Muscle and Anal Sphincter Exercises

Assessment of puborectalis and the EAS is described in Chapters 6 and 22 and patient-specific exercises are recommended depending on the muscle assessment.

The puborectalis is responsible for maintaining the anorectal angle and, as such, is an important continence muscle. As part of the levator ani muscle complex, the puborectalis will be recruited during any exercise producing contraction of the pelvic floor muscles (Chapter 8). Resistance can be applied to the puborectalis per rectum and this can be used to facilitate a voluntary contraction and increase muscle strength.

The EAS is in three parts (see Chapter 20) and is generally recruited when the patient is instructed to squeeze the anal muscles as if preventing the escape of flatus. The deep part of the EAS merges with the puborectalis and so these two muscles generally work together. There is evidence that squeeze duration in excess of 20 s is necessary to control faecal urgency due to liquid stool.[35]

Functionally, both puborectalis and the EAS are recruited to control faecal urgency, and patients should practice "hanging on" and deferring defecation during a bowel retraining programme.

21.4.2 Electrical Stimulation

Chapter 12 describes the theory and practice of electrical stimulation in the management of urinary incontinence, and when treating anal incontinence, the same principles apply. However, in order to ensure maximum stimulation of the perianal musculature, an anal electrode should be used (see Fig. 21.3).

In the selection of electrical parameters, it should be remembered that the anal canal is generally more sensitive than the vagina and so caution should be exercised when increasing current intensity.

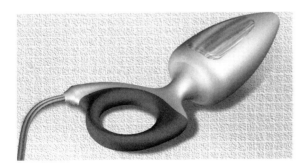

Figure 21.3 Anuform anal electrode (Neen HealthCare, UK for electrical stimulation and EMG biofeedback.

Maximum stimulation at a frequency that produces a comfortable tetanic contraction of the EAS and puborectalis (35–40 Hz), with a non-fatiguing duty cycle, is applied daily (if possible), and the patient instructed to "join in" with the stimulated contraction.

Some small studies have shown a beneficial effect of electrical stimulation used in a hospital setting, or battery-operated units used at home.[36,37]

A further technique has been described by Binnie et al.[38] using the pudendo-anal reflex in the treatment of faecal incontinence due to pudendal nerve damage. A prolonged latency from the stimulus site (mid line at the base of the clitoris) to the anal sphincter, indicates, among other things, the degree of neuropathy. Eight women with incapacitating faecal incontinence and pudendal nerve neuropathy self-administered three 5-min treatments per day for 8 weeks. A submaximal current of 1 Hz and pulse width 0.1 ms was applied through saline-soaked felt electrodes at the base of the clitoris. An immediate effect of stimulation was an increase in anal canal pressures and a significant rise in EAS electromyographic (EMG) activity. At the end of 8 weeks' treatment, an increase in mean resting pressure in the anal canal and increases in reflex and voluntary response to coughing and squeezing actions respectively was demonstrated. The changes led to seven of the eight patients becoming continent.

21.4.3 Biofeedback Training

J.D. Barlow

Biofeedback, in the therapeutic context, is the implementation of a training programme enabling the "feedback" of the biological signal to the patient. In psychological terms this is described as operant conditioning using positive reinforcement of correct behaviour (see also Chapter 10). Functional disorders of the anal sphincter are common, and anal sphincter tone can be poor both at rest, due to problems with the internal anal sphincter (IAS), and during contraction, due to problems with the external anal sphincter (EAS). Several workers have shown that biofeedback generates some degree of symptom relief in adults,[39,40] and improvement in children presenting with congenital disorders has been described.[41,42]

21.4.3.1 Biofeedback Techniques

One of the earlier reported biofeedback training programs utilised the Schuster device,[43] which is a dual-balloon pressure-measuring system housed on a catheter. One balloon is sited within the rectum, the other within the anal canal. As the rectal balloon is inflated, the internal anal sphincter relaxes generating the recto-anal inhibitory reflex (RAIR). As anal pressure drops, resulting from internal sphincter relaxation, the patient is instructed to tighten the voluntary anal muscles.

This type of technique is applicable to patients with loss of co-ordination between rectal sensation and contraction of the external anal sphincter, which generally happens automatically with the "urge" to defecate. It can also be used to re-educate rectal sensation and improve patient awareness of rectal filling. Patients with faecal incontinence, in general, know when they need to squeeze; it is the ability to squeeze strongly, for long enough, that is compromised.

Simple pelvic floor exercises are useful, but patients appear more motivated if they have some form of feedback to inform on correct muscle contraction. Biofeedback in the treatment of patients with faecal incontinence is reviewed by Barlow.[44]

Multiple pressure measurements in the circumferential plane within the anal canal can be used to generate three-dimensional pressure profiles.[45–47] These pressure profiles are markedly more asymmetrical in faecally incontinent patients than in continent patients and controls.[48] This asymmetry may result in reduced sphincteric integrity, despite a mean anal canal pressure falling within the normal range.

Most biofeedback units used in physiotherapy utilise either anal sphincter muscle EMG or anal canal pressure (manometry) to monitor muscle activity during training sessions. At rest, the pressure amplitude is mainly determined by the function of the internal anal sphincter, which is composed of smooth or involuntary muscle. However, during tightening or squeezing of the anal muscles, the augmentation in pressure and EMG activity results from contraction of the external anal sphincter, which is composed of striated or voluntary muscle. The pressure or EMG signal is made visible to the patient and so provides information or feedback of the "correctness" of their responses to contract and relax the voluntary anal musculature. Electrical stimulation and biofeedback using EMG has been used in combination to generate improvement in a patient with imperforate anus.[41]

The main elements to consider prior to commencing the biofeedback training programme include:

- Investigations allowing the correct diagnosis to be made, and an accurate pre-biofeedback evaluation for comparison with the post-biofeedback results, are essential.

- The "trainer" must be able to gain the confidence of the patient and so maintain a high degree of motivation towards the training program.
- Constant reinforcement of the correct responses needs to be made, to ultimately generate a subconscious response to ongoing biological information about rectal sensation and anal canal status and so ensure correct anorectal function.

Enck[49] investigated the long-term efficacy of a biofeedback training program over a 5 year period and showed that improvement could be maintained in the long term. A review of 13 clinical trials of biofeedback for faecal incontinence and 7 trials of biofeedback for constipation demonstrated patient benefit in the majority of cases.[49]

21.4.3.2 Diagnosis

Investigation of patients with faecal incontinence generally shows that they have poor anal sphincter tone on digital examination with low anal canal pressures on manometric assessment. Individual pressure measurements in the circumferential plane often demonstrate significant asymmetry between the measured pressures using the biofeedback catheter shown in Fig. 21.4.

The pressure profile can be displayed as a three-dimensional image illustrating the longitudinal pressure changes along the length of the anal canal and also the circumferential pressure variation. An example of a three-dimensional pressure recording during a continuous pull-through from the rectum to the anal verge in an incontinent patient is shown in Fig. 21.5. Figure 21.5a shows the resting pressure

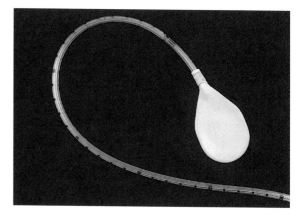

Figure 21.4 Catheter used for biofeedback training illustrating the placement of the eight circumferentially arranged perfusion ports. The catheter used for 3-D pressure images has an identical pressure port configuration but does not have the attached rectal balloon.

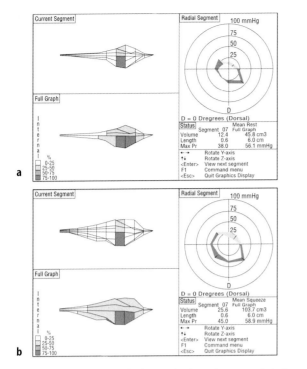

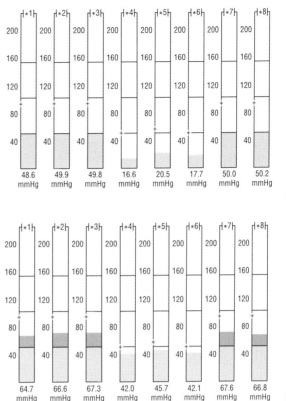

Figure 21.5 Pressure profile from eight channels: **a** at rest; **b** during voluntary contraction.

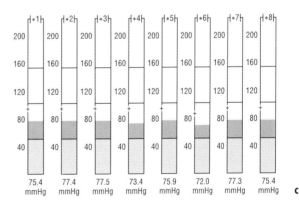

Figure 21.6 Visual display used during the biofeedback training sessions. Each column represents the pressure from one of the pressure ports on the catheter: **a** at rest; **b** during a voluntary contraction. **c** Improvement after biofeedback therapy.

profile and Fig. 21.5b shows the pressure profile while the patient is contracting the anal muscles (squeezing).

A true sphincter injury or division may be suspected during manometry and confirmed on endoanal ultrasound. However, pressure asymmetry in the absence of a defined sphincter defect indicates that sphincter muscle tone is not consistent across the circumferential plane, and this may be a significant factor in the loss of continence in these patients.

21.4.3.3 Training Programme

Training consists of a series of EAS and pelvic floor maximum contractions of increasing duration; the patient is encouraged to maintain a stable contraction during the period of squeezing. The aim of these exercises is to improve the overall strength, endurance and coordination of the continence muscles. Biofeedback training should be aimed at improving not only the squeeze function but also the symmetry of the muscle contraction for improvements in continence to be attained, and for this, three-dimensional imaging is required, as described above.

21.4.3.4 Exercise Regimen

A simple exercise regimen that has been shown to be effective consists of a series of contractions (squeezes), which involve tightening and lifting the muscles around the anal canal. A polyvinyl, multi-lumen catheter with a balloon at the tip for rectal distension is inserted so that the balloon is in the rectum and the eight circumferentialy arranged pressure measuring ports are within the section of the anal canal at which the highest pressure is measured (Fig. 21.4). The patient is instructed to focus on the anal canal and be aware of the muscle around the canal becoming tighter and a feeling of lifting as the pelvic floor contracts, all the time observing the monitor. Attempts to increase both the amplitude and symmetry of their pressures whilst squeezing are encouraged and the patient observes their responses as coloured columns going up and down on the computer screen. The higher the pressure, the higher the column will be. An example of the pressure differences seen in the anterior segment of the anal canal of an incontinent patient at rest is shown in Fig. 21.6a and during a voluntary contraction of EAS (Fig. 21.6b). Each of the eight columns represents the pressure recorded from one of the pressure recording channels. The orientation of each channel within the anal canal is known, and the patient can be specifically instructed to improve their squeeze effort in the particular plane where a pressure deficit is detected. Improvement in the symmetry of the squeeze pressures is shown in Fig.21.6c where all the pressures are equivalent and the pressure anomaly in the anterior plane has been minimised.

Suggested Exercise Sequence   Squeeze held for:

    2 s, repeated 5 times
    5 s, repeated 5 times
    10 s repeated 5 times.

The above sequence may need to be modified in light of the contractility of the EAS. Initially, the squeeze sequence is undertaken with no air in the rectal balloon. The sequence is then repeated with 20, 40 and then 60 ml in the balloon. Over a period of time an improvement in sensory thresholds to rectal distension can be demonstrated. Once the patient has achieved a degree of control over anal sphincter muscle function, a series of 10 1s squeezes can be introduced. This simple exercise protocol is also suitable for using with EMG recording devices although the information about the circumferential variation in muscle tone cannot be determined. The patients would typically attend for five 1h training sessions, during which time discussion would take place about their symptoms and suggestions for the development of coping strategies to help them achieve some degree of bowel control.

References

1. Royal College of Physicians (1995) Incontinence. Causes, management and provision of services. A Working Party of the Royal College of Physicians. J R Coll Physicians Lond 29(4): 272–4.
2. Nelson R, Norton N, Cautley E, Furner S (1995) Community-based prevalence of anal incontinence. JAMA 274(7): 559–61.
3. Drossman DA, Li Z, Andruzzi E et al. (1993) U.S. householder survey of functional gastrointestinal disorders. Dig Dis Sci 38(9): 1569–80.
4. Talley NJ, O'Keefe EA, Zinsmeister AR, Melton LJ (1992) Prevalence of gastrointestinal symptoms in the elderly: a population-based study. Gastroenterology 102: 895–901.
5. Peet SM, Castleden CM, McGrother CW (1995) Prevalence of urinary and faecal incontinence in hospitals and residential and nursing homes for older people [see comments]. BMJ 311(7012): 1063–4.
6. Brocklehurst JC, Dickinson E, Windsor J (1998) Laxatives and faecal incontinence in long term care. Elderly Care 10(4): 22–5.
7. Nakayama H, Jorgensen HS, Pedersen PM, Raaschou HO, Olsen TS (1997) Prevalence and risk factors of incontinence after stroke: The Copenhagen Stroke Study. Stroke 28(1): 58–62.
8. Brocklehurst JC, Andrews K, Richards B, Laycock PJ (1985) Incidence and correlates of incontinence in stroke patients. J Am Geriatr Soc 33: 540–2.
9. Glickman S, Kamm MA (1996) Bowel dysfunction in spinal-cord-injury patients. Lancet 347(9016): 1651–3.
10. Hinds JP, Eidelman BH, Wald A (1990) Prevalence of bowel dysfunction in multiple sclerosis. Gastroenterology 98: 1538–42.
11. Swash M, Snooks SJ, Chalmers DHK (1987) Parity as a factor in incontinence in multiple sclerosis. Arch Neurol 44: 504–8.
12. Jorge JM, Wexner SD (1993) Etiology and management of fecal incontinence. Dis Colon Rectum 36(1): 77–97.
13. Connell AM, Hilton C, Irvine G, Lennard-Jones JE, Misiewicz JJ (1965) Variation in bowel habit in two population samples. Br Med J ii: 1095–9.
14. Heaton KW, Radvan J, Cripps H et al. (1992) Defaecation frequency and timing, and stool form in the general population: a prospective study. Gut 33: 818–24.
15. Whitehead WE, Orr WC, Engel BT, Schuster MM (1981) External anal sphincter response to rectal distension: learned response or reflex. Psychophysiology 19(1): 57–62.
16. Delechenaut P, Leroi AM, Weber J et al. (1992) Relationship between clinical symptoms of anal incontinence and the results of anorectal manometry. Dis Colon Rectum 35: 847–9.
17. Gee AS, Durdey P (1995) Urge incontinence of faeces is a marker of severe external anal sphincter dysfunction. Br J Surg 82(9): 1179–82.
18. Engel AF, Kamm MA, Bartram CI, Nicholls RJ (1995) Relationship of symptoms in faecal incontinence to specific sphincter abnormalities. Int J Colorectal Dis 10: 152–5.
19. Engel AF, Kamm MA, Bartram CI (1995) Unwanted anal penetration as a physical cause of faecal incontinence. Eur J Gastroenterol Hepatol 7: 65–7.
20. van Dam JH, Gosselink MJ, Drogendijk AC, Hop WCJ, Schouten WR (1997) Changes in bowel function after hysterectomy. Dis Colon Rectum 40: 1342–7.
21. Sultan AH, Kamm MA, Hudson CN, Thomas JM, Bartram CI (1993) Anal sphincter disruption during vaginal delivery. N Engl J Med 329: 1905–11.

22. Donnelly VS, O'Herlihy C, Campbell DM, O'Connell PR (1998) Postpartum fecal incontinence is more common in women with irritable bowel syndrome. Dis Colon Rectum 41(5): 586–9.

23. Scott AM, Kellow JE, Eckersley GM, Nolan JM, Jones MP (1992) Cigarette smoking and nicotine delay postprandial mouth-cecum transit time. Dig Dis Sci 37(10): 1544–7.

24. Rausch T, Beglinger C, Alam N, Meier R (1998) Effect of transdermal application of nicotine on colonic transit in healthy nonsmoking volunteers. Neurogastroenterol Mot 10 (3): 263–70.

25. Brown SR, Cann PA, Read NW (1990) Effect of coffee on distal colon function. Gut 31: 450–3.

26. Donnelly V, O'Connell PR, O'Herlihy C (1997) The influence of oestrogen replacement on faecal incontinence in post-menopausal women. Br J Obstet Gynaecol 104: 311–5.

27. Khullar V, Damiano R, Toozs-Hobson P, Cardozo L (1998) Prevalence of faecal incontinence among women with urinary incontinence. Br J Obstet Gynaecol 105: 1211-13.

28. Cukier JM, Cortina-Borja M, Brading AF (1997) A case control study to examine any association between idiopathic detrusor instability and gastrointestinal tract disorder, and between irritable bowel syndrome and urinary tract disorder. Br J Urol 79: 865–78.

29. Wyndaele JJ, Eetvelde B Van (1996) Reproducibility of digital testing of the pelvic floor muscles in men. Arch Phys Med Rehabil 77: 1179–81.

30. Marcello PW, Barrett RC, Coller JA et al. (1998) Fatigue rate index as a new measure of external sphincter function. Dis Colon Rectum 41: 336–43.

31. Frudinger A, Bartram CI, Spencer J, Kamm MA (1997) Perineal examination as a predictor of underlying external anal sphincter damage. Br J Obstet Gynaecol 104: 1009–13.

32. Ardron ME, Main ANH (1990) Management of constipation. Br Med J 300(6736): 1400.

33. Chung BD, Parekh U, Sellin JH (1999) Effect of increased fluid intake on stool output in normal healthy volunteers. J Clin Gastroenterol 28(1): 29–32.

34. Klauser AG, Beck A, Schindlbeck NE (1990) Low fluid intake lowers stool output in healthy male volunteers. Zeitschr Gastroenterol 28: 606–9.

35. Chiarioni G, Scattoloni C, Bonfante F, Vantini I (1993) Liquid stool incontinence with severe urgency: anorectal function and effective biofeedback treatment. Gut 34: 1576–1580.

36. Mills P M, Deakin M Kiff E S (1990) Percutaneous electrical stimulation for ano-rectal incontinence. Physiotherapy 76: 433–8.

37. Pescatori M, Pavesio R, Anastasio G, Daini S (1991) Transanal electrostimulation for faecal incontinence: clinical, psychologic and manometric prospective study. Dis Colon Rectum 34: 540–5.

38. Binnie NR, Kawimbe BM, Papachrysostomou M, Smth AN (1990) Use of the pudendo-anal reflex in the treatment of neurogenic faecal incontinence. Gut 321: 1051–5.

39. Schimbaur W, Barnet J, Wienbeck M (1992) Anal incontinence: evaluation and biofeedback therapy. Mater Med Pol 3(83): 181–4.

40. Chiarioni G, Scattolini C, Bonfante F et al. (1993) Liquid stool incontinence with severe urgency: anorectal function and effective biofeedback therapy. Gut 34: 1576–80.

41. Kirsch SE, Shandling B, Watson SL et al. (1993) Continence following electrical stimulation and EMG biofeedback in a teenager with imperforate anus. J Paediatr Surg 28: 1408–10.

42. Benninga MA, Hoeven CW Van der, Wijers OB et al. (1994) Treatment of faecal incontinence in a child with sacral agenesis: the use of biofeedback training. Dev Med Child Neurol 36: 518–27.

43. Engel BT, Nikoomanesh P, Schuster MM (1974) Operant conditioning of recto-sphincteric responses in the treatment of faecal incontinence. N Engl J Med 290: 646–9.

44. Barlow JD (1997) Biofeedback in the treatment of faecal incontinence. Eur J Gastroenterol Hepatol 9(5): 431–4.

45. Perry RE, Blatchford GL, Christensen MA et al. (1990) Manometric diagnosis of anal sphincter injuries. Am J Surg 159: 112–17.

46. Williamson JL, Nelson RL, Orsay C et al. (1990) A comparison of longitudinal and radial recordings of anal canal pressures. Dis Colon Rectum 33: 201–6.

47. Jorge JMN, Wexford SD (1988) Ano-rectal manometry: techniques and clincial applications. South Med J 86: 924–931.

48. Barlow JD (1994) Biofeedback training for faecal incontinence: functional implications of vector volume analysis. Gut 35 (Suppl)(5): S32.

49. Enck P (1993) Biofeedback training in disordered defecation, a critical review. Dig Dis Sci 39: 1953–1960.

50. Vaizey CJ, Carapetri EA, Cahill JA, Kamm MA (1999) Prospective comparison of faecal incontinence grading systems. GUT 44, 77–80.

22 Constipation

P.E. Chiarelli

22.1 Prevalence of Constipation and Associated Factors

Constipation is a subjective term used to describe difficulty in defecation, either because of the infrequent passage of small hard stools, or because of straining at defecation, or both.[1] In a study of "normality" in bowel function patterns among 789 people not seeking health care, Drossman et al. suggested that constipation might be defined as "straining at stool ≥25 % of the time or passing two or fewer stools per week".[2]

Bowel patterns in individuals change over time, and because prevalence studies have used different definitions of constipation, it is difficult to obtain an accurate estimate of the prevalence of constipation in adult populations. In the United States studies of the self-report of constipation within the last 10 years place the estimation of constipation in population samples in males from 1% to 8%, and in females from 3% to 17%.[3-6] Amongst the elderly population in the USA, the prevalence of constipation using a validated questionnaire was estimated to be about 40%.[7] Australian data suggest that older women report constipation 42% more often than older men.[8]

A large epidemiological study (n = 41,857) allowed for the examination of the prevalence of constipation as well as factors significantly associated with constipation in three age cohorts of Australian women.

- In the *younger cohort (aged 18–22 years)* the prevalence of constipation was estimated to be 14.1%. Parity, haemorrhoids and "other bowel symptoms" were shown to be significantly associated with constipation.
- In the *middle cohort (aged 45–49 years)* prevalence of constipation was estimated to be 26.6%. Haemorrhoids, "other bowel symptoms", going through menopause in the last year, currently taking hormone replacement therapy and having had gynaecological surgery and taking drugs for sleep or for "nerves" were shown to be significantly associated with constipation.
- In the *older cohort* (aged 70–74 years) the prevalence of constipation was estimated to be 27.7%. Haemorrhoids and "other bowel symptoms", having had gynaecological surgery and taking drugs for "sleep" or for "nerves" were shown to be significantly associated with constipation.

Constipation is commonly experienced by women during pregnancy. The overall prevalence during pregnancy is estimated to be about 40%, with 24% of women reporting constipation occasionally, and 16% reporting it often or almost always.[9] Although studies suggest that these disturbances in gastrointestinal motility might be largely attributed to alterations in sex hormones,[10] there are many factors that contribute to constipation during pregnancy.

Constipation is a commonplace symptom, largely self-managed, the impact of which might not be realised by healthcare professionals. Although constipation is not associated with mortality, a significant proportion of women experience it, and the financial costs of its sequelae are great.

22.2 Aetiology and Pathophysiology

Defecation has been succinctly defined as being:

a coordinated process of storage and expulsion of faeces that depends on sensorimotor activity of voluntary and involuntary sphincters. Integration of somatic and autonomic mechanisms, intrinsic gut neural and endocrine systems, cortical and conditioned reflex mechanisms and local and spinal reflex responses are required with voluntary contraction and relaxation of the striated muscles, abdominal wall and respiratory muscles of the diaphragm and rib cage.[11]

Many of the factors identified as being associated with constipation are also associated with dysfunction of the pelvic floor muscles (PFMs). Damage to the PFMs and their innervation, which can occur during childbirth or gynaecological surgery, may contribute to constipation in women.[12–14] Repeated straining at stool is thought to exacerbate the damage, and can result in weakness of the pelvic floor, perineal descent during straining, and secondary anatomical changes. These changes may lead to anorectal dysfunction, difficulties in defecation and, at their worst, faecal incontinence.[12–16] Constant straining at stool has also been implicated in the development of uterovaginal prolapse in the presence of defective uterine supports.[15]

Constipation is a symptom of many diseases and disorders, both physical and psychological. As well as these myriad extracolonic factors, constipation may also have underlying congenital or pharmacological causes.

22.2.1 Functional Constipation

Functional constipation can be divided into constipation caused by colonic inertia (slow transit constipation) or obstructed defecation, which is sometimes referred to as disordered defecation, anismus, paradoxical puborectalis contraction or pelvic outlet obstruction.

22.2.1.1 Slow Transit Constipation

This might be defined as a mechanism of chronic idiopathic constipation in which patients have no organic cause for their symptoms and have delayed transit through the colon and rectum. It is considered to be a neuromuscular disorder, classified as a disorder of the mesenteric plexus. Patients with slow transit constipation have a normal-sized colon.[17] The upper level of normal transit time might be considered to be 72 h.

22.2.1.2 Obstructed Defecation

Obstructed defecation might be defined as having the urge to defecate but being unable to empty the rectum without undue straining. The patients make statements such as "I need to go, but I just can't get it out". A clinical picture such as this might include such syndromes as anterior rectal wall prolapse, intussusception, enteric prolapses, descending perineum (with or without prolapse) and dyssynergia (anismus).

22.2.2 Syndromes Associated with Obstructed Defecation

22.2.2.1 Intussusception

An intussuception is defined as a circular rectal wall infolding of more than 4 mm of the rectal mucosa during straining.[18]

22.2.2.2 Enteric Prolapses

Sigmoidocele and enterocele are prolapses of the colon into the rectovaginal fossa. Rectal prolapse is herniation (procidentia) of the full thickness of the rectum through the anal canal.[18]

22.2.2.3 Anterior Rectal Wall Prolapse (Rectocele)

This is a herniation of the anterior rectal wall through the rectovaginal septum and posterior vaginal wall into the lumen of the vagina. Caused by primary laxity of the rectovaginal septum or by septal damage due to chronic or excessive straining; most are asymptomatic. Women often effect defecation by placing one or two fingers into the vagina during a bowel motion and pressing backward toward the coccyx or by applying firm pressure on the perineum. This has the effect of flattening out the "pouch" of the rectocele, which allows emptying to proceed.

22.2.2.4 Descending Perineum Syndrome

Usually seen only in women, this syndrome is clinically defined as occurring when the plane of the perineum (led by the anal verge) extends beyond the ischial tuberosities during valsalva. Normally, the perineum moves 2–3 cm during a bearing down effort (Valsalva manoeuvre). Sometimes the descended perineum is obvious at rest, patients presenting with the anus sitting in a less defined natal cleft. Pain can be a problematic component of this syndrome. The pain is a poorly localised, deep discomfort brought on by standing for long periods of time and relieved by rest.

The puborectalis muscle plays an important role in supporting the anal sphincter during defecation. It helps to "funnel" the contents as the EAS relaxes and allows for faecal expulsion. When the muscles are overstretched, as in the descending perinum syndrome, this support is lost.

22.2.2.5 Muscle Dyssynergia

The normal co-ordinated action of the muscles of the pelvic floor is often taken for granted. Two types of impaired muscle coordination can affect the act of defecation.

- Some patients contract rather than relax the muscles around the anal canal during expulsive efforts. During a rectal examination, this might be felt as a lack of measurable increase in the anorectal angle (the puborectalis muscle is not felt to relax) or no decrease in anal sphincter tone (the external anal sphincter does not relax) between rest and attempts at expulsion. The anorectal angle at rest is relatively acute. During pelvic floor contraction, this angle should be felt to become more acute, and during attempts at expulsion (simulated defecation), the angle should be felt to widen.
- Some patients are unable to generate an adequate propulsive force within the pelvis.

22.3 Assessment of the Constipated Patient

The comprehensive assessment of a patient complaining of constipation should include a close examination of the symptoms experienced by the patient, examination of the abdomen by palpation and a physical examination of the PFMs and their function. This necessitates a rectal examination, and in women a vaginal examination too. Finally, the patient's straining pattern should be assessed.

Symptoms of constipation often manifest themselves as part of irritable bowel syndrome. It is important that clinicians try to differentiate between slow transit constipation and disordered defecation, while realising that both can be experienced simultaneously.

Clinicians use the term "constipation" to describe infrequent, incomplete, difficult or prolonged evacuation or to describe stools that are too small, too hard or too difficult to pass. Patients, on the other hand, tend to dwell on such symptoms as bloating, abdominal and pelvic pain and nausea. Investigators in the USA have developed a well-validated constipation scoring system (CSS) aimed at obtaining a universally objective definition to assist in the clinical diagnosis and treatment of functionally constipated patients[18] (Table 22.1).

Using the CSS, patients scoring more than 15 (out of a possible 30) are considered to have constipation. Careful evaluation of the pattern of symptoms within the CSS provides information that might allow for clearer differentiation between those

Table 22.1. The constipation scoring system

Symptom	Score
Frequency of bowel movements	
1–2 times per 1–2 days	0
2 times per week	1
Once per week	2
Less than once per week	3
Less than once per month	4
Difficulty: Painful evacuation effort	
Never	0
Rarely	1
Sometimes	2
Usually	3
Always	4
Completeness: Feeling incomplete evacuation	
Never	0
Rarely	1
Sometimes	2
Usually	3
Always	4
Pain: abdominal pain	
Never	0
Rarely	1
Sometimes	2
Usually	3
Always	4
Time: Minutes in lavatory per attempt	
Less than 5	0
5–10	1
10–20	2
20–30	3
More than 30	4
Assistance	
Without assistance	0
Stimulative laxatives	1
Digital assistance or enema	2
Failure: unsuccessful attempts for evacuation per 24 h	
Never	0
1–3	1
3–6	2
6–9	3
More than 9	4
History: duration of constipation (yr)	
0	0
1–5	2
5–10	3
10–20	3
More than 20	4

From Agachan et al.,[18] reprinted with permission from Dr S Wexner.

Table 22.2. Comparison between patient profiles of slow transit constipation and disordered defecation

Constipation group	General comment	Main symptoms	Method used to effect bowel emptying
Slow transit constipation	Predominantly female Many failed treatments	Abdominal pain and bloating No spontaneous bowel movements	Best results with laxatives
Disordered defecation		Feelings of incomplete emptying Often requires digitation	Best results with enemas, suppositories and digitation

Table adapted from studies by Pemberton and Agachan.[18]

patients with slow transit constipation and those experiencing disordered defecation (Table 22.2).

In the present climate of evidence-based practice, the quantitative assessment of patients' symptoms using the CSS allows for valid outcome measurement as well as providing positive input to act as motivation for the patient during what can sometimes be a rather prolonged treatment program.

22.3.1 Physical Assessment of the Constipated Patient

A clear understanding of the normal sequence of events that occur during defecation, together with the clinical significance of dysfunction within any part of the sequence, is essential in the assessment

Table 22.3. Outline of the physical assessment of the constipated woman

Assessment	At rest	During a contraction	During straining
Perineum (visually)	Visible prolapses Scarring or deformity of perineal body Lax introitus Perineal descent	Inward movement Inappropriate accessory muscle action	Pelvic organ prolapse through the vaginal introitus Perineal descent >2–3 cm
Anus (visually)	Observe skin condition and presence of haemorrhoids, skin tags, a sentinel pile Patulous (loose)	Visible contraction around the full circumference. Inward movement and puckering	Descending perineum syndrome
Vagina (digitally)	Resting tone of the muscle Areas of tenderness Volume Pelvic organ prolapses	PERFECT assessment with suggested modifications (see text)	Descensus of pelvic organ prolapses especially rectocele
Anorectum (digitally)	Pull the anus apart gently at the 9 o'clock and 3 o'clock positions to see if it gapes at rest Constant resistance during finger insertion, gradually relaxing. Palpate circumferentially for areas of thinning or absent tissues Anorectal angle should be acute Faecal bolus present? Feel puborectalis as a sling posteriorly Sweep across the bodies of puborectalis, pubococcygeus and iliococcygeus	Muscle deficiencies in EAS usually on anterior wall. Use a sweeping motion with the examining finger and check for areas of atrophy, hypertrophy, unilateral or bilateral elevation Assess proprioception	Ano rectal angle should open and become more obtuse. Puborectalis and EAS should be felt to relax

Table 22.4. Assessment of the defecation pattern

Patient's body	Correct response	Incorrect response
Position		
Arms	Forearms resting on the thighs	Any other position
Legs	Hips at more than 90°, heels raised	Hips at <90°, feet not touching the floor or flat on the floor
Spine	Forward lean with a normal spinal curve	Posterior pelvic tilt, slumping
Muscle actions		
At the waist	The waist widens	No change or the waist narrows
Lower abdomen	The stomach bulges	No change or is pulled inward
Anus	Opens	Tightens, moves up or closes
Breathing		
	Deep, basal, diaphragmatic Intercostal angle increases Breath held with diaphragm held down low	No basal expansion Diaphragm held high

and management of disordered defecation, and is presented here in table form (Table 22.3).

A full physical examination of patients complaining of constipation should include a visual assessment of the perineum and the anus at rest, during contraction and during a Valsalva manoeuvre. Following this, a digital assessment of the vagina and the anorectum and PFM function (at rest during contraction and during straining) should be carried out (Table 22.4).

Explicit details of visual and digital examination and assessment of both the perineum and PFM function have been presented earlier (see Chapter 6.)

22.3.2 Vaginal Assessment of the Pelvic Floor Muscles

PFM function should be tested and the results transcribed following Laycock's PERFECT model (see Chapter 6.7). Additions to this acronym in the management of constipation and prolapse are suggested as follows:

P = power
E = endurance
R = repetitions
F = fast twitch
E = elevation
C = cough response
T = transcribe it all

22.3.3 Assessment of Pelvic Floor Elevation

During a vaginal examination, the woman is asked to contract the PFMs as the examining finger exerts a downward pressure on each side of the levators in turn. Elevation of the muscle can be palpated directly and differences between right and left should be noted. In this way, proprioception can also be assessed.

22.3.4 Anorectal Assessment

A full explanation of why the examination is being carried out should be given at every stage throughout the procedure. A warning should be given that the patient might feel as though she might lose control of her bowels. She should be reassured that this is a normal response and that any "accidents" are highly unlikely to happen.

The woman should be asked to remove any tampons that might be in place. It is recommended that the patient should be placed in side lying with a pillow supporting the upper thigh, and a towel draped over the buttocks to provide a sense of modesty.

A clean glove should be used if a vaginal examination has preceded the rectal examination, and plenty of lubricating gel should be applied to the

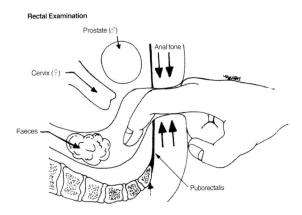

Figure 22.1 Rectal examination.

gloved index finger. The patient should be told when the rectal examination is about to begin, and she should be reassured that no instruments will be used during the examination. The examiner should anticipate the patient's apprehension while placing the index finger flat over the anal sphincter. Gentle pressure is applied on the posterior anal verge until the sphincter yields and the *relaxed* finger glides gently into the anus, the finger tip aiming forwards initially and then in the direction of the coccyx. It is sometimes helpful to ask the patient to bear down to facilitate relaxation of EAS. If resistance is still felt, ask the woman to gently bulge the lower part of her stomach, that part just above her pubic hair line. The relaxed finger should slide gently in past the anal sphincter and will naturally come to rest upon the anorectal angle with the tip of the finger pointing toward the coccyx (see Fig. 22.1). The rectal contents and mucosa within easy reach of the finger are palpated. The prostate or the cervix can be palpated along with any prolapses of the anterior rectal wall. Assessment of the anorectum should follow as described in Table 22.3.

The patient is asked to squeeze up and hold. Anal sphincter contraction is noted. The examining finger can be swept across the right and left levators from anterior to posterior to feel for muscular deficiencies in puborectalis. The patient's proprioception can be assessed by gently applying downward pressure on the levators on each side and asking the patient to describe what they can feel. In constipated patients, there may be little sensation in the presence of overstretched muscles, especially in cases where descending perineum syndrome is evident.

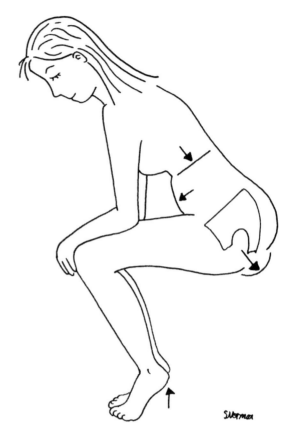

Figure 22.2   The body position and functional pattern for effective defecation.

22.3.5 Assessment of Defecation Pattern

For this assessment, the woman should sit, clothed, on a firm chair without any back support. She is then asked to adopt her usual defecation position. The therapist places one hand upon the woman's lateral abdominal wall at waist level while the other hand is placed suprapubically over the lower abdomen. The woman is asked to simulate defecation and inappropriate responses are noted. This pattern is then corrected, if necessary, according to the guidelines in Fig. 22.2 and Table 22.4.

After the examinations and assessments, the woman should be given a very clear understanding of the findings and exactly how these might impact upon her presenting complaint. Any pre-existing knowledge that the woman has of the condition should be explored, so that any incorrect ideas can be contradicted. This information is best given using anatomical models, diagrams and line drawings.

22.4 Treatment Programmes for the Patient with Constipation

Dietary advice and advice regarding fluid intake are routinely given to patients complaining of constipation (see Chapter 21). PFM rehabilitation will be necessary where muscle weakness, imbalance or lack of co-ordination have been found, and should be directed at the specific area of deficiency. In cases where incorrect defecation patterns have been detected, these patterns will require retraining.

22.4.1 Pelvic Floor Muscle Rehabilitation

Various methods for PFM rehabilitation have been addressed comprehensively in Chapters 8–12.

Many studies have shown that the response to isometric resistance training is very specific to the exercise both in terms of the muscle itself, the muscle length in isometric exercise, the speed of the contractions and the postural specificity of the exercise.[19,20] It has also been suggested that, rather than using conventional exercises to strengthen individual muscle groups, it might be more effective to identify particular functional deficits and then repeatedly practice these, with or without added resistance.[19] There seems little point in restoring muscle strength if this cannot be appropriately utilised in activities of daily life. It is not yet certain whether strength training provided soon after a period of disuse in the form of voluntary muscle contractions can induce a faster or a more complete recovery of muscle strength than that provided by the correct performance of everyday activities alone.[19]

Since the transversus abdominis (TrA) plays an important role in the development of intraabdominal pressure (IAP) as well as enhancing PFM contractions,[20] careful attention should be paid to the co-contraction of TrA during pelvic floor contractions. This is effected by asking the woman to pull in her tummy at the level of her bikini line as she performs any PFM contractions.

22.4.2 Improving Perineal Elevation

Following the assessment of perineal elevation as described earlier, the woman can be encouraged to use the concept of lift during PFM contractions. This can be done using a hand mirror to watch her own perineal elevation during an "un-braced" and then a "braced" cough. Since studies show the urethral and anal sphincters both work maximally during a cough,[20] it seems rational to use this as part of any strengthening program.

22.4.3 Retraining Altered Defecation Patterns

Specialised centres offer biofeedback training for functional constipation using either manometric or electromyographic instrumentation. Many authors have reported good results from biofeedback training programmes[17,21] used in constipation with various functional causes.[22,23] Other studies have favorably compared the outcome of muscle training with and without the aid of biofeedback.[24] Retraining of dysfunctional straining patterns should be specifically directed to individual areas of dysfunction in each woman (see Table 22.4). In retraining patients with disordered defecation, the aim is to increase IAP without increasing the anal sphincter pressure.[20]

- *Correct position:* this should be enhanced by the use of a small stool under the feet.
- *Lower abdominal bulging:* This is taught by asking the woman to relax her tummy and let it bulge out in front. It should be allowed to "fall into her hands". In this position, the lower abdomen should be made to "harden", i.e. the rectus abdominus is contracted in its outer range to increase IAP. TrA is activated to increase IAP as well.
- *Anal sphincter opening:* Relaxation can only be taught following contraction. This can be facilitated using EMG biofeedback or the use of a simple hand mirror, as described above.

When each of the component parts has been mastered, the pattern can be practised as a whole. Thereafter this sequence should be used only on the toilet.

Relaxation of the internal anal sphincter (IAS), the external anal sphincter (EAS) and puborectalis is facilitated by the squatting position and by increased IAP which accompanies straining. An increase in IAP during heavy lifting does not normally produce the same response. In short, during sudden rises in IAP as in coughing, EAS activity is enhanced whereas during defecation EAS is normally inhibited. This activity is mediated by stretch receptors in the PFMs and defecation reflexes. There is a functional interrelationship between the visceral and somatic elements of the sphincter mechanism, but these are not clearly understood.

22.4.4 During Pregnancy

Antenatal education should include information about the impact of constipation on women's health as well as pointing out the causative factors of constipation during pregnancy.

These factors include:[25]

- Stool dehydration resulting from decreased fluid intake which is secondary to nausea, vomiting and peripheral oedema.
- Changes in dietary patterns together with iron supplements.
- Psychological problems.
- Delayed colonic transit: this can be the result of hormonal changes, which include increases in plasma progesterone levels and decreased levels of oestrogen and motilin.
- Pseudo-obstruction: outlet obstruction caused by hemorrhoids, anal fissures, increased pressure arising from the gravid uterus and adhesions from previous deliveries.

22.4.5 Postpartum Period

Focus groups held amongst postpartum women revealed that women do not seek help for constipation from healthcare professionals but feel confident with self-management of their symptoms.[26]

The postpartum continence promotion programme designed using a customer focus includes descent-minimising techniques such as perineal support during defecation, information about the long-term consequences of constipation and checking the straining patterns of women who admit constipation. Information about the importance of diet and fluid intake is given, with special reference to the increased fluid requirements when breastfeeding. PFM integrity underpins the information about the development of good bowel habits in the postpartum. Since women profess confidence in their own management of constipation, the postpartum offers a unique opportunity to give out this valuable information.[26]

22.4.6 Postoperative Urogenital Surgery

In view of the significant association between constipation and urogenital surgery, it seems rational to propose that women routinely be given instructions about avoiding constipation. These might include instruction in correct straining patterns for defecation along with functional PFM exercises and information about pain relief medication, diet and fluid intake before discharge from hospital.

22.4.7 Constipation in Elderly People

The prevalence of constipation is much higher in elderly people than in the rest of the population. Decreases in levels of mobility, concomitant medical conditions and polypharmacy all contribute to this.

22.4.8 In Conclusion

The continence therapist is in a unique position to treat constipation in patients who are suffering its consequences, as well as in patients who do not perceive constipation as a threat to their health or wellbeing. The promotion of good bowel habits should be seen as an important contribution to a holistic approach to the management of patients who are experiencing any form of pelvic floor dysfunction. The assessment and treatment protocols offered here might provide a broader base for primary healthcare professionals of all persuasions, in order that they might make use of every opportunity for the promotion of good bowel health and pelvic floor integrity.

22.5 Abdominal Massage

J. Laycock

Abdominal massage in the management of constipation can be a self-treatment technique or may be carried out by a trained physiotherapist or nurse. The technique can also be taught to carers. It can be especially useful for mothers dealing with babies and children with constipation.

The use of abdominal massage to improve colonic motility[27] has been shown to increase peristalsis and relieve flatulence and have positive psychological effects.[28] The technique involves alternate effleurage and kneading along the line of the colon (Fig. 22.3) using slow, deep movements.[29] Kneading and self-kneading, may be done using the knuckles (all fingers fully flexed).

The depth of massage may be limited by abdominal pain in some patients, so more superficial massage should be carried out initially.

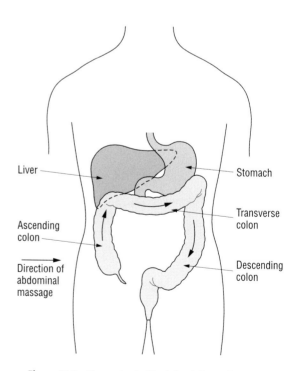

Figure 22.3   The anatomical basis for abdominal massage.

A further self-treatment technique used in some spinal injury units employs a small ball (e.g. a tennis ball); the ball is rolled up the ascending colon, across the transverse colon and down the descending colon.[30]

When applying abdominal massage, the patient should be comfortable and in a warm environment, and the procedure explained; the massage, which generally takes 10–20 min,[27] is more comfortable if oil is used. However, many patients find it more convenient to self-massage over their clothes, in a sitting position.

A study comparing massage and laxative therapy on the colonic motility of profoundly disabled people[27] showed no statistical difference in treatment outcomes, which included transit times, stool frequency, stool size and consistency, and the requirement for enemas. However, the population had grossly abnormal colonic transit times and defecation problems, and so these results are not transferable to all patients presenting with constipation. However, within the limitations of this study it is interesting to note that abdominal massage proved to be as effective as laxative therapy for this profoundly disabled patient group.

General activity, especially bending and stretching, can have a "massage-like" effect on the small and large bowel, and should be encouraged as much as possible. Furthermore, deep breathing, either taught specially or as a result of exercise, may also help to stimulate activity in the gastrointestinal tract.

Abdominal massage should always be used in combination with exercise, dietary and fluid regulation, and laxatives if required, with attention to concomitant medication which may be exacerbating the problem. Further research is needed to identify the effectiveness and appropriateness of this modality in the management of constipation.

22.6 Laxatives

J. Laycock

If constipation is due to an impacted rectum, the preferred treatment is to empty the rectum from below by administering an enema each day until the faecal mass is cleared. Failing this, manual evacuation may be required,[31] although the use of this technique is controversial. If slow transit constipation is the cause, a number of laxatives are available.

The Oxford dictionary describes "laxative" as "tending to stimulate or facilitate evacuation of the bowels"; from Latin laxare 'loosen'". "Purgative" and "cathartic" are alternative terms used to describe medication to stimulate or increase the frequency of bowel evacuation, or to encourage a softer or bulkier stool.

Clearly, many foods can be classified as having a "natural laxative effect", and these should always be considered as part of the overall management of the constipated patient. In particular, foods high in fibre taken with plenty of fluids are recommended. Fibre, non-starch polysaccharides (NSP), is the indigestible part of vegetable foods. Insoluble fibre tends to bind with water and increase the bulk of the stool, which, in turn, stretches the walls of the colon and stimulates peristalsis.[32] The main sources are wheat and corn bran and oat hull. Soluble fibre, found in fruit, vegetables and pulses, is fermented by anaerobic flora in the large bowel with the release of SCFA (short chain fatty acids), carbon dioxide, hydrogen and occasionally methane. SCFA increases the bacteria in the stool (bacteria are 80% water).

However, it is not always advisable to recommend increased dietary fibre as routine for constipated elderly patients as it may cause colonic faecal loading and may add to the constipation that already exists; it may also increase their risk of faecal incontinence.[33]

Prescribed laxatives come in a variety of types depending on their perceived action; they include bulk-forming laxatives, faecal softeners, osmotic laxatives, stimulant laxatives, suppositories and enemas. Many laxative policies generally recommend starting with bulk-forming additives and then progress to stimulant and osmotic preparations if needed.

22.6.1 Bulking Agents

These laxatives consist of plant fibre, e.g. bran or ispaghula, or synthetic alternatives, e.g methylcellulose. Isphaghula husk (Fybogel) or methylcellulose tablets (Celevac) can be taken daily or twice daily, with at least 300 ml of water.

22.6.2 Faecal Softeners

These products ease straining by softening the stool. Liquid paraffin and castor oil have been used in the past but are less popular now because of reported harmful side-effects, including interference with digestion and possible harm to the lungs if inhaled. Each works by stimulating the small bowel, leading to complete bowel clearance,[34] and lubricating the passage of faeces.[35] Docusate sodium acts by lowering the surface tension of faeces, allowing the penetration of water.[31]

22.6.3 Osmotic Laxatives

Whether taken orally or rectally, osmotic laxatives draw fluid into the bowel and so ease the constipation; they should always be taken with plenty of water, as directed by the manufacturer. *Magnesium salts* have an additional effect of stimulating intestinal motility by releasing cholecystokinin.

Lactulose has a microbial and pH effect as well as an osmotic action that increases stool output.[35] Lactulose is metabolised by the colonic bacterial flora to produce SCFA (see above), and its laxative effect may be associated with abdominal pain, bloating and flatus.[36]

Polyethylene glycol (PEG; Movicol) is a mixture of non-absorbable, non-metabolised polymers of high molecular weight that acts as a pure osmotic agent, and is active without increased colonic gas production.[36] Movicol rapidly cleanses the bowel before radiography or colonoscopy and can be used for chronic constipation and faecal impaction.[35]

A multicentre randomised comparative trial of low-dose polyethylene glycol with lactulose for treatment of chronic constipation (n = 115) showed that low-dose PEG (Movicol) was more effective than lactulose and better tolerated. Stool frequency was higher and the median daily score for straining at stool was lower in the Movicol group. Furthermore, the percentage of patients who used suppositories or microenemas was significantly lower in the Movicol group.[36]

22.6.4 Stimulant Laxatives

For patients with a soft or formed stool, stimulant laxatives are required.[31] Stimulant laxatives increase colonic motility and may cause colicky pain; in the long term continued use may cause hypokalaemia or "cathartic colon".[35] Stimulant laxatives should only be taken on specific occasions and avoided in children or pregnancy[35]. *Senna* (Senokot) is an anthracine laxative which is hydrolysed by bacteria in the colon. Its derivatives are absorbed in the colon and stimulate the myenteric plexus, increasing peristaltic activity. Stimulant laxatives are used for bowel clearance before surgery or bowel investigations, or to initiate therapy in severe constipation; they can be administered orally or rectally. Stimulant laxatives should be used for short periods only, as they may cause bowel habituation and adverse effects if used regularly over several months.

22.6.5 Suppositories and Enemas

Of the rectally administered laxatives, the disposable small-volume enemas are the most convenient. *Phosphate enemas* are the most commonly used. They contain 10% sodium acid phosphate and 8% sodium phosphate in a total volume of 128 ml. Sodium acid phosphate is poorly absorbed from the rectum; its osmotic activity increases the water content of the stool, and rectal distension induces defecation by stimulating rectal motility.[31] For patients who cannot retain a phosphate enema, a microenema or suppository should be used. For lesser problems, or in combination with an oral laxative, *glycerine* or *bisacodyl* suppositories may be effective.

Several preparations are available which combine one or two of the above-mentioned drugs. For example, *Manevac* is a mixture of ispaghula and senna, and *Codalax*, containing poloxamer 188 and danthron, is a faecal softener and stimulant. Individual constipated patients respond differently to laxatives and many may need a "cocktail" to ensure regular bowel evacuation.

References

1. Moore-Gillon V. (1984) Constipation: what does the patient mean? Journal of the Royal Society of Medicine. 77: 108–110.
2. Drossman D, Sandler R, McKee D, Lovitz A. (1982) Bowel patterns among subjects not seeking healthcare. Gastroenterology, 83: 529–534.
3. Everhart JE, Go VLW, Johannes RS, Fitzsimmons SC,Roth HP, White LR. (1989) A longitudinal survey of self-reported bowel habits in the United States. Dig Dis Sci. 34: 1143–1162.
4. Sonnenberg A, Koch T. (1989) Epidemiology of constipation in the United States Dis Colon Rectum. 32: 1–8.
5. Sandler RS, Jordan MC,Shelton BJ. (1990) Demographic and dietary determinants of constipation in the US population. Am J Public Health . 80: 185–189.
6. Talley NJ, Weaver AL, Zinsmeister AR, Melton JL. (1993) Functional Constipation and outlet delay: a population-based study. Gastroenterol. 105: 781–790.
7. Talley NJ, Fleming KC, Evans JM, O'Keefe EA, Weaver AL, Zinsmeister AR et al., (1996) Constipation in an elderly community: a study of prevalence and potential risk factors. Am J Gastroenterol. 91(1): 19–25.
8. Mathers C. Health differentials between Australian males and females: a statistical profile. 1994, Australian Institute of Health and Welfare: Canberra.
9. Marshall K, Toterdal D, McConnell V, Walsh D, Whelan M. (1996) Urinary incontinence and constipation during pregnancy and after childbirth. Physiotherapy. 82(2): 98–103.
10. Baron T, Ramirez B, Richter JE. (1993) Gastrointestinal motility disorders during pregnancy. Ann Int Med. 118: 366–375.

11. Uher E, Swash M. (1998) Sacral Reflexes. Physiology and Clinical Application. Dis Col Rectum . 41: 1165–1177.

12. Snooks SJ, Barnes PRH, Swash M, Henry MM. (1985a) Damage to the pelvic floor musculature in chronic constipation. Gastroenterology. 89: 977–981.

13. Swash M, The neurogenic hypothesis of stress incontinence, in Neurobiology of Incontinence. Ciba Foundation Symposium 151, G. Bock and J. Whelan, Editors. 1990, John Wiley and Sons: Chichester.

14. Taylor T, Smith A. Fulton P. (1989) Effect of hysterectomy on bowel function. BMJ. 299: 300–301.

15. Spence-Jones C, Kamm M, Henry M, Hudson CN. (1994) Bowel dysfunction: A pathogenic factor in utero-vaginal prolapse and urinary stress incontinence. Br J Obstet Gynaecol. 101: 147–152.

16. Henry MM, Parks AG, Swash M. (1982) The pelvic floor musculature in the descending perineum syndrome. Br J Surg. 69: 470–472.

17. Mollen R, Claasen A, Kuijpers J. (1997) The evaluation and treatment of functional constipation. Scand J Gastroenterol. 32 Suppl 223: 8–17.

18. Agachan F, Chen T, Pfeifer J, Reissman P, Wexner S. (1996) A constipation scoring system to simplify evaluation and management of constipated patients. Dis Col Rectum . 39: 681–685.

19. Herbert R, ed. Human strength adaptations – implications for therapy. Key Issues in Musculoskeletal Physiotherapy, ed. J.A.M. Crosbie, J. 1993, Butterworth Heinemann: London.

20. Markwell S, Sapsford R, Physiotherapy Management of Pelvic Floor Dysfunction, in Women's Health . A Textbook for physiotherapists., R. Sapsford, J. Bullock-Saxton, and S. Markwell, Editors. 1998, WB Saunders Company Limited: London. 383–411.

21. Basmajian, Muscles Alive. Their functions revealed by electromyography . 3rd ed. 1974, Baltimore: Williams and Wilkins.

22. Fleshman J, Dreznik Z, Meyer K, Carney R, Kodner I. (1992) Outpatient protocol for biofeedback therapy of pelvic floor outlet obstruction. Dis Col Rectum . 35: 1–7.

23. Karlbom U, Hallden M, Eeg-Oloffsen K, Pahlman L, Graf W. (1997) Results of biofeedback in constipated patients. Dis Col Rectum . 40: 1149–1155.

24. Koutsomanis D, Lennard-Jones J, Roy A, Kamm M. (1995) Controlled randomised trial of visual feedback versus muscle training without visual display for intractable constipation. Gut. 37: 95–99.

25. Cappell M, ed. Pregnancy and Gastrointestinal Disorders . Gastroenterology Clinics of North America, ed. H. Cullen. Vol. 27. 1998, WB Saunders: Philadelphia. 197–211.

26. Chiarelli P, Cockburn J. (1999) The development of a physiotherapy continence promotion program using a customer focus. Aust J Physiother. 45(2): 111–120.

27. Emly M, Cooper S and Vail A (1998) Colonic motility in profoundly disabled people. A comparison of massage and laxative therapy in the management of constipation. Physiotherapy. 84: 4: 178–183.

28. Beard G and Wood E C (1964) Massage: principles and techniques. Saunders, Philadelphia.

29. Emly M (1993) Abdominal massage. Nursing Times: 89: 34–36.

30. Richards A (1998) Hands on help. Nursing Times. 94: 69–72.

31. Barrett J A (1992) Faecal incontinence. In (Ed) B Roe. Clinical Nursing Practice. Prentice Hall, London. 208–211.

32. Chiarelli P and Markwell S (1992) Let's Get Things Moving. ISBN 1 875531 23 8. 32–37.

33. Ardron M E and Main A N H (1990) Management of Constipation. British Medical Journal. 300; 1400.

34. Irvine L (1996) Faecal Incontinence. In (Ed) C Norton. Nursing for Continence. Beaconsfield, UK.246–248.

35. MIMS (Monthly Index of Medical Specialities) (1998) 22–25.

36. Attar A, Lemann M, Ferguson A et al (1999) Comparison of low dose polyethylene glycol electrolyte solution with lactulose for treatment of chronic constipation. GUT. 44: 226–230.

IV Pelvic Pain

23 Prevalence of Pelvic Pain

B. Shelly, S. Knight, P. King, G. Wetzler, K. Wallace, D. Hartman and G.C. Gorniak

23.1 Definition and Management

Pelvic pain is a poorly defined condition, which often becomes chronic in nature. It is difficult to

Table 23.1. Terminology associated with hypertonus of the pelvic floor[11]

Condition	Signs and symptoms
Levator ani syndrome[11,12] Pelvic floor tension myalgia[13]	Poorly localized pain in the perivaginal, perirectal, suprapubic or coccyx regions, possibly down the posterior thigh. PFM spasm
Non-relaxing puborectalis, puborectalis syndrome[14] Paradoxical puborectalis contraction (PPC)[15]	Bowel movement dysfunction, constipation
Proctalgia fugax[16]	Sharp fleeting rectal pain (seconds to 20–30 min)
Coccygodynia[17,18]	Coccygeal pain and tenderness noted primarily when seated
Vaginismus[10]	Spasm or active holding of introital muscles, dyspareunia
Urethral syndrome[19,20]	Urinary urgency, frequency and suprapubic pelvic or perineal pressure. Urethral pain, burning or sensitivity. Pain after volding
Chronic pelvic pain (CPP)	Pelvic pain of 6 months or more duration with an episode of pain occurring in the past 3 months
Vulvodynia[21]	Chronic genital burning, pain and rawness
Pudendal neuralgia[22]	Constant localized burning, itching sensations

diagnose, and may have a multifactorial origin.[1] It may be divided into several categories, including chronic pelvic pain (CPP) with a musculoskeletal component, specific pelvic floor pain syndromes and vulvodynia (see Table 23.1).

The nature and severity of the pain may bear little or no relationship to the actual physical findings. In many cases extensive investigation still reveals no obvious pathology.[2] Lack of a specific diagnosis and continuation of symptoms has a severe effect on the quality of life for the sufferer; many women with CPP show evidence of mental distress and depressive illnesses. Pelvic pain is often defined as being non-cyclical.[2] However, many sufferers report concurrent symptoms of dyspareunia and dysmenorrhea which may affect the overall pain process. Irritable bowel syndrome and endometriosis may also give rise to pain patterns similar to those found in pelvic pain syndromes, and may coexist with pain of musculoskeletal origin, giving a complicated presentation.

Management of CPP is variable. Patients may be referred to gynaecologists, urologists, colorectal specialists, pain specialists, undergo multiple tests and invasive procedures only to be told "nothing is wrong". Others may be given a specific medical diagnosis, or clustered into "syndromes". The musculoskeletal system is rarely considered during medical evaluation of pelvic pain. A significant amount of literature exists to support the role of the physiotherapists on the CCP team.

23.2 Prevalence

Because of inconsistency in definitions and differential diagnoses the prevalence of pelvic pain is not clearly known, and available data are few and confusing. A recent meta-analysis of published data on pelvic pain[3] found only one community-based population study before 1998, conducted in the USA.[4] Other types of pelvic pain have been studied in the general population, but definitions are inconsistent, and as conditions may coexist and produce similar symptoms, estimated prevalence may not provide a clear picture. There have been several community-based studies reporting a prevalence for both abdominal pain and irritable bowel syndrome, but the definitions used are not specific enough to isolate CPP as a distinct category. As with other pain syndromes, the focus is currently placed on quality of life issues. There is a need for continued study of the effect of CPP on the patient's general health and well-being and the cost to healthcare resources.

A community-based study by a telephone survey in the US reported prevalence for CPP of 15%, in 5263 women aged 18–50 years.[4] The study group consisted of women with a history of pelvic pain of 6 months or longer, unrelated to the menstrual cycle, with an episode occurring in the past 3 months. A similar definition was used in a clinic-based study[5] and a prevalence of 14% was reported. A questionnaire survey to determine the prevalence of dysmenorrhea, dyspareunia, pelvic pain and irritable bowel syndrome was performed in obstetric and gynaecologic clinics in the USA.[6] The prevalence of pelvic pain was reported as 39% (n = 581). However, the definition of CPP was at variance with the previously mentioned studies, and although a group of non-patients completed the questionnaire, the results of patients attending the clinic for treatment and the non-patients were all included together for analysis. An extensive community based study in the UK[7] reports a CPP prevalence of 21 in 1000, slightly less than asthma (37 in 1000).

In the one community-based study in the USA,[4] 61% of the CPP group (n = 773) had pain of unknown aetiology. Those with a definite diagnosis had a variety of conditions, including endometriosis, pelvic inflammatory disease and irritable bowel syndrome. Musculoskeletal problems were not cited amongst the diagnostic findings. The study focused on quality of life and cost issues. The total annual direct costs in the USA were estimated to be $2.8 billion dollars. Respondents had significantly lower general health scores and higher scores for depression and other quality of life measures. Those with a definite diagnosis visited a physician or other healthcare professional more frequently than patients with pelvic pain of undiagnosed origin. Eighty-two (15%) of women in full or part-time employment (n = 548) reported one or more lost work hours per month because of pelvic pain. Single women are less likely to report pelvic pain. This finding was substantiated in a recent UK study.[8] A controlled questionnaire study of demographic and other variables was administered to women with idiopathic pelvic pain of at least 6 months duration[2]. In this study the CCP group took three times more prescription medications than the pain-free control group. Additionally, the total number of minor and major surgical procedures performed on the study group was significantly higher, indicating a large financial cost to healthcare resources.

Women with CPP tend to have a higher lifetime prevalence of sexual abuse.[9] Reiter found 48% of women with pelvic pain reported molestation, incest or rape, as opposed to 6% in the control group.[2] Collett[8] also compared women with CPP, pain not related to the pelvic area and a pain-free control group. The CPP group had a significantly higher history of sexual abuse than the comparison pain group or the control group. Interestingly, these patients had also consulted their general practitioner with other symptoms more frequently than either of the comparison groups.

In a review of the literature on the prevalence of sexual dysfunction, vaginismus and dyspareunia have been the subject of many studies.[10] There are no data for the prevalence of vaginismus in the general population, but estimates range from 5.1% to 17% in women attending sexual dysfunction clinics.[11,12] The prevalence of dyspareunia ranges from 3% to 5.1% in clinical settings, compared to prevalence rates from 8% to 23% in community-based studies.[10] No published studies have been found to estimate the prevalence of other discreet categories of pelvic pain. There is a need for continued community-based studies to include a variety of clearly defined pelvic pain syndromes.

References

1. Steege JF (1998) Scope of the problem. In: Steege JF, Metzger DA, Levy BS (eds) Chronic Pelvic Pain An integrated approach. WB Saunders, Philadelphia, pp. 1–4.
2. Reiter RC, Gambone JC (1990) Demographic and historic variables in women with idiopathic chronic pelvic pain. Obstet Gynecol 75(3): 428–32.
3. Zondervan KT, Yudkin PL, Vesey MP et al. (1998) The prevalence of chronic pelvic pain in women in the United Kingdom: a systematic review. Br J Obstet Gynaecol 105: 93–9.
4. Mathias SD, Kupperman M, Liberman RF et al. (1996) Chronic pelvic pain: prevalence, health-related quality of life, and economic correlates. Obstet Gynecol 87(3): 321–7.
5. Walker EA, Katon WJ, Jemelka R et al. (1991) The prevalence of chronic pelvic pain and irritable bowel syndrome in two university clinics. J Psychosom Obstet Gynecol 12 (Suppl): 65–75.
6. Jamieson DJ, Steege JF (1996) The prevalence of dysmenorrhea, dyspareunia, pelvic pain and irritable bowel syndrome in primary care practices. Obstet Gynecol 87(1): 55–8.

7. Zondervan KT, Yudkin PL, Vessey MP et al. (1999) Prevalence and incidence of chronic pelvic pain in primary care: evidence from a national general practice database. Brit J Obstet Gynaecol 106(11): 1149–55.

8. Collett BJ, Cordle CJ, Stewart CR, Jagger C (1998) A comparative study of women with chronic pelvic pain, chronic nonpelvic pain and those with no history of pain attending general practitioners. Br J Obstet Gynaecol 105: 87–92.

9. Walling MK, Reiter RC, O'Hara MW et al. (1994) Abuse history and chronic pain in women: 1. Prevalences of sex abuse and physical abuse. Obstet Gynecol 84(2): 193–9.

10. Spector IP, Carey MP (1990) Incidence and prevalence of the sexual dysfunctions: a critical review of the empiric literature. Arch Sex Behav 19(4): 389–408.

11. Wallace K (1997) Hypertonus dysfunctions. In: Wilder E (ed) The Gynecological Manual. Section on Women's Health, American Physical Therapy Association, Alexandria, pp. 127–40.

12. Salvati E (1987) The levator syndrome and its variants. Gastroenterol Clin N Am 16: 71–78.

13. Sinaki M, Merrit J, Stillwell GK (1977) Tension myalgia of the pelvic floor. Mayo Clin Proc 52: 717–22.

14. Wasserman IF (1964) Puborectalis syndrome. Dis Colon Rectum 7: 87–98.

15. Wexner S, Cheape J, Jorge JMN, Heyman S, Jagelman DG (1992) Prospective assessment of biofeedback of the treatment of paradoxical puborectalis contraction. Dis Colon Rectum 35(2): 145–50.

16. Schuster MM (1990) Rectal pain. Curr Ther Gastroenterol Liver Dis 3: 378–379.

17. Thiele GH (1963) Coccygodynia: cause and treatment. Dis Colon Rectum 6: 422–36.

18. Thiele GH (1937) Coccygodynia and pain in the superior gluteal region. J Am Med Assoc 109: 1271–4.

19. Berstein AM, Phillips HC, Linden W, Fenster H (1992) A psychophysiological evaluation of female urethral syndrome: evidence for a muscular abnormality. J Behav Med 15(3): 229–312.

20. Summitt RL, Ling FW (1991) Urethral syndrome presenting as chronic pelvic pain. J Psychosom Obstet Gynecol Suppl 12: 77–86.

21. Davis DD, Hutchison CV (1999) Clinical management of vulvodynia. Clin Obstet Gynecol 42(2): 221–33.

22. Turner MLC, Marinoff SC (1991) Pudendal neuralgia. Am J Obstet Gynecol 165: 1233–6.

24 Anatomy

B. Shelly, S. Knight, P. King, G. Wetzler, K. Wallace, D. Hartman and G.C. Gorniak

The pelvis is a major attachment site for the muscles of the abdomen, spine, pelvic floor, hip and thigh. Actions of these muscles generate motion and stabilise the lumbosacral joints, sacroiliac joints, pubic symphysis and hip joints. Dysfunctions of these musculoskeletal elements have been identified as possible sources of pelvic pain.[1] A sound knowledge of the musculoskeletal as well as the urogenital anatomy of the pelvis is therefore important for clinicians managing women with pelvic pain.

24.1 Sources of Pelvic Pain

For purposes of anatomical description, the musculoskeletal elements of the pelvic girdle associated with pelvic pain will be categorised as either external or internal anatomic sources of pelvic pain. Faulty postures and muscle imbalances that alter joint mechanics and produce joint- and muscle-related pains in the area of the pelvis are considered to be external sources. Any type of pelvic floor or connective tissue dysfunction may be an internal source of pain. Visceral displacement, as well as fibrosis of the pelvic fascia may entrap, compress, and stretch pelvic nerves and vessels causing somatic and visceral pain.

24.2 Sacroiliac Joint

The sacroiliac (SI) articulation is formed by the auricular surface of the sacrum and the ilium. Both articular surfaces are covered with a thin layer of hyaline cartilage and show an irregular, somewhat interdigitating pattern of ridges and grooves. The ilial surface is covered with fibrocartilage, indicative of the load-bearing functions of the joint.

Some classify the SI joint as a synovial joint, others as a synchondrosis. It is innervated by spinal nerve root levels L4–S3 and stabilised by three sacroiliac and three accessory ligaments. The three sacroiliac ligaments are the interosseous, dorsal sacroiliac and ventral sacroiliac (Fig. 24.1). The interosseous and dorsal sacroiliac ligaments are both very strong. The ventral sacroiliac ligament is thin, with fibres running horizontally across the SI articulation, and is commonly thought to be torn during childbirth.

The iliolumbar, sacrospinous and sacrotuberous ligaments are accessory ligaments of the SI joint. The iliolumbar ligament stabilises the superior part of the sacrum through its attachment to the fourth and fifth lumbar vertebrae. The sacrospinous and sacrotuberous ligaments stabilise the inferior sacrum at their respective attachments to the posterior iliac spine and the ischial tuberosity.

Sacroiliac joint movement occurs via the action of the muscles of the hips and trunk. The iliopsoas,

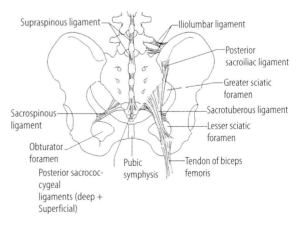

Figure 24.1 Pelvic ligaments – posterior view.

which anteriorly rotates the ilium, is often shortened in clients with CPP.[1] The hip adductors generate a downward or caudal force on the pubic rami when the hip is fixed. Contraction of the piriformis with a fixed hip can nutate or forward bend the sacral base. It can be hypothesised that changes in the length/tension relationships in these muscle groups, associated with trauma or faulty postural habits, may generate asymmetrical forces on the sacroiliac joint, altering its movement and possibly creating a painful dysfunction.

24.3 Pubic Symphysis

The pubic symphysis is a slightly mobile fibrous joint that connects the anterior margins of the pubic bones. Both bony pubic surfaces are lined with a thin layer of hyaline cartilage, between which is the fibrocartilage interpubic disc. The symphysis is stabilised by a thin superior pubic ligament which runs transversely between the pubic tubercles and a thick arcuate ligament which follows the pubic arch and attaches to the interpubic disc.

The width of the pubic symphysis varies markedly. For primiparous females and for males the average width is approximately 4.4 mm. During late pregnancy, the average symphyseal width is about 7.7 mm but has been reported to reach up to 20 mm.[2,3] Motion at the pubic symphysis, as determined from radiographs, is very limited.[3] However, several muscle groups may produce vertical shear forces and torsion on the symphysis when there are muscle imbalances. Unilateral hamstring or abdominal muscle tightness can generate an ipsilateral upward force on the symphysis. Unilateral tightness of the hip adductors can apply an ipsilateral downward force. If shear forces are large, collagen fibres in ligaments can tear, resulting in inflammation and pain. With repetition of this pattern, a chronic inflammatory condition may develop.

24.4 Sacrococcygeal Joint

The sacrococcygeal joint lies between the apex of the sacrum and the base of the first coccygeal segment (CS1). These bony surfaces are separated by a fibrocartilage disc, which is thick centrally and thin on the periphery. Several thin ligaments maintain joint stability. Arising from the coccyx is the anococcygeal ligament. This midline ligament attaches to the posterior rectoanal junction and provides the medial attachment for the levator ani muscles.

Motion at the sacrococcygeal joint is very limited.[4] Ventral movement of the coccyx occurs with shortening contraction of the coccygeus and levator ani.

24.5 Muscles of the Pelvis

Many muscles of the hip and trunk attach to the pelvis. Short or weak muscles may lead to pelvic dysfunction and pelvic pain. Travell and Simons[5] have outlined the referral pain patterns for trigger points throughout the body. These referral patterns point out the relationship of pain symptoms to muscle dysfunction (Fig. 24.2).

24.6 Vestibule

The vestibule of the vagina is considered part of the female external genitalia and frequently a source of discomfort in pelvic pain syndromes. The vestibule of the vagina is a ring of tissue located between the labia minora surrounding both the vaginal and urethral orifices. The pudendal nerve innervates the vestibule, clitoris, labia and perineum (Fig. 24.3).

24.7 Pelvic Nerves

The nerves of the pelvic area originate from the lumbar and sacral nerve roots. Knowledge of cutaneous innervation helps to identify possible nerve involvement (Fig. 24.4).

Scar tissue, fascial restrictions, and muscle compression along any part of the nerve pathway can contribute to pelvic pain. Just inferior to the tendinous arch on the medial side of the ischial tuberosity is the pudendal canal (also called Alcock's canal), carrying the pudendal nerve and the internal pudendal artery and vein to the perineum. The obturator internus fascia also forms this canal. Horizontal tension on the tendinous arch may tense the obturator fascia thus reducing the size of the pudendal canal. This compresses the neurovascular contents giving rise to perineal pain.

24.8 Pain Pathways

Pelvic pain can be transmitted from the pelvic muscles and joints along general somatic afferents associated with the lumbar and sacral plexus (Fig. 24.5). Because of this, pelvic pain from exter-

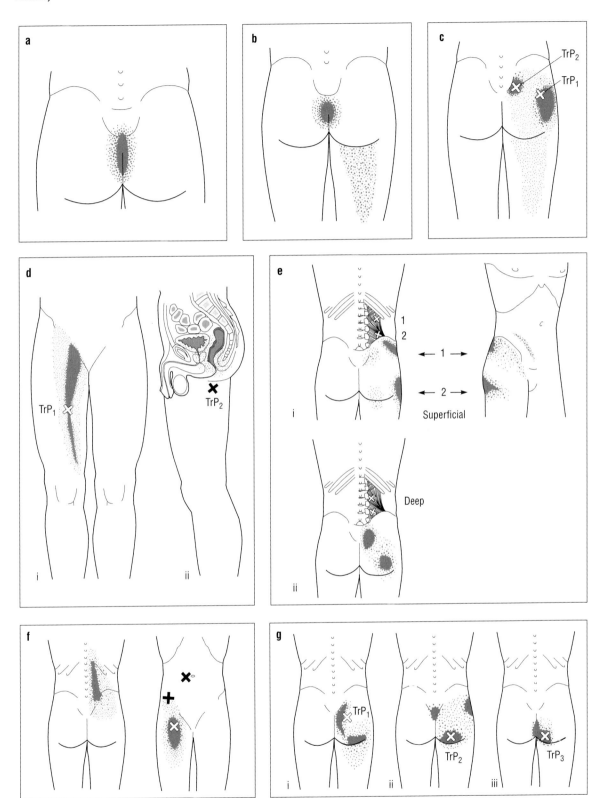

Figure 24.2   Trigger point referral patterns:[5] **a** Levators ani **b** Obturator internus **c** Piriformis **d** Adductors **e** Quadratus lumborum **f** Iliopsoas **g** Gluteus maximus.

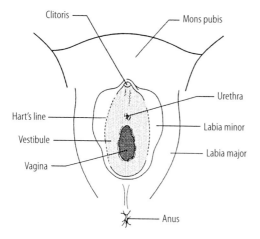

Figure 24.3   The vulva.

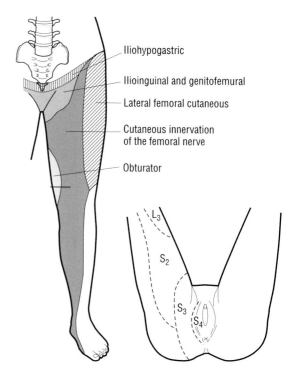

Figure 24.4   Sensory nerve innervation of the lower limb and perineum.

nal sources can refer to the low back, lower abdomen, thigh and pelvic floor muscles (PFM).[1] Pelvic pain can also be transmitted from pelvic viscera and fascia along general visceral afferents associated with sympathetic and parasympathetic efferents to the pelvic viscera.[6] These visceral afferents are carried from visceral plexuses by:

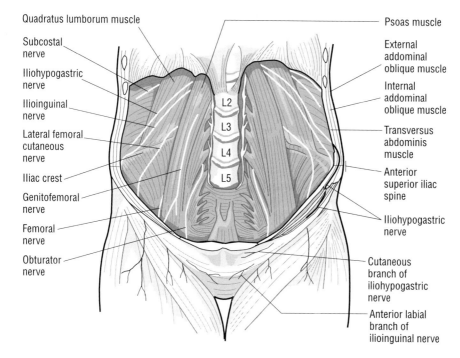

Figure 24.5   Lumbar plexus.

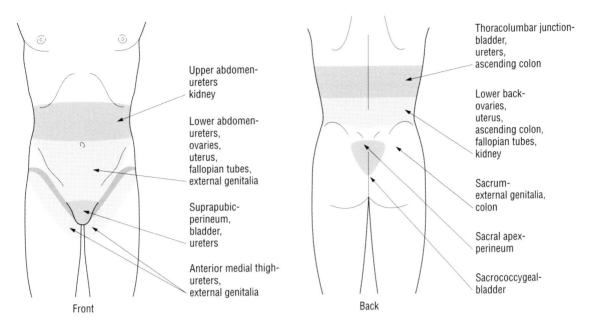

Figure 24.6 Pain referral patterns of lower quadrant visceral structures.

- sacral splanchnic (sympathetic) nerves through the sympathetic chain to the level of T10–L2
- visceral sympathetic afferent nerves through the inferior hypogastric plexus to the superior hypogastric plexus
- visceral parasympathetic afferents of the vagus and pelvic splanchnic nerves.

Organ pain is often dull and poorly defined. Organ referral patterns, shown in Fig. 24.6, often overlap muscle trigger point referral patterns.[5] Therapists are encouraged to become familiar with symptoms of organ dysfunction for appropriate referral to other medical professionals.

References

1. Baker TK (1993) Musculoskeletal origins of chronic pelvic pain. In: Ling FW (ed) Contemporary Management of Chronic Pelvic Pain, Obstet Gynecol Clin N Am 20: 719–42.
2. Abramson D, Roberts SM, Wilson PD (1934) Relaxation of the pelvic joints in pregnancy. Surg Gynecol Obstet 58(3): 595–613.
3. Walheim GG, Seluik G (1984) Mobility of the pubic symphysis. Clin Orthop Relat Res 191: 129–35.
4. Hollingshead WH, Rosse C (1985) Textbook of Anatomy (4th ed). Harper & Row, New York.
5. Travell JG, Simons DG (1992) Myofascial Pain and Dysfunction, Vols 1 and 2. Williams & Wilkins, Baltimore, Md.
6. Rogers RM (1998) Basic pelvic neuroanatomy. In: Steege JF, Metzger DA, Levy BS (eds) Chronic Pelvic Pain: An integrated approach. WB Saunders, Philadelphia, pp. 31–58.

25 Aetiology of Pelvic Floor Muscle Pain Syndromes

B. Shelly, S. Knight, P. King, G. Wetzler, K. Wallace, D. Hartman and G.C. Gorniak

A significant population of urological, gynaecological and colorectal patients present with pain of unknown aetiology. The emphasis of this chapter is on the musculoskeletal system and describing PFM hypertonus dysfunction caused by musculoskeletal, psychogenic, visceral or systemic, iatrogenic and neurological factors. The most common pain diagnosis related to the pelvic floor muscles (PFM) are outlined in Chapter 23. The aetiology of vulvar pain syndromes is discussed in a Chapter 27.5.

25.1 Pelvic Muscle Pain and Vaginismus

Pelvic floor hypertonus is a muscle impairment in which an increase in PFM tension or active spasms cause musculoskeletal pain or dysfunction of the urogenital or colorectal system. Numerous components, presentations and diagnoses are associated with this condition. Muscle pain differs from cutaneous and visceral pain in that it is difficult to localise, refers pain to other deep somatic tissues and is usually perceived as aching and cramping.

Vaginismus is one example of a diagnosis that includes PFM dysfunction. It is defined as the recurrent or persistent involuntary muscle spasm of the musculature of the distal one-third of the vagina that interferes with sexual function. The prevalence of vaginismus in clinical samples has been estimated to be between 12% and 17%.

25.2 Musculoskeletal Factors

King et al.[1] examined 132 patients with CPP, most of who had undergone unsuccessful gynecological and psychological treatment. Of those patients 75% were found to have a typical pattern of faulty posture. The musculoskeletal components of hypertonus dysfunction discussed here will include joint, muscle or movement dysfunctions.

25.2.1 Joint Dysfunction

In an overview article, Mense[2] describes the mechanism of reflex inhibition and reflex atrophy of muscles from changes in normal joint input. He acknowledges that there is no generally accepted concept that could explain why muscles react with spasm to one lesion and inhibition to another. He summarises that clinical experience suggests that postural muscles tend to become hypertonic and phasic muscles more inhibited. Trauma to the coccyx or pelvis from childbirth or direct falls can create pelvic floor muscle changes or hypertonus in response to ligament injury or joint malalignment. Coccygodynia is a common diagnosis where the coccyx joint can cause pain or spasm in the pelvic floor, specifically the coccygeus muscles. In addition, sacroiliac, pubic symphysis, lumbar and hip joint dysfunction or pathology can affect the PFM causing reflex spasm or limitations in strength and muscle length.

Maigne[3] defines thoracolumbar junction pain syndromes as painful clinical manifestations involving low back, hip and pubic pain, which mimic gynaecological, urological, and lower gastrointestinal pain and can create autonomic disturbances.

25.2.2 Muscle Dysfunction

Myofascial pain is recognised as one of the aetiologies of chronic pelvic pain. Muscle pain aetiologies in the pelvic floor can come from direct trauma to the perineum and the PFM. Falls, sexual abuse, vaginal delivery, surgery or episiotomy can cause soft tissue and muscle injury to the pelvic floor region with residual pain. Myofascial pain syndrome may be due to trigger points or soft tissue dysfunction. The general term 'regional myofascial pain syndrome' should be used to describe pain from scar, ligaments or trigger points. Muscle spasm is due to non-voluntary motor nerve activity that affects an entire muscle and cannot be controlled by voluntary relaxation. It may or may not be painful. A taut band is a section of tense muscle, which usually contains a trigger point (See Figure 25.1).

25.2.3 Trigger Points

A central myofascial trigger point (TP) is defined as a hyper-irritable spot in skeletal muscle that is associated with a hypersensitive, palpable nodule in a taut band. The spot is painful on palpation and can give rise to characteristic referred pain, referred tenderness, motor dysfunction and autonomic phenomena. An active TP is always tender, prevents full lengthening of the muscles, weakens the muscle, and mediates a local twitch response of muscle fibre when adequately stimulated.

The aetiological definition of a central trigger point is

> a cluster of electrically active loci each of which is associated with a contraction knot and dysfunctional motor endplate in skeletal muscle.[4]

The onset of symptoms is related to some degree of muscle overload which may be acute, sustained or repetitive. Causes of TPs parallel those of hypertonus impairments as they may stem from musculoskeletal, psychogenic, visceral or systemic, iatrogenic, and neurological origin. Hypertonic muscles may or may not have trigger points.

Travell and Simons[5] have identified TPs in specific muscles of the pelvic region (see Chapter 24). Slocumb[6] found trigger points in 131 (74%) of 177 patients referred for evaluation of CPP. In addition, Reiter and Gambone[7] reported abdominal trigger points in approximately 55% of women referred for CPP following negative laparoscopy.

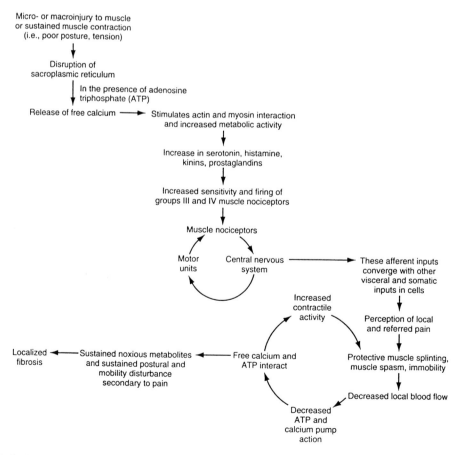

Figure 25.1 Pathophysiology of myofascial pain syndromes. [Rachlin ES (Ed.) Myofascial Pain and Fibromyalgia. St. Louis. CV Mosby 1994. P. 152.]

25.2.4 Movement and Muscle Recruitment Dysfunction

Movement dysfunction can occur with learned abnormal use patterns of the PFM. An example of abnormal use is chronic holding of the muscles due to a 'falling out feeling' or fear of bladder leakage. Dysfunctional use patterns such as contraction of a muscle rather than relaxation may also develop.

Surface electromyography (SEMG) biofeedback is a helpful tool in assessing recruitment and coordination of the PFM and can be used to identify recruitment and the lack of co-ordination. White et al.[8] report poor and delayed relaxation responses to muscle work in the PFM of patients with vulvar pain.

25.3 Psychogenic Factors

Lifestyle and stress issues, as well as sexual abuse, can cause physiological muscle tension to be held in the PFM. In many cases it is difficult to distinguish whether a concurrent or previous medical problem has caused tension or spasm or if a chronic holding of the muscles has created a tension–pain cycle.

Weiss[9] describes how the PFM evolved. In the animal, the actions of the tail are controlled by the PFM. Often an animal holds its tail tightly in fear and relaxes it with joy. He suggests the same action of the PFM in humans; the PFM are perhaps the ultimate representation of the mind–body connection.

25.4 Visceral or Systemic Factors

Pelvic inflammation, infection or disease may give rise to chronic holding patterns in the pelvic musculature. Concurrent diagnoses of CPP, interstitial cystitis, irritable bowel syndrome, fibromyalgia, endometriosis, dysmenorrhea or premenstrual syndrome, vulvodynia, dermatological conditions of the vulva and perineal infections, including sexually transmitted diseases, can trigger hypertonus as a muscle response to pain or irritability. In addition, systemic influences of the endocrine and metabolic function such as oestrogen hormone imbalance and thyroid deficiencies can lead to vulnerability of trigger points.

25.5 Iatrogenic Factors

Urogenital or rectal surgery may result in painful inhibition associated with guarding of the PFM. Adhesions or scar tissue can create pain or muscle tenderness in the PFM. The surgical position may be traumatic to the pelvic structures contributing to CPP. A case report by Alevizon and Finan[10] identified pudendal nerve entrapment after sacrospinous colpopexy as the aetiology of postoperative perineal and buttock pain.

25.6 Neurological Factors

Neurologic factors can contribute to painful urogynecologic or colorectal symptoms. The ilioinguinal nerve (L1) and the genitofemoral nerve have pain distribution patterns in the region of the medial groin, mons, labia and inner thigh. The character of this pain varies from constant burning to sharp and jabbing and can be aggravated by lifting movements of the ipsilateral leg, walking or coughing. Nerve entrapment is an often misdiagnosed postoperative sequelae. The ilioinguinal nerve can be injured during needle urethropexy. A Pfannenstiel's incision can cause postoperative adhesions restricting the iliohypogastric and genitofemoral nerves and referring pain to the genital region. In a study of a group of patients suffering from chronic perineal pain in the seated position, Robert et al.[11] describe three sites of potential entrapment of the pudendal nerve. These sites include a constriction between the sacrotuberous and sacrospinous ligament, in the pudendal canal of Alcock and during the straddling of the falciform process of the sacrotuberous ligament by the pudendal nerve. They considered idiopathic perineal pain as an entrapment syndrome. Pudendal neuralgia is one painful diagnosis of neurologic origin.

The upper lumbar levels of disc herniation and protrusion also can refer pain to the pelvic region.

It is important to also consider complex regional pain syndrome (CRPS), previously termed reflex sympathetic dystrophy, as an aetiology of pelvic floor pain and hypertonus. Imamura et al.[12] report that CRPS may develop after visceral diseases, and central nervous system lesions or, rarely, without an obvious antecedent event. The causalgia present in CRPS is a result of partial injury of a nerve or one or more of its major branches.

In summary, pelvic floor symptoms may be affected by either musculoskeletal conditions, psychogenic or iatrogenic causes, neurological pain or systemic diseases, or the PFM may be the primary source of pain.

References

1. King PM, Myers CA, Ling FW et al. (1991) Musculoskeletal factors in chronic pelvic pain. J Psychom Obstet Gynaecol 12: 87–98.
2. Mense S (1997) Pathophysiologic basis of muscle pain syndromes. Phys Med Rehab Clin N Am 8(1): 23–53.
3. Maigne R (1997) Pathophysiologic basis of muscle pain syndromes of the thoracolumbar junction. A frequent source of misdiagnosis. Phys Med Rehabil Clin North Am 8(1): 87–100.
4. Simons DG, Travell JG, Simon LS (1999) Myofascial Pain and Dysfunction. Trigger Point Manual (2nd ed) Vol. 1. William & Wilkins, Baltimore, Md.
5. Travell JG, Simons DG (1992) Myofascial Pain and Dysfunction, Vols 1 and 2. Williams & Wilkins, Baltimore, Md.
6. Slocumb JC (1984) Neurological factors in chronic pelvic pain syndrome. Am J Obstet Gynecol 149: 536.
7. Reiter R, Gambone J (1991) Nongynecoligic somatic pathology in women with chronic pelvic pain and negative laparoscopy. J Reprod Med 36: 253.
8. White G, Jantos M, Glazure H (1997) Establishing the diagnosis of vulvar vestibulitis. J Reprod Med 42: 156–60.
9. Weiss J (1998) A holistic approach to treating pelvic pain. National Vulvodynia Association News, Winter.
10. Alevizon SJ, Finan MA (1996) Sacrospinous colpopexy: management of postoperative pudendal nerve entrapment. Obstet Gynecol 88(4): 713–15.
11. Robert R, Prar-Pradal D, Labat JJ et al. (1998) Anatomic basis of chronic perineal pain: Role of the pudendal nerve. Surg Radiol Anat 20(2): 93–8.
12. Imamura ST et al. (1997) The importance of myofascial pain syndrome in reflex sympathetic dystrophy (or complex regional pain syndromes). Phys Med Rehab Clin North Am 8(1): 207–11.

26 Assessment of Pelvic Pain

B. Shelly, S. Knight, P. King, G. Wetzler, K. Wallace, D. Hartman and G.C. Gorniak

26.1 Integrated or Holistic Approach

The role of the physical therapist in the evaluation of pelvic pain is principally to identify and clarify neuromusculoskeletal factors contributing to this multifactorial condition. However, it is important that therapists approach the examination of these complicated patients holistically. The examination process must extend beyond the musculoskeletal system. Additional findings should be included in the decision-making process. Peters et al.[1] supported integrated models of care delivery for pelvic pain patients. Their successful integrated model included multidisciplinary management by physical therapists, psychologists, and physicians and surgeons. They emphasised the importance of evaluation by all professions from the beginning of care. When such a 'team' is not involved from the outset, it is important that practitioners use appropriate screening procedures to ensure that adequate referrals are made. In all cases, ongoing communication is necessary to provide seamless multidisciplinary care and to assess responses to treatment. Therapeutic plans based on evaluations that integrate musculoskeletal impairment information with other client characteristics (such as personal, social, occupational and medical attributes) are likely to be more effective than those treating impairments in isolation.[1–3]

The components of the physical therapy examination are set out in the following three categories: history, systems review, and tests and measures.[4] This chapter reviews history, tests and measures specific to CCP. These components are added to the standard musculoskeletal evaluation of the lower quadrant (see Table 26.1). The urogenital and gastrointestinal systems also require extensive evaluation. Therapists are encouraged to seek additional references to complete the systems review portion of the examination.[5] References are given so that therapists can seek additional information when needed.

Table 26.1. Structures to include in a complete lower quadrant evaluation

Skin and superficial fascia	Scars, adhesions, mobility, fluid exchanges – trunk, lower extremity and perineum[6–8]
Muscles	Muscle length and strength, play, tone, insertions into bony contours, neuromuscular control, trigger points – trunk, lower extremity and perineum[9–11]
Articular	Alignment, stability, laxity, biomechanics – all lower extremity joints including the pelvis and spine[12]
Organs	Mobility, motility, function, displacements – digestive, gynecological, urinary[13,14]
Lymphatic	Drainage, compression syndromes – lower body
Neurovascular	Pressures, exchanges, compression syndromes, disease – lower body, central nervous system[6,15]
Patient habits	Sleep, exercise, movement patterns, static postures, stress reaction

26.2 History – Initial Interview

The examination usually begins with the therapist–patient interview. Levy[16] points out the dual purpose of the history interview in the examination process – to gather information and to establish a therapeutic relationship with the patient. Levy[16] and Grace[3] both emphasise the importance of allowing women with pelvic pain to "tell their story", as much as possible without interruption. History-taking should be collected within the context of the woman's "need to share".

Women are not always certain why they are being referred to physical therapy, and may fail to keep the appointment as a result of fear, anxiety or lack of confidence about the relevance of therapy to their condition. Introductory letters, if utilised, should be informative about the purpose of physical therapy but above all be brief and clear. Patients are encouraged to prepare a history of symptoms, treatments and tests before coming to the initial evaluation by completing a questionnaire. The review of such information before the interview may facilitate the process. Body diagrams denoting pain location, as well as self-administered pain questionnaires, are also appropriate for pre-interview completion. A clear understanding of the aetiology of pelvic floor muscle (PFM) spasm is necessary in order to develop and interpret these questionnaires. A history of all systems is collected, with focus on musculoskeletal, genitourinary and gastrointestinal function.

26.2.1 Subjective Reports of Pain

Location, duration, nature and intensity of symptoms should be recorded; body diagrams completed by the patients are also useful. Patient's verbal descriptions of pain location (i.e. "hip" or "pelvis") are easily misinterpreted. Whole-body diagrams and detailed diagrams of the perineum are needed to document exact pain locations. Pain intensity may be measured by visual analogue or numeric ranking (0–10) scales.[17] It is not uncommon to see pain ratings remain constant while functional ability scores increase. This shows improvement in overall function and indicates need for continued treatment. It is essential to differentiate primary organ pain from musculoskeletal pain; often there is identifiable organ pathology with associated musculoskeletal impairments. Systems review questionnaires should help identify possible organ dysfunction.

It is clear from many research studies that the clinical manifestation of pelvic pain is related to attributes that cross the physical, emotional and social dimensions of the women affected. The Bates model[18] can be useful to therapists attempting to understand the relationship between the various dimensions of the whole person presenting for treatment of pelvic pain. Common pain and func-

tional evaluation tools can be used to assess the multidimensional nature of pain.[17,19–22] There are no validated pain scales specific to pelvic pain.

26.2.2 Dyspareunia

Questions about dyspareunia can help identify dysfunction and impairment location. Frequency of sexual interaction varies widely in the general population and there is no "normal" frequency of intercourse. Current dysfunction should be compared to the frequency of intercourse before the dysfunction occurred. This may be easy to estimate in married couples, but is very difficult for single women where other factors influence sexual interactions. Women with primary dyspareunia have difficulty judging symptoms, as they have never experienced pain-free intercourse. General questions such as "Can you have intercourse whenever you like?" may be used to assess function (see Box 26.1). Lack of desire and limited arousal are common problems with pelvic pain patients and may require intervention from a sexual counsellor. During arousal, lubrication and engorgement of the vaginal tissues prepare the vagina for penetration. Penetration before these physical changes have occurred can be uncomfortable even in women without classic CPP.

Box 26.2

Symptoms of sexual abuse[28]

Low self-esteem, feeling of loss of control

Poor body awareness, often not trusting their own physical or emotional feelings

Difficulty with anger and violence

Difficulty with sexuality and intimacy; may avoid sex completely or compulsively seek sex

Denies and forgets instructions or appointments

Self-mutilating or addictive behaviours

Controlling of environment, treatment, or your time

Multiple personalities

Disassociation (i.e. avoidance of eye contact, distant look), an unconscious defence mechanism to separate the mind from the body and protect the mind from impending trauma; may occur during the treatment sessions.

Box 26.1

Specific questions about dyspareunia with interpretation

1. Do you have pain on penetration or deeply?
   Penetration pain is usually associated with adhered introital scars (episiotomy, vaginal surgery) or dermatological lesions. Vulvodynia can also result in penetration pain. Deep pain can be related to PFM spasm or organ dysfunction/adhesions.

2. How much pain do you have and how long does it last?
   Pain is usually rated on a visual analogue or numeric scale. Length of pain after intercourse can give some indication of the irritability of the tissues

3. Complex scales can be used to determine sexual function. However, physical therapists usually find simple scales, like the one listed below,[23] to be adequate:
   0 – no pain or limitation of intercourse
   1 – some pain with intercourse but no limitation in frequency of sexual activity
   2 – significant pain with intercourse and limitation in frequency of intercourse
   3 – severe pain and inability to tolerate any penetration
   Level 2 may be further clarified with percent of successful intercourse.

4. Does intercourse position affect pain? What positions make it less painful? More painful?
   Many women find differences in pain with varying positions. Discussion of sexual positions can be simple or very complex, requiring referral to other professionals.
   Some possible concerns with common positions include:
   "man on top" – most pressure on the posterior structures of the vagina
   "woman on top" –deepest penetration, but the women has more control over the depth
   "doggie style" (quadruped with rear entrance) – least organ trauma/movement
   "spoon" (side lying with the man behind) – least penetrating

5. Can you achieve orgasm? Does it increase pain?
   Orgasm is a complex process and is seldom easily interpreted. Pain with orgasm may indicate PFM spasm. Lack of orgasm (anorgasmia) may indicate PFM weakness. However, there are many reasons for pain with orgasm and anorgasmia. These symptoms may change with physical therapy treatment of other identified impairments.

26.2.3 Depression

Depression can affect the physical therapy treatment of pelvic pain. Rosefeld[24] reports chronic pain and sexual dysfunction as two risk factors for depression. Other risk factors include prior incident or family history of depression, chronic illness and severe medical illness. Symptoms of depression include: fatigue, loss of interest in usual activities, weight change, sleep disturbances, and difficulty concentrating. Referral to appropriate professionals is indicated if depression appears to be affecting treatment.

26.2.4 Sexual Abuse

Unfortunately, sexual abuse is common in pelvic pain patients. Therapists should watch for symp-

toms of sexual abuse (Box 26.2) and modify treatment accordingly.[25,26] The Abuse History[27] is a tool for eliciting history of sexual and physical abuse in children and adults. Survivors of sexual abuse often need to progress slower and may take longer to achieve therapy goals. Working with the patient's counsellor often enhances patient outcomes.

26.3 Tests and Measures

Tests and measures for the pelvic pain patient are divided into posture assessment, joint integrity, muscle length and strength, and palpation.

Adaptations commonly found in pelvic pain patients are listed in Box 26.3.

Box 26.3

Adaptations commonly found in pelvic pain patients

Sleeping with the legs curled up in hip and knee flexion

Poor breathing pattern – shallow and upper chest

Intolerant of tight clothes at the waist or pelvis

Sneeze in trunk flexion or with one hip flexed

Increased muscle tension in response to pain throughout the body

Dietary changes in response to changes in the digestive system – flatulence, belching and fatigue may indicate lack of proper digestion

Typical pelvic pain posture (TPPP) (see text)

Relaxation of the abdominal wall to protect from abdominal pain leading to a pendulous abdomen

---

26.3.1 Postural Assessment

King et al.[29] identified a common pattern of faulty posture in a sample of 132 pelvic pain patients that was labelled "typical pelvic pain posture" (TPPP). This was described as having exaggerated lordotic curve in the lumbar spine, an anterior tilt of the pelvis and associated joint integrity problems of diminished hip rotation range of motion and decreased iliopsoas length, among others.

Before landmark examination begins, it is useful to note the position the individual chooses for standing. Is weight bearing equal on both lower extremities? Is the weight shifted to one side in relationship to pain or habit? It is of particular importance in pelvic pain populations to note internal/external rotation placement of the lower extremity. Often, individuals who rest with one lower extremity in external rotation have a tight hip and hypomobile sacroiliac on that side. A standard musculoskeletal evaluation of the pelvic and lower extremity landmarks should be completed including lumbar, sacroiliac, pubic symphysis, hip, knee and ankle joints.

The position of the coccyx, pubis and sacrum can impact on the length of the PFM and thus contribute to painful dysfunctions in that muscle group. It may be less obvious but is no less true that faulty positions of the lumbar spine, hip and even other lower extremity joints can contribute to asymmetry of length/tension relationships in the PFM. For example, an anatomically short lower extremity often results in unilateral standing habits that place torsion or rotational stresses on the sacroiliac joints and pubic symphysis. In unilateral standing, it is most likely that a posterior rotation position will develop at the ilium of the weight-bearing side as well as an external rotation position of the hip.

26.3.2 Joint Integrity/Range of Motion

It is important to screen active and passive range of motion (ROM) in the lumbar spine, hips and sacroiliac articulations at a minimum. Before specific ROM tests, a general screening for pelvic stability should be conducted. The Trendelenberg test in standing is useful. If positive, it indicates a need for careful testing of sacroiliac stability and especially gluteus medius strength.

26.3.2.1 Hip Range of Motion

An examination of hip rotation is recommended to determine if further ROM testing is necessary. End feel testing is used to determine if rotation limitation is by muscle or capsule. Capsular restrictions typically present with a hard, but not harsh, resistance to passive force. Muscle end feels are firm but with a slight elastic rebound.

26.3.2.2 Lumbar Range of Motion

Typical testing of the lumbar spine mobility and function should be conducted, including forward bending and side bending in standing. Lordotic lumbar curves should fully reverse equally at all segments during mobility tests. Active lumbar side bending may be limited by lateral soft tissue restriction including the quadratus lumborum and psoas muscle lengths. Active range of motion tests should be followed by passive testing of lumbar intervertebral motion to clarify joint mobility in the region. Special attention is given to the T11–L1 level where the sympathetic hypogastric innervation originates.

26.3.2.3 Sacroiliac Range of Motion

Many tests are used to evaluate sacroiliac (SI) joint dysfunction. Some patients will require more extensive tests, and therapists are encouraged to use advanced tests as indicated. Simple sacroiliac tests include the march test, sacral flexion/extension test in sitting, and passive mobility tests.

26.3.3 Muscle Strength and Length Tests

Normal length and strength of all hip and trunk muscles is necessary for pain-free function of the pelvis. A quick screening test for trunk stability is the quadruped position test in which patients are asked to maintain lumbar spinal neutral while raising alternate arms and legs. Inability to carry out this manoeuvre is indicative of trunk stability problems. All pelvic and trunk muscles require testing in the usual manner. Hip internal rotation with hip flexion, in the supine or sitting position, tests the length of the piriformis muscle. The obturator internus is tested with the hip in extension, usually in prone. Muscles to be tested include: gastrocnemius, soleus, iliopsoas, quadratus lumborum, abdominal corset, piriformis, obturator internus, lumbar paraspinals, adductors, gluteus maximus and medius.

26.3.4 Palpation

Palpation may be the most important part of the evaluation in some patients, and great time and care is taken in careful evaluation of all soft tissue structures. Palpation of joint structures for oedema, tenderness and temperature change is important to complete the examination of these structures. Soft-tissue palpation also includes muscles and their associated tendons, fascia including skin and scars, organs of the abdomen and pelvis, and lower extremities. All the muscles and tendons of the pelvic area, including the pelvic floor, are assessed for play, tone, trigger points and scar mobility.

26.3.4.1 Abdominal Palpation

Abdominal palpation requires knowledge of visceral structure anatomy. With practise, a therapist can develop the ability to feel organ position, mobility and motility. Abdominal muscle impairments can be more easily felt if the patient performs a head lift during palpation. The psoas muscle can be palpated through the abdomen, with care taken not to compress organ structures. Any mass in the abdomen should be reported to the physician.

26.3.4.2 External Palpation of the Pelvic Floor Muscles

The patient is placed in side lying with the top leg approximately in 60–80 degrees of hip flexion with the knee flexed comfortably. Two or three pillows are placed under the top leg to provide stability in

neutral and allow the patient to relax the leg fully, as total patient relaxation is necessary for deep PFM palpation. The therapist is positioned behind the patient and finds the ischial tuberosity on the uppermost ilium. The palpation may be done through the patient's underwear, but is more effective if the fingers are on bare skin. The therapist should wear latex gloves because of the proximity to the anus and perineum. The hand should be in supination with the palm facing upwards and the fingers extended and adducted. The hand should be parallel to the table, the fingertips on the skin medial to the ischial tuberosity, lateral to the anus. Gentle inward pressure should be applied directed towards the anterior superior iliac spine (ASIS) of the upper ilium. The closeness of the ischial tuberosity may result in the skin being pulled taught, restricting deep palpation. If this happens, reposition the fingers more medial to the ischial tuberosity, taking up some skin slack. The levator ani muscles are rather deep; their depth from the skin varies greatly and can be more than 4 cm (1.5 inches). When a firm resistance is felt, ask the patient to contract their PFM. You should feel a firm contraction pushing your fingers outwards. With the PFM at rest, assess for pain, hypertonia and connective tissue restriction in the usual manner. Angling the fingers anteriorly and posteriorly can give information about different areas of the PFM.

The obturator internus is a little more difficult to palpate. A review of anatomy is necessary to orientate yourself to the location of the muscle in the side lying position. Keep the palpating hand in the position previously described and gently change the angle of the hand so that the elbow drops and the fingers move upward into the tissue above. The obturator internus is located in this area and should feel soft. To test the muscle, have the patient lift their top knee upwards while keeping their foot on the supporting surface. The therapist gives resistance to the movement by placing a hand on top of the moving knee. A small isometric movement should result in a palpable muscle tension. The palpation depth is important, shallow palpation results in palpation of the medial ischial tuberosity. In this case continue straight inwards until the tissue releases to a deeper level and then angle the elbow down and the fingers upwards. Myofascial release of muscle or connective tissue can be carried out in this position if impairments are identified.

It is also important to fully evaluate the external perineal structures at the pubic arch, lateral to the clitoris, around the ischial tuberosity and coccyx. External palpation of the sacrotuberous ligament is also performed in this position.

26.3.4.3 Internal Palpation of the Obturator Internus and Piriformis

The obturator internus can be palpated through the vagina and rectum by palpating slightly more cephalad and more lateral than the PFMs. The piriformis can be reached through the vagina but is more easily palpated through the rectal canal slightly lateral to the sacrum and cephalad to the coccygeus. The sacrospinous tendon is located just behind the coccygeus muscle. Pain and dysfunction of the sacrospinous ligament may result following sacrospinous fixation.[30]

References

1. Peters AA, Dorst E van, Jellis B et al. (1991) A randomized clinical trail to compare two different approaches in women with chronic pelvic pain. Obstet Gynecol 77: 5.
2. Myers CA, Baker PK, Ling F (1998) Musculoskeletal screening in the pelvic pain patient. In: Sanfilipo JS, Smith RP (eds) Primary Care in Obstetrics and Gynecology: A handbook for clinicians. Springer, New York.
3. Grace VM (1995) Problems women patients experience in the medical encounters for chronic pelvic pain: A New Zealand study. Health Care Women Int 16: 509–19.
4. American Physical Therapy Association (APTA) (1997) Guide to physical therapy practice. Phys Ther 77: 11.
5. Boissonault WG (1995) Examination in Physical Therapy Practice – Screening for medical diseases. Churchill Livingstone, Edinburgh, UK, pp. 105–50.
6. Upledger J, Vredevoogd JD (1983) Craniosacral Therapy. Eastland Press, Seattle, Wa.
7. Barnes JF (1989) Myofascial Release: The search for excellence. Myofascial Release Treatment Centers and Seminars, Pioli.
8. Johnson G (1991) Soft tissue mobilization. In: White AH, Anderson R (ed) Conservative Care of Low Back Pain. William & Wilkins, Baltimore, Md.
9. Simons DG, Travell JG, Simon LS (1999) Myofascial Pain and Dysfunction. Trigger Point Manual (2nd ed) Vol. 1. William & Wilkins, Baltimore, Md.
10. Hall C (1999) Therapeutic exercises for the lumbopelvic region and the hip. (in Brody L) In: Hall CM, Thein Brody L (eds) Therapeutic Exercises: moving toward function. Lippincott Williams & Wilkins, Philadelphia, Pa.
11. Steege JF, Metzger DA, Levy BA (1998) Chronic Pelvic Pain: An integrated approach. WB Saunders, Philadelphia.
12. DeFranca GG (1996) Pelvic Locomotor Dysfunction: A clinical approach. Aspen Publications, Gaithersburg, Md.
13. Barral JP (1993) Urogenital Manipulation. Eastland Press, Seattle, Wa.
14. Barral JP, Mercier P (1988) Visceral Manipulation. Eastland Press, Seattle, Wa.
15. Weiselfish-Giammatteo S (1998) Integrative Manual Therapy. North Atlantic Books, Berkeley, Ca.
16. Levy BS (1998) History. In: Steege JF, Metzger DA, Levy BS (eds) Chronic Pelvic Pain: An integrated approach. WB Saunders, Philadelphia, pp. 59–63.
17. Jacob MC (1998) Pain intensity, psychiatric diagnosis, and psychosocial factors: assessment rationale and procedures. In: Steege JF, Metzger DA, Levy BS (eds) Chronic Pelvic Pain: An integrated approach. WB Saunders, Philadelphia, pp. 67–76.
18. Bates MS (1996) Biocultural Dimensions of Chronic Pain – Implications for treatment of multi-ethnic populations. State University of New York Press, Albany.
19. Melzack R (1975) The McGill pain questionnaire: major properties and scoring methods. Pain 1: 277.
20. Kerns RD, Jacob MC (1992) Assessment of the psychosocial context of the experience of chronic pain. In: Turk DC, Melzack R (ed) Handbook of Pain Assessment. Guilford Press, New York.
21. Kerns RD, Haythornthwaite J, Rosenburg R et al. (1991) The pain behavior check list (PBCL): factor structure and psychometric properties. J Behav Med 14: 155.
22. Fairbanks JCT et al. (1980) The Oswestry low back pain disability questionnaire. Physiotherapy 66: 8.
23. Marinoff S (1991) Vulvar vestibulitis syndrome: an overview. Am J Obstet Gynecol 165: 1228–33.
24. Rosefeld JA (1997) Women's Health in Primary Care. Williams & Wilkins, Baltimore, Md.
25. Bass E, Davis L (1994) The Courage to Heal: A Guide for Women Survivors of Childhood Sexual Abuse, 3rd ed. Harper & Row, New York.
26. Schacter CL, Stalker CA, Teram E (1999) Toward sensitive practice: Issues for physical therapists working with survivors of childhood sexual abuse. Phys Ther 79(3): 248–69.
27. Drossman DA, Leserman J, Nachman G et al. (1990) Sexual and physical abuse in women with functional organic gastrointestinal disorders. Ann Intern Med 113: 828.
28. Shelly B (1999) The pelvic floor. In: Hall C, Thein Brody L (ed) Therapeutic Exercises: moving toward function. Lippincott Williams & Wilkins, Philadelphia, Pa.
29. King PM, Myers CA, Ling FW et al. (1991) Musculoskeletal factors in chronic pelvic pain. J Psychom Obstet Gynaecol 12: 87–98.
30. Barksdale PA, Gasser RF, Gauthier CM, Elkins TE, Wall LL (1997) Intraligamentous nerves as a potential source of pain after sacrospinous ligament fixation of the vaginal apex. Int Urogynecol J 8: 121–5.

27 Treatment of Pelvic Pain

B. Shelly, S. Knight, P. King, G. Wetzler, K. Wallace, D. Hartman and
G.C. Gorniak

This section describes interventions used by physical therapists and assumes that the therapist will work in collaboration with other appropriate health professionals while these treatments are employed. The key to successful outcomes from interventions is a therapeutic plan with specific goals based on examination findings. Therapists should remember that treating a PFM dysfunction in isolation without also addressing other musculoskeletal imbalances is fruitless. Chronic pain in one part of the body can cause manifestation of other disorders elsewhere in the body. A holistic approach is best.

This chapter describes patient education, stress management, therapeutic exercise treatments, modalities and manual treatments (summarised in Box 27.1). Treatments for vulvodynia are presented later in the chapter.

Adherence or compliance to a therapeutic programme is influenced by several factors, one of which is the patient's understanding of the purpose of the prescribed interventions. Explaining physical therapy interventions is particularly important in the management of pelvic pain. The possible cause of pain and potential interventions should be included in the initial interview. Therapy will be less successful if the patient's expectations are unrealistic, or they believe that therapy will not help.

27.1 Posture and Body Mechanics

Interventions aimed at posture impairments in pelvic pain patients have been reported to be successful by many clinicians.[2-7] The primary goal is to have spinal curves in neutral to reduce strain on lengthened tissues and joints.

27.1.1 Standing Positions

A diagonal stance with feet comfortably shoulder width apart and knees in slight flexion is recommended. For women who spend prolonged periods of time in standing, slight oscillatory movements shifting weight from one foot to the other are useful. These oscillations increase muscle co-ordination and minimise muscle tension (via the gate control mechanism). The diagonal position may be used to address asymmetries of sacroiliac joint (for example, with a left posterior rotation of the ileum, the preferred stance may be on a diagonal with the right foot forward). Care is taken to place equal weight on both feet and avoid the drop hip asymmetrical stance (as used in holding a baby on one hip).

Attention to pelvic neutral is important for optimal abdominal function and to reduce strains on the pelvic floor and sacroiliac articulations. Pelvic neutral includes anterior–posterior pelvic tilt as well as right-to-left weight shifts. Flattened medial foot arches may cause a medial rotation of the femur. Arch supports for the shoes are helpful in minimising medial rotation strain if foot dysfunctions are contributing to the hip malposition. Complex foot dysfunctions need referral to an orthotist (podiatrist).

27.1.2 Sitting Positions

Prolonged sitting often increases coccyx pain.[8] Proper sitting instruction is the most important posture education for patients with PFM spasms, levator ani syndrome and coccygodynia. Sinaki et al.[2] reported marked improvement or complete resolution in 19 out of 35 patients receiving posture instruction for tension myalgia of the PFM. Pressure on the coccyx seems to contribute to the

Box 27.1

Summary of impairments and possible treatments for hypertonus dysfunction[1]

Altered tone of the PFM: muscle spasm and trigger points
Biofeedback for training the PFM to relax
Rhythmic contraction and relaxation of the PFM (quick PFM exercises)
Soft tissue mobilisation, vaginally or rectally
Electrical stimulation on the perineum, vaginally or rectally
Relaxation training, autonomic nervous system balancing
Vaginal or rectal dilators
Ultrasound at the insertion of the PFM at the coccyx
Heat over the perineum

Altered tone of the associated muscles of the hip, buttock and trunk: muscle spasm
Soft tissue mobilisation
Therapeutic exercises for stretching
Modalities such as ultrasound, electrical stimulation, heat, and cold

Muscle impairments and coordination impairments of the associated muscles of the hip, buttock and trunk
Muscle imbalance around the trunk and hip joint
Therapeutic exercises for strengthening and stretching
Coordination training of the muscles around a joint (i.e. around the hip) or between several areas (hip and trunk)

Mobility impairment of scar and connective tissue of the perineum, inner thighs, buttock, and abdominals
Soft tissue mobilisation, scar mobilisation
Visceral mobilisation
Modalities such as ultrasound, heat and microcurrent
Mobility impairments (e.g. hypermobility, hypomobility) of the pelvic joints: sacroiliac, pubic, lumbar, hip and sacrococcygeal joints
Joint mobilisation, muscle energy techniques, strain and counterstrain, craniosacral therapy
Posture and body mechanics education
Therapeutic modalities such as ultrasound, heat, cold, electrical stimulation and
Transcutaneous electrical nerve stimulation (TENS).

Faulty posture leading to undue stress on the pelvic structures
Instruction in proper sitting and standing posture and body mechanics
Use of cushions, lumbar rolls and modified chairs

Pain in the perineum with hypersensitivity of the skin and mucosa
Modalities such as cold, heat, ultrasound and electrical stimulation
Education on avoiding perineal irritants (vaginal creams, douching, laundry detergent, menstrual pads, soaps)

perpetuation of PFM spasm and sacrococcygeal joint dysfunction. The mechanism of this perpetuation is not understood; nonetheless, it is clear that decreasing pressure on the coccyx is necessary for correction of these dysfunctions. In sitting, posterior pelvic tilt markedly increases pressure on the coccyx. Patients should be instructed to sit fully back in the chair with the sacrum pressed against the seat back and both feet flat on the floor (avoiding crossing legs) with a normal lumbar lordosis (use of a lumbar roll is recommended). This sitting position shifts the weight forward onto the ischial tuberosities and posterior thighs and off the coccyx.[1,9] Patients often adopt asymmetrical sitting postures in an attempt to reduce pressure and pain at the tailbone. Faulty sitting postures may also result from torsion asymmetry of the pelvis (forward or backward ilial rotations or sacral asym-

Avoid chairs with excessive cushion and poor support

Avoid hard chairs without a cushion

Doughnut cushions increase pressure on the coccyx and should be avoided by most patients

Doughnut cushions may give some relief for perineal wound pain

Special coccyx cushions increase anterior pelvic tilt and relieve pressure on the coccyx area

Vulvodynia patients typically do not benefit from any special type of cushion

All patients are instructed to change positions frequently

metries). This asymmetry will strain the sacroiliac joints as well as soft tissue structures of the pelvic floor. Patients should have the weight evenly distributed over both ischial tuberosities. (See summary in Box 27.2.)

27.1.3 Recumbent Positions

Restful sleep is essential for all chronic pain patients. A supportive mattress will give the patient better potential to rest in spinal neutral. Patients should be educated in standard positioning for supine, side lying and prone sleeping. No specific position is contraindicated in all patients, although patients will often show preference for one or two postures. Travell and Simons[10] advocate the use of pillows between the knees in side lying with piriformis and quadratus lumborum dysfunction. The pillow(s) should support the uppermost leg with the hip, knee and ankle in the same plane, horizontal to the sleeping surface.

27.1.4 Body Mechanics

Understanding the patient's daily activities will help in body mechanics education. Neutral spine and a symmetrical pelvis are taught during activities of daily living (ADL) to protect the pelvic joints, lumbar joints, hip and trunk muscles. Functional trunk stability education is very useful. These instructions are the same as those given to a back pain patient. It is important to have the patient

perform detailed practise of body mechanics to ensure transfer into daily activity.[11] Loads should be evenly distributed to reduce asymmetrical pull on the trunk. Patients with sacroiliac or pubic symphysis dysfunction should avoid prolonged or repeated unilateral standing and bending. Clinically, patients have reported changes in perineal pain with changes in lumbar alignment during ADL.

27.2 Relaxation and Stress Management

Linton[12] and others have identified the importance of relaxation training in the management of chronic pain. The physiological responses to stress, such as muscle tension and hypertension, are well known. Excessive muscle tension in the PFM, low back and hips is known to be associated with pelvic pain. In many cases it is important that the patient achieves relaxation before other interventions can be effectively applied or carried out (for example, posture adjustments, mobility exercises, strengthening exercises, coordination exercises, etc.). Rest periods with moist heat may be used to achieve relaxation at intervals during the day. Diaphragmatic breathing and progressive relaxation are useful methods of relaxation training. Biofeedback (see Chapter 10) is also helpful in achieving relaxation of specific muscle groups. Relaxation and stress management should be emphasised as part of a healthy lifestyle and must be continued as part of daily routines to manage pelvic pain after discharge. This is particularly true for people with high stress levels or ongoing personal difficulties. Assistance from counselling or psychology professionals may be useful. Referral to complimentary therapists (see Chapters 31–34) for continued care after skilled intervention is complete can minimise recurrences. Consultation with a doctor is necessary if conservative means of relaxation are not gaining the desired effect.

27.2.1 Therapeutic Exercise

A complete evaluation will identify muscles in need of therapeutic exercise. Three categories of exercise are important in pelvic pain patients: general aerobic capacity, trunk stability and muscle balance around the hip. Pain often encourages a sedentary lifestyle, with chronic pain patients becoming very deconditioned. General aerobic exercise helps to enhance overall body health and cardiovascular condition, increase circulation, decrease daily stress and depression, aids in pain relief (due to endorphin release) and can prevent reoccurrence of myofascial pain.[13] Therapists are often challenged to find aerobic exercises that are tolerated by chronic pain patients. Many patients with PFM spasm and vulvodynia find walking to be very helpful in decreasing pain. In some cases, any lower extremity movement increases pain. These patients can exercise aerobically with the upper extremities. Swimming is a good alternative to upright exercise and is tolerated by most patients except those with vulvodynia who are irritated by the chlorinated water.

Trunk stability is necessary for pelvic pain patients. Richardson et al.[14] present EMG studies of the interaction of the PFM with the tranversus abdominis. Poor functioning of the tranversus could disrupt this interaction and result in dysfunction of the PFM. Trunk stability is also necessary for lumbar and pelvic joint alignment, as well as protection of hip and trunk muscles. The Swiss Ball is often used in trunk stability exercise. Bouncing on the ball results in reactive muscle contraction of the PFM.[15] Rhythmical bouncing may enhance PFM relaxation and decrease pain in some patients. However, there is potential for this bouncing to increase PFM spasm. The sitting ball position is similar to the cushion used for coccyx pain and may be helpful in those patients. However, many patients find the pressure on the perineum too great and do not tolerate sitting ball exercise well.

Muscle balance around the hip joint simply means that all the hip muscles are the correct length and strength. Hall[16] provides an excellent reference for exercises to balance the hip and lumbopelvic complex. Single leg standing is a good isometric stability exercise for the hip. Decreased hip rotation is one of the primary biomechanical correlates to pelvic pain.[3]

For continued benefit, patients should be encouraged to adhere to a home exercise programme. Patients should be instructed in a comprehensive programme including posture and body mechanics, relaxation and stress management and therapeutic exercise. Empowering self-pain relief with exercise, positioning or other modalities (to be discussed in detail later in this chapter) gives the patient a sense of control over the pain and increases emotional well-being. Treatment of PFM spasm requires ongoing active participation from the patient.

27.3 Manual Therapies

Using an integrative manual therapy approach, five different treatment philosophies are described in this section and examples of their techniques for

Box 27.3

Summary of manual techniques for pelvic pain

Soft tissue mobilisation
Myofascial release
Visceral mobilisation
Craniosacral therapy
Proprioceptive neuromuscular facilitation
Strain-counterstrain
Muscle energy and joint mobilisation
Manual lymphatic drainage

application to pelvic muscle spasms, dysfunction or pain are presented.

The urogenital tissues are among the most physically stressed in the body, because of the effects of constant internal pressure changes, intestinal or digestive disorders, lumbosacral dysfunction, lower extremity restrictions, emotional or mental holding patterns, menstruation, pregnancy, delivery, menopause or prostate functions. An introduction to connective tissue and the craniosacral system is therefore included here.

Manual therapy has become a highly specialised skill with many diverse modes. Therapists should apply their current skills to this area (see Box 27.3).

27.3.1 Connective Tissue

Complete evaluation often identifies multiple areas of dysfunction that have a relationship to each other. This "relationship" is primarily sustained by connective tissue.

The connective tissue system, the largest tissue system in our body, includes ground substance, elastin, collagen, bone, cartilage, and adipose tissue.[17] Connective tissue is sometimes referred to as a space filler between other tissues, but in reality it is a tissue that houses blood, lymphatic vessels and nerve bundles and stores fat for the nourishment and communication of the other major tissues.

Loose connective tissue or fascia spreads in a three-dimensional web from head to toe. Every muscle, bone, organ, nerve and vessel is wrapped in fascia. The purpose of fascia is to separate, support, bind, connect and defend.

Fascia is frequently overlooked as a potential for dysfunction. However, treatment of fascial restrictions is essential to restoring pain free function. Improved fascial mobility may follow manual

Box 27.4

Effects of fascial mobilisations

An alteration of adhesive/scar tissue matrix

A redistribution of interstitial fluids

Improved lubrication and hydration

The breaking of restrictive intermolecular crosslinking

The mechanical and viscoelastic elongation of existing collagenous tissues through the phenomena of creep

A neuroreflexive response that may alter vascular, muscular and biomechanical factors related to immobility[18]

therapy release techniques as a result of the factors listed in Box 27.4.

27.3.2 Craniosacral System

The craniosacral system is a semi-closed hydraulic system contained within a tough, waterproof membrane (the dura mater) which envelops the brain and spinal cord. Dysfunction in this system has a profound effect on the neurological system as well as on other systems such as the endocrine, respiratory, lymphatic, vascular and musculoskeletal systems.[19] The meningeal membranes are firmly attached to the foramen magnum and sacrum. During treatment, mobilisation of the occiput and sacrum can effect the system's function and the extensibility of the meningeal membranes. The craniosacral system with points of attachment of the dura can be seen in Figure 27.1.

The production, circulation and reabsorption of cerebrospinal fluid within the dura mater produces a continuous rise and fall of fluid pressures within the craniosacral system. Limitation in extensibility of the system results in a build up of pressure and can contribute to dysfunction.[20]

27.3.3 Techniques

Many manual therapy techniques are used on pelvic pain patients. These techniques are difficult to describe and are best learned with practical demonstration and practice.

27.3.3.1 Joint Mobilisation and Manipulation

Skilled passive stretching of accessory joint movements are often indicated in pelvic pain patients with impaired joint mobility in the lumbar spine, hips, pubic symphysis and sacroiliac as well as sacrococcygeal articulations.

Restricted hip rotation and reduced spinal forward bending are common findings in pelvic pain patients.[3] It is important to restore accessory movements in the lumbar spine to achieve full lumbar forward bending in these patients. Joint manipulations to restore lateral glide of the femur restore full hip rotation and stretch the external rotator muscles.

27.3.3.2 Soft Tissue Mobilisation for Levator Ani Syndrome

In patient with levator ani syndrome, digital rectal examination of the levator ani muscles can reproduce sharp pain in the sacral region, myofascial trigger areas, local soreness, tight fibrous bands, decreased fascial glide and a hard end feel of the muscles and fascia. Findings are similar in the PFM of patients with coccygodynia.

Thiele[21] introduced massage of the levator ani and coccygeus muscles via the rectum. This tech-

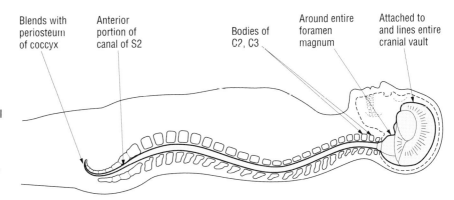

Figure 27.1 The craniosacral system with points of attachment to the dura. [Upledger JE, CranioSacral Therapy 1 study guide. Seattle, Eastland Press, UI Publishing, 1987; 129.]

Blends with periosteum of coccyx

Anterior portion of canal of S2

Bodies of C2, C3

Around entire foramen magnum

Attached to and lines entire cranial vault

nique involves rubbing the muscle fibres from origin to insertion with a stripping motion 10–15 times on each side.[21] Other methods of intravaginal or intrarectal palpation and treatment are listed below and can provide greater specificity in the individual muscles.

The foundational concept of soft tissue mobilisation is to treat according to the specific layer of tissue restriction and direction of motion barrier. The goal is to achieve the desired results while using the least amount of force. Evaluation should determine the three-dimensional direction of tissue fibre restriction. The tissue is compressed to evaluate for depth of dysfunction. Direction of dysfunction is assessed by directing force across the fibres as if touching the numbers on a clock. Dysfunction is noted by restriction of fascial movement; this may or may not be the most painful area. To release a myofascial trigger point, maintain depth and direction on the dysfunctional area. Place sufficient force upon the restriction, in a precise depth, direction and angle to take the dysfunctional tissues to their end range. As the tissue "lets go", follow the pathway of the release. The patient can assist the treatment with conscious relaxation and appropriate feedback. Contraction and relaxation of the pelvic floor muscles with sustained pressure can augment soft tissue mobilisation.

These techniques can be performed on any connective tissue component, including scar tissue. Patients with adhered episiotomies and abdominal scars should be taught these techniques.

27.3.3.3 Visceral Mobilisation for Urethral Syndrome

Healthy organs have physiological motion and need room to expand, displace and rotate with various phases of digestion or elimination. Any restriction, fixation or adhesion to another structure implies functional impairment of the organ.[22] Visceral manipulation restores normal organ movements. During or after inflammation, infection or surgery, the urethra may remain adherent to the vaginal wall or pubourethral ligaments. Urethral syndrome with urethral pain, and urinary frequency with slow and hesitant micturition, can result from these adhesions. Urethral stretching in the longitudinal direction loosens the striated and elastic fibres.

27.3.3.4 Craniosacral Therapy for Pudendal Nerve Entrapment

Pudendal neuralgia is often associated with sacral immobility. Lumbosacral release through traction and subsequent stretching of the dural tube may improve sacral mobility. Lower abdominal tension is

easily treatable with gentle pelvic diaphragm release. This is often an easy way to begin overall tension reduction in the region of the pelvis. Because it is an external technique, it may be the first technique used.

This section has presented a sample of the multitude of effective techniques for pelvic pain. Proficiency in this area requires continued commitment to developing skills. Our tissues carry the knowledge that guides the route of correction and the destination of resolution.

27.4 Modalities for Pelvic Floor Muscle Spasms

The use of modalities to relieve pelvic floor spasm has two main objectives: to directly treat and heal the spasm, and to decrease or mask pain so the patient can participate in activities that will help in the healing of the spasm. It is important to reduce pain immediately, if possible, to give the patient some hope that treatment will be effective. Return to social interactions and an increased feeling of usefulness enhances the patient's psychological well-being and helps to motivate the patient to participate fully in physical therapy treatment. Increased overall activity also increases circulation and decreases time spent in poor recumbent postures. Modalities may also be used before or after manual therapy or exercise. Modalities used before treatment help to prepare the tissue for stretching. Modalities applied after manual treatment or exercise may help to reduce post-treatment soreness. A summary of modalities is given in Table 27.1.

27.4.1 Application of NMES, TENS and Interferential Therapy– External Electrode Placements

A crossing pattern over the sacral nerve roots seems to be the most effective placement for perineal pain, and a crossing pattern over the abdomen is often effective for abdominal pain. Some iliopsoas spasm and trigger points can be treated by placing electrodes unilaterally on the abdomen and back. Placing the electrodes on the perineum, or perianally, often results in unsatisfactory pain relief. Rectal or vaginal electrodes may also be used.

27.4.2 Biofeedback

Early surface electromyography (sEMG) research[40,41] clearly showed that muscle tension may be present

Table 27.1. Modalities for treating pelvic pain

Modality	Uses
Moist heat	Reduce muscle spasms and trigger points[10] Enhance the effects of muscle stretching, scar mobilisation and myofascial treatments[23,24] General muscle soreness and post-exercise soreness Total body warmth and relaxation, decreased sympathetic output
Cold	Acute joint trauma: pubic symphysis, coccyx, sacroiliac Acute perineal swelling: postpartum, haemorrhoids Trigger point referral treatment Muscle spasm, decrease muscle excitability[25] Anaesthetic effects, decreased excitability of free nerve endings Elongation of hip and trunk muscles with spray and stretch method
Ultrasound	Scar pain or adhesions: surgery, episiotomy, trauma,[26–28] before or after massage techniques Muscle spasm and trigger points:[10] (vaginismus, anismus, pelvic girdle muscles, piriformis syndrome,[29] levator ani syndrome[30] Perineal swelling (postpartum, post surgical): haemorrhoids Joint pain: coccygodynia, pubic symphysis disruption Wound healing: episiotomy, surgical
High-voltage pulsed current	Levator ani syndrome[31–34] Muscle fatigue, overstimulation, motor neuron suppression, accommodation, adaptation of CNS pathways[31] Rhythmical contractions, increased blood flow and equalized sarcomere length[10]
NMES, TENS, interferential	Muscle spasm, levator ani syndrome, coccygodynia Generalized pelvic pain, vulvodynia, adhesions, pain gate theory[35] Increase circulation with submotor stimulation Endometriosis, dysmenorrhea,[36] interstitial cystitis[37–39] Muscle strengthening Pain management: increase functional ability, break from the pain during or after exercise for full participation, decrease post treatment soreness
Microcurrent	Trigger points, muscle spasms Scar restriction, painful keloids Fibromyalgia, chronic pain, RSD, sympathetically mediated pain, neuralgia Generalized relaxation
Pulsed electromagnetic energy	Painful perineum after delivery[28]
Iontophoresis	Sacrococcygeal joint pain in coccygodynia
Biofeedback	Muscle re-education and rhythmical contraction: up training and contract relax Enhanced relaxation of a particular muscle: down training Enhanced total body relaxation: decreased sympathetic output

NMES, neuromuscular electrical nerve stimulation; RSD, reflex sympathetic dystrophy (complex regional pain syndrome); TENS, transcutaneous electrical nerve stimulation.

even when the patient or therapists cannot feel it. This is especially true in the PFM, as nerve input is often disrupted. A high resting baseline with high variability and occasional spasms are often seen in pain patients. Ideally the patient will gain the ability to recognise the difference between relaxation and contraction. Using sEMG biofeedback to enhance muscle relaxation is referred to as *down training* (See Box 27.5). Teaching a muscle to relax is often more difficult than teaching it how to contract (*up training*), as the feeling of relaxation is small. Good body awareness and persistence is necessary. Some patients never gain the conscious ability to recognise relaxation, but they can be effectively trained with EMG home trainers (see Chapter 10).

Learned muscle tension refers to high resting tone in a muscle as a result of inappropriate voluntary muscle contraction. DeLancey et al.[42] reported two case studies in which the women created levator ani myalgia by performing excessive PFM exercises to reduce incontinence. Excessive holding of the PFM can lead to spasm. In some cases this excessive resting tone is created unconsciously. Stressful events or thinking about a stressful event may

Box 27.5

Down training methods

1. Practice 20–30 min twice a day. Build relaxation into daily activities
   Many patients need home sEMG units to perform relaxation effectively
   Experiment with several different techniques
2. Diaphragmatic breathing: contraction and relaxation of the respiratory diaphragm can encourage relaxation of the PFM
3. Visualisation – a relaxing place, the ischial tuberosities separating, heavy warmth, a hole getting larger
4. Perineal bulging
   Have patient place a hand over the anal cleft with the middle finger in the cleft
   Gently push out as if expelling gas. The patient should feel the tissues bulge into the finger
   Remind patients to be gentle, not to bear down.
5. Quiet environment, soft music, relaxation audio tapes, low lights, comfortable position, warmth
6. A picture of the muscle may help visually oriented patients to visualise the sagging of a hammock
7. Total body relaxation from head to toes, or toes to head, progressive relaxation
8. Body scanning: patients learn to scan (or bring attention to) the PFM often during the day for stress and tension. When tension is recognised, the patient performs a brief relaxation exercise.
9. Advanced training: progresses to more stressful environmental situations.
   Visualise a stressful event, keep the bright lights on in the treatment room, distract your patient during sEMG practice, relaxation in standing or sitting.
10. Dilator practice
    "Practise" intercourse. External anal electrodes allow the patient to insert the dilator while monitoring the PFM. This give the women control over the situation, she can stop without worrying about her partner's reaction.
    Start by inserting the dilator slowly then progress to moving the dilator, simulating intercourse.
    Visualising her partner during this exercise also helps in the transition to actual intercourse.

Table 27.2. Possible types of vulvodynia

Vulvar vestibulitis	Pain and erythema localised to the vestibule and its glands
Cyclic vulvovaginitis	Vestibule pain which cycles with hormonal changes of menses, pregnancy, oral contraception, and menopause
Dysesthetic vulvodynia	Severe pain in many areas of the perineum and pelvis, often associated with other chronic pelvic pain conditions
Vulvar dermatoses	Non cyclic progressive symptoms usually including itching and burning, visual skin changes are evident although special instrumentation may be needed in some patients, biopsy confirms diagnosis including: squamous cell hyperplasia, lichens sclerosis/ planus, hyperkeratotic changes

trigger excessive tension and eventually spasm. After several painful intercourse experiences, the woman may begin to anticipate that intercourse will hurt. This anticipation often results in muscle contraction, spasm and eventually pain. This cycle perpetuates the muscle dysfunction without conscious awareness. Biofeedback can bring muscle tension to a conscious level and also reverse the effects of excessive learned muscle activity.

Not all vaginal pain is related to PFM spasm and it is important to complete an accurate sEMG evaluation to confirm the presence of PFM spasm. EMG equipment with a band width of 25 Hz or lower is needed to accurately measure microvolt output of

Box 27.6

Possible aetiology of vulvodynia

Difficulty in metabolism of oxylates
Connective tissue changes leading to thin skin
Bacterial vaginosis with pH changes in the vagina
Decreased or absent lactobacilli
Hormone imbalances including oestrogen, thyroid and others
Autoimmune disorders (immunoglobin A)
Pelvic floor muscle instability
Myofascial pain and trigger points
Sympathetically mediated pain

the PFM. If high resting tone is not seen on initial measurement, it may be necessary to simulate the circumstances in which pain occurs (at the end of the day in standing, after lifting or sitting in a certain way). Provoking the muscle with activities of daily living (ADL) may be a more accurate measure of the muscle function.

In conclusion, the use of modalities for pelvic pain can greatly enhance the effect of treatment.

27.5 Vulvodynia

27.5.1 History and Definition

Vulvodynia is a chronic vulvovaginal pain disorder that was noted in the medical literature in the early 1900s and not again for nearly 50 years. Pellisse and Hewitt[43] described similar symptomology in 1976, with numerous articles to follow. In 1983, the Seventh Congress for the International Society for the Study of Vulvar Diseases accepted a standard definition of vulvodynia as "chronic vulvar discomfort, especially that characterised by the patient's complaint of burning, stinging, irritation, or rawness".[44] Studies of the disorder continued and, in 1987, a second diagnostic term, vulvar vestibulitis syndrome (VVS), was suggested as a more appropriate description of the disorder.[45] Friedrich[45] detailed a constellation of symptoms including severe pain on vestibular touch or attempted vaginal entry, tenderness to light pressure localised within the vulvar vestibule, and gross physical findings limited to vestibular erythema of various degrees. In 1989, five subsets of vulvodynia were identified, including vulvar dermatoses, cyclic vulvitis, vulvar papillomatosis, vulvar vestibulitis and essential vulvodynia[46] (see Table 27.2). Vulvar vestibulitis syndrome, cyclic vulvovaginitis, and dysesthetic vulvodynia ("dysesthetic" replaced "essential" in 1995) have recently been sited as those most commonly seen.[47] It is widely agreed that all disorders are multifactorial problems, aetiologically and psychologically.[48]

27.5.2 Aetiology

The aetiology of vulvar dermatoses are often clearly identifiable; however, most types of vulvodynia are considered idiopathic with many possible aetiologies. Onset of symptoms may occur after yeast infection, sexually transmitted diseases such as chlamydia or human papilloma virus, vulvar or pelvic surgery, a stressful period of time, or pregnancy. Testing of vulvodynia patients has identified conditions that may be possible aetiologies (see Box 27.6).

Patients are often sensitive to environmental irritants, which may also be related to the aetiology of the condition.[49-52] Glazer et al.[53] have proposed a theory based on instability of the PFM. They propose that the original insult (whatever that may be) results in an unstable resting tone. Unstable tone can be seen on an EMG tracing as increased "jumpiness".

Some EMG manufactures have included standard deviation as a measure of instability, thus making it easy to quantify this measure and track improvements. The theory goes on to state that PFM instability perpetuates irritated nerve impulses which in turn cause physiological changes related to pain in the vestibule.

27.5.3 Prevalence

Diagnostic criteria for vulvodynia are complex and poorly standardised. This makes prevalence studies difficult to compare. Goetsch[54] reported that at one clinical site 15% of all gynecological patients seen in a 6-month period were found to satisfy the diagnosis of VVS. Denbow and Byrne[55] found 13% of consecutive new patients attending a genitourinary medicine clinic were found to have vulvar pain, with more than half (55%) demonstrating candidiasis, 20% diagnosed with genital herpes and only two of the five with no active infections were diagnosed with VVS.

The National Vulvodynia Association is a nonprofit organisation run by lay people to provide support and information to women with vulvar pain. The association has no way of knowing if these women have vulvodynia, but the current membership of this organisation is approximately 2000 (with about 80 international members). The group receives approximately 1800 hits per month on their web site and 400 phone and mail inquiries per month for further information.

27.5.4 Clinical Presentation

Multiple chronic pain syndromes are often present in vulvodynia patients. Some practitioners feel there is a relationship between vulvodynia, interstitial cystitis, irritable bowel syndrome and fibromyalgia.[48]

The National Vulvodynia Association reported in 1997[56] on a survey of 500 of their membership diagnosed with either VVS or dysesthetic vulvodynia. There was an age range of 12 to 90 years (mean 43 years). The average onset of vulvar pain was 5 years and they had all consulted at least five physicians. Forty-three per cent had other concurrent chronic pain syndromes, and 58% suffered with low back pain. Irritable bowel syndrome and interstitial cystitis was suffered by 51% and sexual functioning was markedly impaired in more than 60%.

Clinically, the physical therapist will most likely see women diagnosed with either vulvar vestibulitis syndrome or dysesthetic vulvodynia, as other vulvar pathologies (as identified in the subsets above) are successfully diagnosed and treated medically.

27.5.4.1 Vulvar Vestibulitis Syndrome

Patients with VVS often complain of varying degrees of dyspareunia (painful intercourse) and an inability to use tampons. Often, there is a complaint of vaginal pain and pressure when wearing tight-fitting jeans, or of an inability to ride a bicycle or horse. Other activities of daily living may not be affected by the symptoms. Physical evaluation findings are localised to the vestibule with severe

pain to light touch (the cotton swab test) at 3 and 9 o'clock. Erythema is also noted at the vestibule and gland openings.

27.5.4.2 Dysesthetic Vulvodynia

Patients with dysesthetic vulvodynia present with complex case histories, often reporting a number of associated and pre-existing chronic pain disorders. Patients' symptoms are often more severe than in VVS, including dyspareunia, an inability to wear tight-fitting clothes, limitation in social activities, and inability to work, sit or stand for any length of time as a result of severe vaginal pain. Patients describe the symptoms with words like "stabbing", "burning", "itching", or "throbbing" occurring in and around the

a Threshold determination: assessment of one (10s) contraction

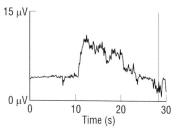

	Avg	Std Dev
Rest 1	4.0 µV	0.2 µV
Work	8.5 µV	1.0 µV
Rest 2	3.6 µV	1.0 µV

| Ch1 threshold: | 4.4 mV |
| Ch1 duration of 40 % peak: | 9.4 s |

b Assessment of four work/rest cycles (work: 5 s, rest: 5 s)

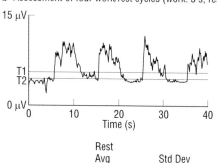

	Rest Avg	Std Dev	Work Avg	Std Dev	Peak
Channel 1	4.2 µV	0.2 µV	8.2 µV	1.1 µV	11.7 µV

Ch1 average onset:	0.6 s
Ch1 average release:	5.0 s
Ch1 %time above threshold:	100.0 %

Figure 27.2 Before treatment sEMG recordings.

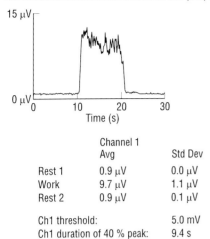

a Threshold determination: assessment of one (10s) contraction

	Channel 1 Avg	Std Dev
Rest 1	0.9 μV	0.0 μV
Work	9.7 μV	1.1 μV
Rest 2	0.9 μV	0.1 μV

Ch1 threshold:	5.0 mV
Ch1 duration of 40 % peak:	9.4 s

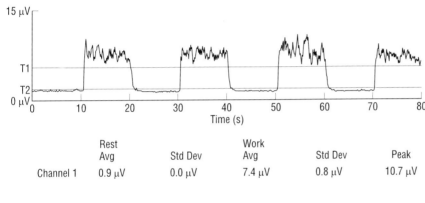

b Assessment of four work/rest cycles (work: 10 s, rest: 10 s)

	Rest Avg	Std Dev	Work Avg	Std Dev	Peak
Channel 1	0.9 μV	0.0 μV	7.4 μV	0.8 μV	10.7 μV

Ch1 average onset:	0.7 s
Ch1 average release:	0.6 s
Ch1 %time above threshold:	100.0 %

Figure 27.3 After treatment sEMG recordings.

vaginal opening. Historically, reports of chronic vaginal yeast or urinary tract infections are common. In many cases, these patients have seen many healthcare professionals who have attempted diagnosis and treatment, and, all too often, fallen short of both. In contrast to the VVS patients, these patients have widespread dysfunction with multiple musculoskeletal dysfunctions of the pelvis and lumbar spine, trigger points in many hip and trunk muscles as well as pelvic floor muscle dysfunction and vestibular pain.

27.5.5 Physical Therapy Assessment

The physical assessment of both groups begins with a complete examination of historical events, beginning with pertinent past history. By utilising a detailed and in depth questioning procedure, factors possibly lending to the disorders may become apparent, helping to lead the therapist in the appropriate direction for treatment of the cause of the problem, rather than treatment of the symptoms alone. A comprehensive assessment (as described in the assessment section of this chapter) is essential for vulvodynia.

27.5.6 Vulvar Assessment

The vulvar region should be checked visually as well as physically for erythema, oedema and discharge, and for sensitivity to pressure or to light touch. The presence of inflammation in the vestibule should be noted. Be aware, however, that the presence or intensity of the inflammation may not be in proportion to the subjective complaints. Sensory testing should be performed in the saddle area. This can be accomplished using a cotton-tipped swab applied to dermatomal regions and compared bilaterally. Reflex testing should also be completed by brief stroking of the clitoris (bulbocavernosus reflex) and of the perineal body (anal wink). A normal response to both would be a visual and reflexive contraction of the superficial pelvic floor vaginally and anally, respectively.

Physicians often perform a cotton swab test, assessing for presence of pain within the vestibule. This is performed using a moistened swab. Pressure is exerted at the introitus in three areas (3, 6, and 9 o'clock, where the clitoris indicates 12 o'clock). A positive test is recorded when the patient complains of pain with gentle inward pressure.

27.5.7 Physical Therapy Treatment

Awareness of the patient as a whole is essential when treating vulvar pain. Therapists should work in a team, realising the limitations of only treating mechanical dysfunctions and musculoskeletal imbalances. Appropriate referrals are especially important in vulvodynia. Treatment of this difficult group of patients follows the impairments identified during the initial assessment, as noted earlier in this chapter. Attention must first begin with the correction of abnormal postures, both sitting and standing, and of problematic gait patterns. Joint restrictions should be noted, with appropriate therapeutic exercises and manual treatment prescribed.

Visceral restrictions should be addressed both externally and internally.[22] External visceral release also begins to address the additional problems of bladder and bowel irritability and spasm. Vaginal and rectal therapeutic approaches can prove to be highly effective. Internal techniques include myofascial release, soft tissue mobilisation, muscle reeducation, sEMG and urogenital mobilisation.

Multiple modalities are appropriate for use in this population, including biofeedback, TENS and ultrasound. Surface EMG biofeedback has been successfully used in the treatment of vulvar vestibulitis syndrome.[53] Glazer et al.[53] instruct the patient in twice-daily exercises that renew the strength, stability, and resting tone of the PFM (Figures 27.2 and 27.3). Patients are encouraged to maintain a steady contraction of the PFM. This protocol involves long-term (6–10 months) of work with an EMG home trainer.

References

1. Shelly B (1999) The pelvic floor. In: Hall C, Thein Brody L (ed) Therapeutic Exercises: Moving toward function. Lippincott Williams & Wilkins, Philadelphia, Pa.
2. Sinaki M, Merrit J, Stillwell GK (1977) Tension myalgia of the pelvic floor. Mayo Clin Proc 52: 717–22.
3. King PM, Myers CA, Ling FW et al. (1991) Musculoskeletal factors in chronic pelvic pain. J Psychom Obstet Gynaecol 12: 87–98.
4. Slocumb JC (1984) Neurological factors in chronic pelvic pain syndrome. Am J Obstet Gynecol 149: 536.
5. Peters AA, Dorst E van, Jellis B et al. (1991) A randomized clinical trail to compare two different approaches in women with chronic pelvic pain. Obstet Gynecol 77: 5.
6. Hunter W, Zihlman AL (1970) Abdominal pain from strain of intrapelvic muscles. Clin Orthop Rel Res 130: 279.
7. Paradis H, Marganoff H (1969) Rectal pain of extrarectal origin. Dis Colon Rectum 12: 306.
8. Caldwell G (1951) Minor injuries of the lumbar spine and coccyx. Surg Clin North Am 31: 1345.
9. Livingstone L (1998) Post-natal management. In: Sapsford R, Bullock-Saxton J, Markwell (eds) Women's Health: a text book for physiotherapists. WB Saunders, London.
10. Travell JG, Simons DG (1992) Myofascial Pain and Dysfunction, Vols 1 and 2. Williams & Wilkins, Baltimore, Md..
11. Linton SJ (1994) Activities training and physical therapy. Behav Med 20(3): 105–11.
12. Linton SJ (1994) Chronic back pain: integrating psychological and physical therapy: an overview. Behav Med 20: 3.101–4.
13. Costello K (1998) Myofascial syndromes. In: Steege JF, Metzger DA, Levy BS (eds) Chronic Pelvic Pain: An integrated approach. WB Saunders, Philadelphia, pp. 251–66.
14. Richardson C, Jull G, Hodges P, Hides J (1999) Therapeutic exercises for spinal segmental stabilization in low back pain. Churchill Livingstone, Edinburgh, pp. 52–3.
15. Carriere B (1998) The Swiss Ball. Springer-Verlag, Berlin.
16. Hall C (1999) Therapeutic exercises for the lumbopelvic region and the hip. In: Hall CM, Thein Brody L (eds) Therapeutic Exercises: moving toward function. Lippincott Williams & Wilkins, Philadelphia, Pa.
17. Williams PL, Warwick R (1980) Gray's Anatomy (36th ed). Churchill Livingstone, Edinburgh, UK.
18. Johnson G (1991) Soft tissue mobilization. In: White AH, Anderson R (ed) Conservative Care of Low Back Pain. William & Wilkins, Baltimore, Md.
19. Barnes JF (1989) Myofascial Release 1. The Myofascial Release Treatment Centers and Seminars, Paoli.
20. Upledger J, Vredevoogd JD (1983) Craniosacral Therapy. Eastland Press, Seattle, Wa.
21. Thiele GH (1963) Coccygodynia: cause and treatment. Dis Colon Rectum 6: 422–36.
22. Barral JP (1993) Urogenital Manipulation. Eastland Press, Seattle, Wa.
23. Micklovitz SL (1990) Thermal Agents in Rehabilitation, 2nd ed. FA Davis, Philadelphia.
24. Prentice W (1998) Therapeutic Modalities for Allied Health Professionals. McGraw-Hill, New York.
25. Creates V (1987) A study of ultrasound treatment to the painful perineum after childbirth. Physiotherapy 73(4): 162–5.
26. Everett T, McIntosh J, Grant A (1992) Ultrasound therapy for persistent post-natal perineal pain and dyspareunia. Physiotherapy 78(4): 163–7.

27. Ferguson HN (1981) Ultrasound for the damaged perineum. Newsletter, Association of Chartered Physiotherapists in Obstetrics and Gynaecology, London.

28. Grant A, Sleep J, McIntosh J, Amherst H (1989) Ultrasound and pulsed electromagnetic energy treatment for perineal trauma: a randomized placebo-controlled trial. Br J Obstet Gynecol 4: 434–9.

29. Hallin RP (1983) Sciatic pain and the piriformis muscle. Postgrad Med 74: 69–72.

30. Lilius HG, Valtonen EJ (1973) The levator ani spasm syndrome: a clinical analysis of 31 cases. Ann Chiropractic Gynecol Fenn 62: 93–7.

31. Sohn N, Weinstein MA, Robbins RD (1982) The levator syndrome and its treatment with high volt electrogalvanic stimulation. Am J Surg 144(11): 580–2.

32. Nicosia JF, Abcarian J (1985) Levator syndrome: a treat that works. Dis Colon Rectum 28: 406–8.

33. Morris L, Newton RA (1997) Use of high voltage pulsed galvanic stimulation for patients with levator ani syndrome. Phys Ther 67(10): 1522–5.

34. Oliver GC, Rubin RJ, Salvati EP, Eisenstat JE (1985) Electrogalvanic stimulation in the treatment of levator ani syndrome. Dis Colon Rect 28: 662–3.

35. Melzack R, Wall P (1965) Pain mechanisms: a new theory. Science 150: 971–9.

36. Daywood MY, Raymos J (1990) Transcutaneous electrical nerve stimulation for treatment of primary dysmenorrhea: a randomized cross over comparison with placebo TENS and ibuprofen. Obstet Gynecol 75(4): 656–60.

37. Fall M (1987) Transcutaneous electrical nerve stimulation in interstitial cystitis. Urology 29 (Suppl)(4): 40–2.

38. Fall M (1985) Conservative management of chronic interstitial cystitis: trancutanous electrical nerve stimulation and transurethral resection. J Urol 133: 774–8.

39. Fall M, Carlsson C, Erlandson B (1980) Electrical stimulation in interstitial cystitis. J Urol 123: 192–5.

40. Basmajian JV (1979) Muscles Alive. William & Wilkins, Baltimore, Md.

41. Basmajian JV (1983) Biofeedback: Principles and practice for clinicians (2nd ed.). William & Wilkins, Baltimore, Md.

42. DeLancey JO, Sampselle CM, Purch MR (1993) Kegel dyspareunia: levator ani myalgia caused by overexertion. Obstet Gynecol 82: 658–9.

43. Pellisse M, Hewitt J (1976) Erythematous vulvitis enplaques. Proceedings of the Third Congress of the International Society for the Study of Vulvar Disease, 1976, Cocoyoc.

44. ISSVD (1984) Burning Vulvar Syndrome: Report of the ISSVD. J Reprod Med 29: 457.

45. Friedrich EG Jr (1987) Vulvar vestibulitis syndrome. J Reprod Med 32(2): 110–14.

46. McKay M (1989) Vulvodynia: a multifactorial clinical problem. Arch Derm 125(2): 256–62.

47. Paavonen J (1995) Vulvodynia: a complex syndrome of vulvar pain. Acta Obstet Gynecol Scand 74(4): 243–7.

48. Steege JF, Metzger DA, Levy BA (1998) Chronic Pelvic Pain: An integrated approach. WB Saunders, Philadelphia.

49. Marinoff S (1991) Vulvar vestibulitis syndrome: an overview. Am J Obstet Gynecol 165: 1228–33.

50. Spadt S (1995) Suffering in silence: Managing vulvar pain patients. Contemporary Nurse Practitioner Nov/Dec.

51. Secor M (1992) Vulvar vestibulitis syndrome. Nurse Practitioner Forum 3(3): 161–8.

52. Gordon DD, Hutchison C (1999) Clinical management of vulvodynia. Clin Obstet Gynecol 42(2): 221–33.

53. Glazer HI, Rodke G, Swencionis C, Hertz R, Young AW (1995) Treatment of vulvar vestibulitis syndrome with electromyographic biofeedback of pelvic floor musculature. J Reprod Med 40(4): 283–90.

54. Goetsch MF (1996) Simplified surgical revision of the vulvar vestibule for vulvar vestibulitis. Am J Obstet Gynecol 174(6): 1701–6.

55. Denbow ML, Byrne MA (1998) Prevalence, causes and outcome of vulvar pain in a genitourinary medicine clinic population. Int J STD AIDS 9(2): 88–91.

56. National Vulvodynia Association (1997) Report. National Vulvodynia Association, PO Box 4491, Silver Springs, Md.

V Pelvic Organ Prolapse

28 Background

C.A. Glowacki and L.L. Wall

28.1 Definitions

- *Genital prolapse* or *pelvic organ prolapse* refers to a loss of fibromuscular support of the pelvic viscera that results in a vaginal protrusion. The prolapse is usually described according to the area of the vagina in which it occurs.

- An *anterior vaginal prolapse* generally involves the bladder (*cystocele*), and often involves hypermobility of the urethrovesical junction as well (*cystourethrocele*).

- A *posterior vaginal prolapse* often involves protrusion of the rectum into the vaginal canal (*rectocele*) and/or protrusion of a loop of small bowel in a peritoneal sac (enterocele).

- *Procidentia* refers to a complete protrusion of the uterus and vagina.

- The term *vaginal vault prolapse* refers to a complete or partial inversion of the vaginal apex, most commonly occurring in patients who have had a hysterectomy.

- The term *pseudorectocele* was introduced to describe an inadequate or defective perineum resulting in exposure of the midportion of the posterior vaginal wall. It mimics the appearance of a rectocele, but does not involve creation of a rectal pouch that incorporates both the rectal and vaginal walls with loss of vaginal rugation.

- An *enterocele* is the herniation of a peritoneal sac (usually filled with small bowel) through the vaginal apex. An enterocele may be further classified as a traction enterocele or a pulsion enterocele.

- A traction *enterocele* is a protrusion of the posterior cul-de-sac that is pulled down by the prolapsing cervix or vaginal cuff.

- A pulsion *enterocele* is a protrusion of the cul-de-sac through the vagina resulting from chronically increased intra-abdominal pressure. Pulsion enteroceles are frequently large and always contain small bowel. Enteroceles are usually encountered as they dissect through the rectovaginal septum, but may also occur in the space between the bladder and anterior vaginal wall.[1]

28.2 Prevalence

Estimates suggest that 50% of parous women have some degree of genital prolapse, but only 10–20% seek evaluation and treatment for their condition.[2] Most women with prolapse are parous; nulliparous women account for only 2% of prolapse cases in North America. The incidence and prevalence of prolapse increases with age, and 29% of women who undergo repair will subsequently undergo another operation. Factors which predispose women of all ethnic groups to the development of prolapse include vaginal delivery, chronic increases in intra-abdominal pressure, obesity, cigarette smoking, advancing age and oestrogen deficiency.[3-6] A strong family history of genital prolapse is also a risk factor, and this is probably related to differences in collagen structure in different subpopulations.[4] Pelvic trauma and pelvic surgery may damage the neurovascular structures, connective tissue and muscles of the pelvic floor, and vaginal delivery leads to stretching, dislocation, tearing and avulsion of pelvic tissues. Neurological injury to the pudendal nerve may also occur, as has been demonstrated in women with stress incontinence and pelvic organ prolapse.[7,8] There is some evidence that women who had an episiotomy or a perineal laceration at delivery were less likely to develop urinary stress incontinence or pelvic organ prolapse, perhaps by directing obstetric trauma in other directions. Chronic straining may also damage the pudendal nerve and lead to subsequent pelvic floor dysfunction by compromising neuromusular function.[9]

Post-hysterectomy vaginal vault prolapse is a distressing and increasingly common problem. It may occur following vaginal or abdominal hysterectomy and often results from inattention to the proper reconstruction of vaginal apex support following removal of the uterus.[10]

28.3 Symptomatology

Pelvic organ prolapse can present with many symptoms, depending on the organs involved. The most frequent symptom is a complaint of a protrusion or "bulge" from the vagina that worsens with prolonged standing or walking. In some cases the prolapse may be large enough to impair ambulation. Other common symptoms include low back pain, urinary incontinence, voiding difficulty and difficulty emptying the rectum. Changes in the vaginal epithelium are frequently present in women with prolapse. In younger women the vaginal skin may be hypertrophic, but in older women it will be atrophic, particularly if they are not receiving oestrogen replacement therapy.[11] Patients may report impaired faecal evacuation, faecal incontinence, or a need to reduce or manually "splint" the prolapse in order to empty the rectum.[12,13]

Sexual dysfunction may also be present in women with prolapse due to alterations in vaginal anatomy and pelvic organ function. Although most sexually active women with prolapse have sexual function that is comparable to women of similar age without prolapse, advanced forms of prolapse may interfere with coitus on a purely mechanical basis.

28.4 Anatomy and Physiology

The endopelvic fascia, attaching the bladder, uterus, vagina and rectum to the pelvic side walls, is a fibrous connective tissue layer extending diffusely throughout the pelvic floor to form a continuous sheet-like mesentery. It is subdivided into the parametrium and paracolpium. The parametrium consists of the cardinal and uterosacral ligaments, which provide part of the structural support of the uterus. These so-called "ligaments" are really only two different parts of a single mass of loose tissue. The paracolpium attaches the upper two-thirds of the vagina to the pelvic wall and is continuous with

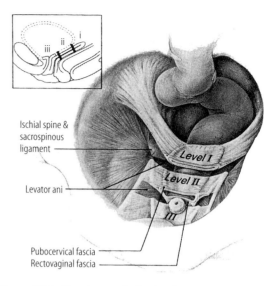

Figure 28.1 The three main levels of vaginal support. [From Delancey JOL Anatomic aspects of vaginal eversion. Am J Obstet Gynecol 166; 1992: 1719.]

the parametrium when the uterus is in situ. It helps suspend the vaginal apex after hysterectomy. The vagina has three main levels of support:[10]

- Level I support includes the vaginal apex and the paracervical vagina, which is suspended by the long connective tissue fibres of the superior paracolpium (see Figure 28.1).
- The midportion of the vagina (level II) is attached laterally, stretching between the bladder and the rectum and supported by the inferior portion of the paracolpium. At this level the anterior vaginal wall and the endopelvic fascia merge to form the pubocervical fascia, which underlies the bladder. Posteriorly, the endopelvic fascia merges with the posterior vaginal wall to form the rectovaginal fascia. This layer prevents the rectum from protruding through the posterior vaginal wall.
- The lowest portion of the vagina (level III) is found at the vaginal introitus and has no intervening paracolpium to suspend it. At this level the vagina fuses directly with the levator ani muscles laterally, the urethra anteriorly and the perineum posteriorly.

Injury to the suspensory fibres at level I may result in vaginal and uterine prolapse and enterocele formation. Damage to the pubocervical fascia or rectovaginal fascia (the supportive fibres of level II), leads to the development of cystocele and rectocele, respectively. Injury often occurs at both levels and results in a combination of defects. Another import-

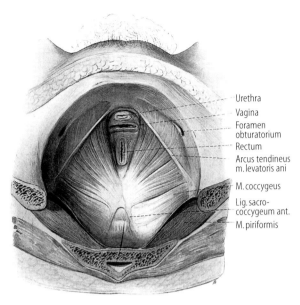

Figure 28.2   The levator ani muscles. Also demonstrated is the arcus fascia tendineus pelvis. [From Peham HV, Amreich J (ed), Operative Gynecology, JB Lippincott, Philadelphia, p 167.]

ant component of the pelvic floor is the levator ani muscles, which may be subdivided into a pubo-coccygeal or 'pubovisceral' portion, and an iliococcygeal portion (see Figures 28.2 and 28.3, and Chapter 2).

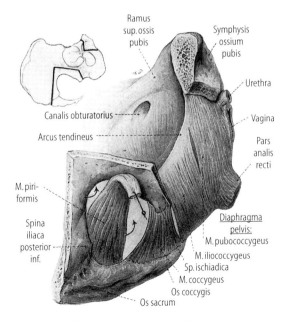

Figure 28.3   The pubococcygeal and iliococcygeal portions of the levator ani muscles. [From Anson BJ, An Atlas of Human Anatomy. WB Saunders, Orlando, 1950, p 367.]

28.5 Aetiology and Pathophysiology

Pelvic floor dysfunction and genital prolapse result from the interaction of many different aetiological factors. Bonney suggested that prolapse originates from a process similar to that used by a surgical scrub nurse who must evert the invaginated finger of a surgical glove. By compressing the air within the glove, the invaginated finger is forced outwards. In a similar way, increases in intraabdominal pressure may force the uterus and vagina to prolapse if their supports are defective.[14]

DeLancey, inspired by Bonney, suggests that the uterus and vagina are maintained in their normal position by three mechanical principles:

- First, the endopelvic fascia suspends the uterus and vagina through its attachments to the pelvic side walls.
- Secondly, the levator ani forms an occlusive and supportive layer on which the pelvic organs rest.
- This anatomic structure creates a flap-valve effect, which is the third mechanical force at work in maintaining normal pelvic support.

Suspended by the endopelvic fascia, the uterus and vagina rest against the adjacent supporting wall. Increases in abdominal pressure force the pelvic organs against the wall, pinning them in place.

These principles can be visualised at work by thinking of the uterus and vagina as analogous to a boat in a dry dock (Figure 28.4). The uterus and

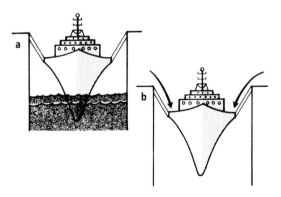

Figure 28.4   **a** The uterus and vagina (the boat) anchored in place by the pelvic ligaments and endopelvic fascia (the mooring), supported by the pelvic musculature (the water). **b** Defects in or weakening of the pelvic floor musculature may strain the ligaments beyond their capacity to support the uterus and vagina. [From Norton PA (1993) Pelvic Floor Disorders: The Role of Fascia and Ligaments. JB Lippincott, Philadelphia, p 927.]

vagina (the boat) are anchored in place by the ligaments and endopelvic fascia, which serve as a mooring to keep them from drifting out of place, but the real support is provided by the musculature, analogous to the water under the boat. If the moorings are cut or stretched the boat will be displaced. If the water level drops, the moorings are strained past their capacity to support the boat. Although gynaecological surgeons tend to think of ligaments as the main factors important in pelvic organ support, the real bulk of the work is done by the muscles of the pelvic floor. Injury to these structures predisposes women to the development of pelvic organ prolapse.[15]

The levator ani muscles are critical in pelvic floor support. These muscles maintain a constant basal tone that maintains the uterus and vagina in place. Above the levator ani, the ligaments and fascia stabilise the organs in position. Constant adjustments in muscular activity prevent the stretching of the pelvic ligaments. Contraction of the pubovisceral muscle pulls the rectum toward the pubic bone, closing the urogenital hiatus and compressing the urethra, vagina and uterus. The pelvic floor should be seen as a dynamic trampoline that is constantly expanding and contracting in response to changing stimuli, rather than a static slab.[16] The levator muscles contract reflexively during periods of increased intra-abdominal pressure (coughing, sneezing, etc.). In this process the urethra, vagina and rectum are compressed against the levator plate, maintaining their normal positions in the pelvis. Any stretching or laceration of the levator muscles or endopelvic fascia can result in widening of the urogenital hiatus and a rotation in the axis of the levator plate with the subsequent development of a predisposition to uterine or vaginal prolapse.

Connective tissue, which holds the body together, is composed primarily of collagen and elastin.[15] Over 12 different types of collagen have been identified; type I collagen is the most common.[17] It forms large strong fibres and is found in large amounts in ligaments, fascia and tendons. Type II collagen is more prone to degradation by collagenase and is found in higher proportions in flexible tissues such as skin, blood vessels, uterus and fascia.

The ligaments and fascia of the pelvic floor contain visceral connective tissue, which provides a flexible capsule for the pelvic organs. The visceral connective tissue contains important neurovascular structures, smooth muscle cells, elastin and collagen. The connective tissue of the supportive ligaments of the uterus (the cardinal and uterosacral) is similar to that of vessel walls. Ligaments such as the arcus tendineus fascia pelvis or the iliopectineal (Cooper's) ligament are composed of stronger, more fibrinous collagen. Collagen abnormalities have been found to be more common among patients with pelvic floor dysfunction and genital prolapse than among normal women without these problems.[18] This strongly suggests that intrinsic collagen abnormalities ("poor tissue") are involved as one factor in the development of disorders of pelvic support.

References

1. Harris TA, Bent AE (1990) Genital prolapse with and without urinary incontinence. J Reprod Med 35: 792–8.
2. Beck RP (1983) Pelvic relaxational prolapse. In: Kase NG, Weingold AB (ed) Principles and Practice of Clinical Gynecology. John Wiley & Sons, New York, p. 677.
3. Smith AR, Hosker GL, Warrel DW (1989) The role of partial denervation of the pelvic floor in the aetiology of genitourinary prolapse and stress incontinence of urine: a neurophysiological study. Br J Obstet Gynaecol 96: 24–8.
4. Davila GW (1996) Vaginal prolapse: Management with non-surgical techniques. Postgrad Med 99: 171–6.
5. Dwyer PL, Lee ETC, Hay DM (1988) Obesity and urinary incontinence in women. Br J Obstet Gynaecol 95: 91–6.
6. Bump RC, McClish DK (1992) Cigarette smoking and urinary incontinence in women. Am J Obstet Gynecol 167: 1213–18.
7. Wall LL (1999) Childbirth trauma and the pelvic floor: Lessons from the developing world. J Women's Health 8: 149–55.
8. Gilpin SA, Gosling JA, Smith ARB, Warrell DW (1989) The pathogenesis of genitourinary prolapse and stress incontinence of urine. A histological and histochemical study. Br J Obstet Gynaecol 96: 15–23.
9. Wall LL (1993) The muscles of the pelvic floor. Clin Obstet Gynecol 36(4): 910–25.
10. DeLancey JOL (1992) Anatomic aspects of vaginal eversion after hysterectomy. Am J Obstet Gynecol 166: 1717–24.
11. Fidas A, MacDonald HL, Elton RA et al. (1989) Prevalence of spina bifida occulta in patients with functional disorders of the lower urinary tract and its relation to urodynamic and neurophysiological measurements. BMJ 298: 357–9.
12. Nager CW, Kumar D, Kahn MA, Stanton S (1997) Management of pelvic floor dysfunction. Lancet 350: 1751.
13. Jackson SL, Weber AM, Hull TL, et al (1997) Fecal incontinence in women with urinary incontinence and pelvic organ prolapse. Obstet Gynecol 89: 423–7.
14. Bonney V (1934) The priniciple that should underlie all operations for prolapse. J Obstet Gynaecol Br Emp 4: 669–83.
15. Norton PA (1993) Pelvic floor disorders: the role of fascia and ligaments. Clin Obstet Gynecol 36: 926–38.
16. Huguosson C, Juroff H, Lingman G, Jacobsson B (1991) Morphology of the pelvic floor. Lancet 337: 367.
17. Lapiere C, Nusgens B, Pierard G (1997) Interaction between collagen type I and type III in conditioning bundles organization. Connect Tiss Res 5: 21–9.
18. Norton P, Boyd C, Deak S (1992) Abnormal collagen ratios in women with genitourinary prolapse. Neurourol Urodyn 11(2): 300–1.

29 Evaluation of Prolapse

C.A. Glowacki and L.L. Wall

The evaluation and classification of pelvic organ prolapse is a crucial component in the initial assessment of the patient. An accurate initial description of pelvic anatomy allows observers to assess the stability or progression of prolapse over time, and also allows an accurate assessment of treatment outcomes. This is particularly important in evaluating the outcome of surgical operations designed to correct pelvic organ prolapse. The International Continence Society (ICS) has developed a standardised system for describing the anatomic position of the pelvic organs to allow reproducibility and comparison of physical examinations and establishment of the clinical significance of different grades of prolapse.[1] It utilises clear anatomic reference points defined in terms of vaginal wall segments rather than the organs lying behind the vagina. The hymeneal ring provides an easily identifiable fixed landmark, even though the actual plane of the hymen may vary according to the degree of levator ani dysfunction. Six defined points in the anterior, superior and posterior vagina are located in reference to the hymen and measured in centimetres (Figure 29.1). A negative number denotes a point proximal to the hymeneal ring. For example, –2 indicates a point 2 cm above the hymeneal ring. A positive number indicates a point protruding beyond the hymen. Measurements are made with a ruler or appropriately marked measurement device such as a cotton-tipped swab.

The first two points are located on the anterior vaginal wall. Point Aa is 3 cm proximal to the external urethral meatus in the midline. It corresponds approximately to the "urethrovesical crease", which is often obliterated in postmenopausal patients. Its measurement ranges between –3 and +3. Point Ba, the second anterior vaginal wall point, represents the most distal or dependent portion of the upper vaginal wall from the anterior vaginal fornix or the posthysterectomy vaginal cuff. In the absence of vaginal prolapse it is approximately 3 cm proximal to point Aa.

Two additional points are identified on the superior vagina. Point C represents the most distal edge of the cervix or the vaginal cuff in the posthysterectomy patient. In a woman with a cervix, point D indicates the position of the posterior fornix or pouch of Douglas at the level of the uterosacral ligaments. Comparison between points C and D allows differentiation between cervical elongation and suspensory failure of the uterosacral-cardinal ligament complex (possible enterocele). Elongation of point C in comparison with point D indicates cervical elongation.

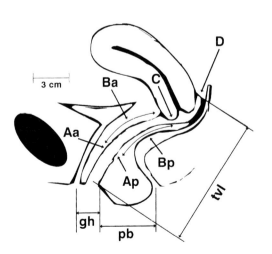

Figure 29.1   The six points (Aa, Ba, C, D, Ap, Bp), total vaginal length (tvl), genital hiatus (gh) and perineal body (pb) utilised in quantification of pelvic organ prolapse. From Bump RC, Mattiasson A, Bø K et al. The standardization of terminology of female pelvic organ prolapse and pelvic floor dysfunction. Am J Obstet Gynecol 1996; 175:12.

The points along the posterior vaginal wall are analogous to those of the anterior vaginal wall. Point Ap is in the midline 3 cm proximal to the hymenal ring. As with point Aa, it ranges from –3 cm to +3 cm relative to the hymen. The most distal or dependent portion of the upper posterior vaginal wall is point Bp. In the nonprolapsed vagina, point Bp is approximately 3 cm superior to point Ap.

Additional measurements, also in centimetres, include the genital hiatus, the perineal body, and the total vaginal length. The distance between the middle of the external urethral meatus to the posterior midline hymen is the genital hiatus. The firm palpable tissue of the perineal body is used as a reference point if the location of the hymeneal ring is unclear. The length of the perineal body is measured from the posterior midline hymeneal ring (the posterior margin of the genital hiatus) to the midanal opening. The total vaginal length is the greatest depth of the vaginal canal in its normal position.

Although this system may appear complicated at first sight, it is easy to use in practice. Understanding the system is greatly aided by an instructional videotape.[2] Once the quantitative description of the prolapse has been completed, a stage may be assigned according to ICS criteria. Allowance is made for the distensibility of the vagina and the inherent imprecision in the measurement of vaginal length by allowing a 2 cm buffer. The ICS defines five stages of prolapse, as follows:

Stage 0:   No prolapse is demonstrated. Points Aa, Ba, Ap, and Bp are all at –3 cm. Point C or D is between the total vaginal length or the total vaginal length minus 2 cm.

Stage I   The most distal portion of the prolapse is >1 cm above the hymeneal plane.

Stage II   The most distal portion of the prolapse is ≤1 cm proximal or distal to the hymen.

Stage III   The most distal portion of the prolapse is >1 cm below the level of the hymen, protruding no greater than 2 cm less than the total vaginal length.

Stage IV   Complete eversion of the total vaginal length, protruding at least ≥2 cm less than the total vaginal length (TVL – 2). Generally, the leading edge of the prolapse will be the cervix or the scar left at the vaginal cuff by prior hysterectomy.

Measurements should be made using a Sims speculum with the patient in either the dorsal lithotomy or the left lateral decubitus position. When a point of reference has been identified, the patient is asked to bear down. The extent of the descent is measured with a ruler or other calibrated measuring device. Nine separate measurements (eight if post-hysterectomy) are made of the six reference points, total vaginal length, genital hiatus and perineal body. Once all measurements are recorded a diagrammatic vaginal profile may be drawn (see Figure 29.2).

A more common, but less precise, classification system has been recommended by the American College of Obstetrics and Gynecology.[3] This examination is also performed with a Sims speculum as previously described, also without the use of traction, attempting to duplicate the patient's daily symptoms. The presence of prolapse is classified into four degrees of severity:

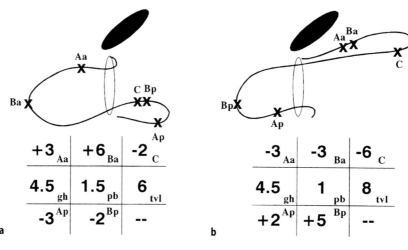

Figure 29.2   Predominant defect of anterior vaginal support denoted in grid and line diagrams. Stage III prolapse with the leading edge of the defect at point Ba. Predominant defect of posterior vaginal support, with leading edge of defect at point Bp. There is minimal descent of the vaginal cuff. (–8 to –6). This is also a stage III defect. [From Bump RC, Mattiasson A, Bo K et al. The standardization of terminology of female pelvic organ prolapse and pelvic floor dysfunction. Am J Obstet Gynecol 1996; 175: 12.]

First degree | On depression of the perineum, the prolapse extends to the mid-vagina.

Second degree | The prolapse approaches the hymeneal ring.

Third degree | The prolapse is at the hymeneal ring.

Fourth degree | The prolapse extends beyond the hymeneal ring.

Accurate grading of prolapse depends on the patient's ability to strain vigorously during clinical examination. Prolapse tends to worsen as the day progresses, particularly if the patient stands upright for long periods. Patients should be examined in the supine or Sims position as well as in the standing position, in order to accurately assess the degree of prolapse that is present. Every attempt should be made to reproduce the maximal degree of prolapse experienced by the patient.

References

1. Bump RC, Mattiasson A, Bø K et al. (1996) The standardization of terminology of female pelvic organ prolapse and pelvic floor dysfunction. Am J Obstet Gynecol 175: 10–17.
2. Video available at nominal charge from the American Urogynecology Society, Suite 300, 1200 Nineteenth Street, NW; Washington, DC 20036-2422, USA.
3. American College of Obstetricians and Gynecologists (1995) Pelvic Organ Prolapse. ACOG Technical Bulletin No. 214. American College of Obstetricians and Gynecologists, Washington, DC.

30 Treatment and Prevention of Prolapse

C.A. Glowacki and L.L. Wall

30.1 Therapeutic Options for the Patient with Prolapse

Unless the patient is symptomatic, mild degrees of prolapse may not require treatment. Symptomatic prolapse may be managed conservatively or surgically. Non-surgical therapies that may benefit the patient with prolapse include oestrogen replacement therapy, pelvic muscle exercises ("Kegels") and biofeedback, and support of the prolapse with a pessary. Surgery may be performed by either the vaginal or abdominal route.

Many women with pelvic organ prolapse are perimenopausal or postmenopausal, so evaluation of the patient's oestrogen status is essential. Oestrogen replacement therapy will help reverse changes in the tissues and improve the patient's tolerance of the use of a pessary. It will also improve the quality of tissues with which the surgeon has to work if surgical treatment is undertaken.

Pelvic muscle exercises (see Chapter 8) may help prevent the development of prolapse in normal women, as well as delay its progression in women with early symptoms.

Patients with mild symptoms associated with an early stage prolapse will often get temporary relief by using a tampon or diaphragm in specific situations that are associated with their symptoms such as exercising or standing for long periods of time. With more severe degrees of prolapse and more significant symptomatology, patients may obtain relief by using a pessary. A pessary is a prosthetic device that is inserted into the vagina to support the prolapse. Most pessaries are now made of soft, flexible silicone that allows them to be inserted and removed easily, without irritation. Many pessaries permit drainage and minimise the development of vaginal discharge. Pessaries are useful devices for patients who are poor candidates for surgery or who do not wish to undergo an operation for their condition. They also offer temporary relief of symptoms in cases where definitive surgical correction of the prolapse must be delayed.

Pessaries may also be used as a tool for the evaluation of urinary incontinence. Patients with high-stage prolapse will often develop a "kinking" of the urethra and bladder neck as the prolapse descends to or beyond the hymen. If the prolapse is reduced, previously undetected ("occult") incontinence may be demonstrated. This finding often requires the addition of a specific anti-incontinence procedure at the time of surgical correction of the prolapse.

A wide variety of pessaries are available (see Figure 30.1). Identifying the best type for any specific patient is a process of trial and error.

Ring pessaries, with or without platform support, and doughnut pessaries, are readily accepted by patients because of their similarity to contraceptive diaphragms. These pessaries are most useful in the treatment of uterine prolapse, particularly stage I or II prolapse.[1] The platform type of pessary avoids the rare complication of a uterus being incarcerated by protruding through an opening in a pessary.

A *platform pessary* is built to be folded in half, then inserted into the vagina, where it then springs back into its previous shape (see Figures 30.1, 30.2). When in position, these pessaries rest below the cervix and above the pubic symphysis in a position similar to that occupied by a contraceptive diaphragm. This usually allows intravaginal pressure to be distributed equally throughout the vagina, aiding reduction of the prolapse. Sexual intercourse is possible while these pessaries are in place.

The *Gellhorn pessary* provides more support for patients with severe uterine or vaginal prolapse and is useful where there is a large prolapse of the anterior vaginal wall. They hold their position better if

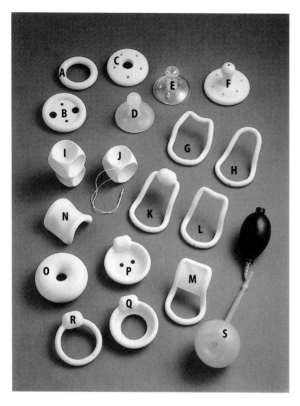

Figure 30.1 Pessaries: **A** Ring , **B** Ring with support, **C** Shaatz, **D–F** Gellhorn, **G** Risser, **H** Smith, **I** Tandem cube, **J** Cube, **K** Hodge with knob, **L** Hodge, **M** Hodge with support, **N** Gehrung, **O** Donut, **P** Incontinence dish with support, **Q** Incontinence dish, **R** Ring incontinence, **S** Inflatoball latex. Courtesy of Milex Products, Inc., Chicago, IL.

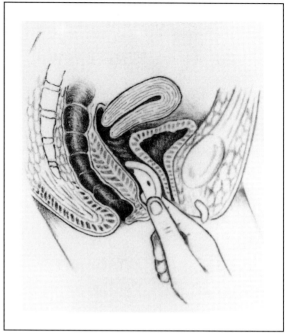

Figure 30.2   Insertion of ring with support. Courtesy of Milex Products, Inc., Chicago, IL.

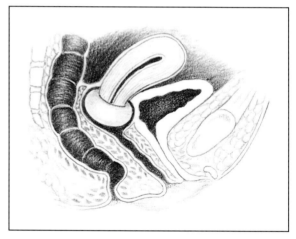

Figure 30.3   Donut pessary in position. Courtesy of Milex Products, Inc., Chicago, IL.

the patient has an intact perineal body. These pessaries are usually made of a rigid material, and may be more difficult to insert (Figure 30.4). A Gellhorn pessary should be removed before sexual intercourse is attempted.

Inflatable pessaries are doughnut-shaped devices with an attached stem. The stem protrudes through the vagina, where it is accessible for inflating and deflating the device (see Figure 30.5). Use of this device requires manual dexterity, so it is not suitable for all women. Protrusion of the stem beyond the vaginal introitus may create uncomfortable vulvar irritation.

Cube pessaries are constructed with six concave surfaces that create a suction effect with the vaginal walls and hold the pessary in place (see Figure 30.6). Pessaries of this type are particularly useful in patients with vaginal eversion or complete uterine prolapse. Unless the suction is broken periodically, however, ulceration of the vagina may occur. Ideally these pessaries should be removed, cleaned and reinserted on a daily basis. Unless patients are able

to do this themselves they require careful monitoring and frequent pessary checks by a knowledgeable clinician.

Smith–Hodge pessaries elevate the bladder neck into a retropubic position and provide support similar to that obtained by bladder neck suspension surgery (see Figure 30.7). This type of pessary may be useful in helping predict the likelihood of incontinence after surgery for the correction of prolapse, as

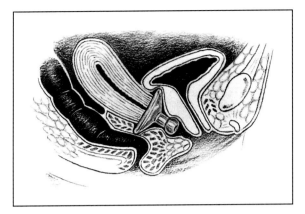

Figure 30.4 Gellhorn pessary in position. Courtesy of Milex Products, Inc., Chicago, IL.

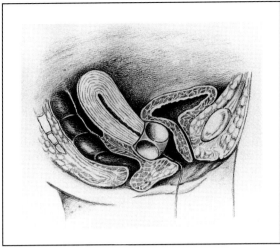

Figure 30.6 Cube pessary in position. Courtesy of Milex Products, Inc., Chicago, IL.

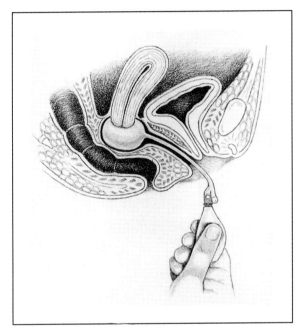

Figure 30.5 Inflatable pessary being inflated. Courtesy of Milex Products, Inc., Chicago, IL.

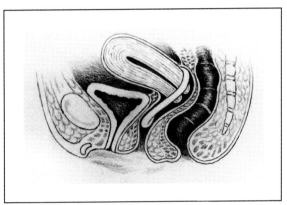

Figure 30.7 Hodge pessary in position. Courtesy of Milex Products, Inc., Chicago, IL.

well as in helping predict if reconstructive surgery will help restore normal urinary continence.[2]

Proper fitting of the pessary will minimise the development of complications. The optimal pessary provides support of the prolapsed vaginal segment and fits snugly but not too tightly. A pessary should not interfere with normal voiding. Three or four sizes of a variety of types of pessary should be available during a pessary fitting session. If the pessary is too large, it may create a sensation of pelvic fullness

and possibly pelvic pain. Pessaries that are fitted improperly may cause urinary retention and vaginal irritation, ulceration, or bleeding. Pessaries that are neglected, particularly those placed in the vaginas of elderly women and forgotten, can become entrapped or embedded in the vagina or erode through the vagina to create vesico-vaginal or recto-vaginal fistulas, or form a focus of chronic irritation that contributes to the development of a vaginal or cervical cancer. Neglected pessaries also commonly lead to an abnormal or excessive vaginal discharge. If the pessary is too small, it may simply fall out or be expelled by the patient with a cough, or during defecation or urination.

When a pessary is placed for the first time, the patient should be encouraged to wear it around the office or clinic for a brief period of time to make sure that it is comfortable and provides adequate support. If this is satisfactory, the patient may go home with the pessary in place, but should return in a few days to have it checked and to review instructions for its insertion, removal and care. Under ideal conditions, a patient with good manual dexterity should be encouraged to remove her pessary twice a week, wash it with soap and water, and reinsert it using a water-soluble lubricant. Some pessaries, such as Gellhorn or doughnut pessaries, can safely be left in place for 3 months or longer. Half an applicator of vaginal oestrogen cream is extremely useful in maintaining optimal condition of the vaginal epithelium. Patients with pessaries should have a pelvic examination after 3 months, and at periodic intervals thereafter.[1] Patients who have poor manual dexterity should have the pessary removed, washed and reinserted during a clinic visit every 3–4 months, depending on the type of pessary and the patient's clinical history. Pessary use should be discontinued if erosion or ulceration of the vagina occurs. Patients who develop a heavy vaginal discharge while using a pessary may find periodic vaginal douching with a dilute solution of vinegar and water helpful. Bowel or bladder dysfunction should be investigated.

30.2 Surgical Options

Patients with more severe grades of prolapse or particularly troubling symptoms frequently require reconstructive pelvic surgery.

Prolapse of the vaginal vault may be repaired either vaginally or abdominally. The vaginal approach may limit surgical access to some types of defects, and there is some debate about the long-term efficacy of certain vaginal operations compared to abdominal operations, particularly with regard to the treatment of stress incontinence.

Traditionally, anterior vaginal wall prolapse was thought to be due to a thinning or stretching of the vagina. Attempts at surgical correction were therefore directed towards the excision and plication of weak, redundant vaginal tissue. This operation is called an *anterior colporrhaphy* and has undergone many modifications over time. Probably the most widely utilised technique is the Kelly plication of the bladder neck. A midline vertical incision is made in the anterior vagina from the urethra to a point just distal to the urethrovesical junction. The vaginal epithelium is dissected away from the pubocervical

fascia laterally, and the proximal urethra and urethrovesical junction are plicated with vertical mattress sutures placed in the underlying fascia laterally to the midline on each side. When tied down, these sutures pull the redundant vagina and fascia into the midline, elevating the bladder base. Any excess vaginal tissue is excised and the epithelium is then reapproximated in the midline (see Figure 30.8).

A further theory proposed that cystoceles were due not to stretching of the vagina, but rather due to specific anatomical defects. Richardson et al.[2] described isolated lateral, transverse or superior and midline breaks in the pubocervical fascia that they felt were responsible for cystocele formation. The most common pathology, occurring in more than 75% of patients, is a lateral break in the fascia that creates a paravaginal support defect. This probably results from avulsion of the anterolateral vaginal sulcus from its attachment to the arcus tendineus fascia pelvis along the pelvic sidewall.[2,3] A mild to moderate cystocele with a loss of urethrovesical support and, frequently, the development of stress incontinence, commonly occurs in this situation. Repair of anterior vaginal wall prolapse should be

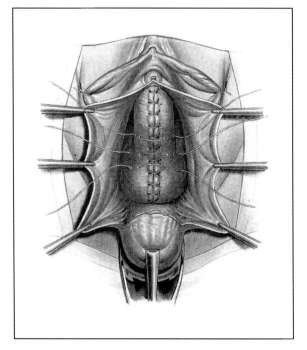

Figure 30.8 Kelly plication sutures placed in the region of the bladder neck. [From Hoskin, J. ed. (1968) Shaw's Textbook of Operative Gynecology. Lippincott; Williams; Menefee SA, Miller KF, Wall LL (1999).]

directed at the identification and repair of the underlying site-specific defects.

Lateral and central defects of the anterior vagina may be differentiated during physical examination. A tongue blade or similar instrument is placed along each lateral sulcus of the anterior vagina, and the vagina is re-approximated to the pelvic sidewall. If the cystocele disappears, it is most likely due to a lateral paravaginal defect; however, if the cystocele persists after this manoeuvre has been performed, the defect is most likely due to a central separation of the fascia. This latter defect can be repaired with a standard anterior colporrhaphy as described.

Paravaginal or lateral vaginal defects may also be repaired through a vaginal incision, although this approach is rather more difficult. A persistent central defect may also require concomitant anterior colporrhaphy.

Repair of posterior vaginal prolapse ("rectocele") has traditionally proceeded along the lines of the anterior colporrhaphy. Traditionally, this defect has been ascribed to "stretching" of the vagina and repaired by plication of the redundant tissues posterior to the vagina, much as is done in anterior colporrhaphy. This operation is often combined with a perineorrhaphy to rebuild a relaxed perineal body. If either of these operations is performed in an overly vigorous fashion, a shelf of tissue may be created in the posterior vagina that may cause pain with sexual intercourse.

Newer concepts regarding the aetiology and pathogenesis of posterior vaginal prolapse have evolved, just as they have changed with regard to anterior vaginal prolapse. The rectovaginal septum is a dense layer of tissue underlying the posterior vaginal wall. It separates the ventral rectal compartment from the posterior urogenital compartment.[4] As with the anterior vagina, Richardson[5] was able to demonstrate that isolated tears in the rectovaginal septum produced similar forms of prolapse posteriorly. The most common defects are a transverse separation of the tissue immediately above the perineal body where the septum is normally attached, and a vertical midline defect. Both defects may be related to previous trauma during vaginal delivery. A transverse defect commonly results in a low rectocele that presents as a bulge just inside the vaginal introitus; midline defects may extend higher, and there may be lateral defects or higher transverse separations. Correction of the defects involves opening the posterior vagina and dissecting it off the underlying rectovaginal fascia. By pushing up through the rectum with a gloved finger, the surgeon can isolate the uncovered rectal muscularis from areas covered by the rectovaginal fascia, thereby isolating the defects. The edges of the defect are then reapproximated with a series of interrupted sutures.

Poor perineal support, which manifests itself as a slack perineal body with an apparent rectal bulge over the top, may mimic a rectocele. This condition is called a pseudorectocele, and it is corrected by perineorrhaphy rather than a rectocele repair. Perineal defects are generally caused by obstetric trauma which has either not been repaired or which has been repaired inadequately. Care must be taken not to narrow the vaginal opening excessively or to build up too much of a shelf; both conditions may result in dyspareunia.

Uterine prolapse is a descent of the uterus from its usual position at the top of the vagina. Mild uterine prolapse generally does not require treatment. More severe degrees of prolapse may be symptomatic, and this often requires a hysterectomy and vaginal resuspension of some form. The hysterectomy may be done vaginally or abdominally, depending on coexisting disease processes as well as the nature of the planned reconstructive procedure. It is crucial to understand that removal of the uterus alone is only half of the operation: the vagina must be suspended after the uterus is removed or the patient will suffer a recurrent prolapse that may be worse than her original problem. Before surgery, postmenopausal patients should if possible be placed on some form of oestrogen replacement to maximise the quality of tissues involved at the time of surgery.

Several approaches for suspension of the vagina have been described. Selection of the appropriate operation depends on the presence of any coexisting pathology, the nature of the anatomic defects present, as well as the personal preference and experience of the operating surgeon.

A transvaginal approach to vaginal suspension has several advantages. It avoids the increased morbidity of an abdominal incision, which may shorten both the patient's hospital stay and her time to recovery. It also allows correction of any coexisting cystocele or rectocele without a separate incision.

The most common transvaginal approach to vaginal vault prolapse is suspension of the prolapsed vaginal apex to the sacrospinous ligament, which runs between the ischial spine and the sacrum. This operation usually provides good vaginal depth and capacity for future coitus, although this is somewhat dependent on the configuration of the pelvis and the location of the ischial spines.

Complications of the sacrospinous ligament suspension include haemorrhage from the pudendal vessels, buttock pain or numbness from nerve entrapment or injury, bladder or rectal lacerations, voiding difficulty, granulation tissue at the site of suture attachment and point tenderness over the ischial spine.[6,7] Recurrent prolapse in the form of cystocele or rectocele formation sometimes occurs, and recurrent prolapse of the vaginal vault is also reported in 4–23% of patients undergoing this operation.[8–13]

Another, less popular, vaginal operation for vaginal vault prolapse involves attachment of the uterosacral ligaments to the prolapsed vaginal cuff. The uterosacral ligaments can easily be identified during vaginal hysterectomy, and they should routinely be reattached to the vaginal cuff during this operation. Patients who have had a previous hysterectomy often have thin, attenuated cardinal and uterosacral ligaments, which may be distorted by an enterocele. This operative approach seeks to secure the vagina to its original point of attachment, thereby recreating the normal vaginal axis, obliterating the cul-de-sac of Douglas, and decreasing the change of a recurrent vaginal vault prolapse.

Abdominal sacral-colpopexy carries a relatively higher morbidity than the vaginal operations, because of the neeed for an abdominal incision. This increased morbidity is offset by an extremely high and very consistent long-term success rate.[14–17] In a prospective study by Benson and colleagues comparing vaginal and abdominal approaches to vaginal vault and cervical prolapse, abdominal sacral colpopexy was found to be twice as likely to result in optimal suspension as was sacrospinous ligament fixation performed vaginally.[18] Complications associated with sacral-colpopexy include possible erosion of artificial mesh through the vagina, infection, recurrent prolapse (usually posterior), injury to bowel, bladder or ureters, haemorrhage from injury to the presacral vessels, as well as the standard complications of any abdominal operation.

In any operation for pelvic organ prolapse, it is essential to repair any enterocele that is present to avoid the problem of recurrent prolapse. In particular, prophylactic culdoplasty at the time of hysterectomy is recommended to close an enterocele and obliterate the rectouterine peritoneal cul-de-sac (pouch of Douglas).

Some patients with significant uterovaginal prolapse are frail, often elderly women who are not sexually active and who do not wish to pursue future sexual activity. Such women often have significant medical problems that make them poor candidates for extensive reconstructive operations. In such women an operation either to close off the vagina or to remove it completely may be a suitable solution to their prolapse. A LeFort colpocleisis preserves the uterus and allows drainage of cervical

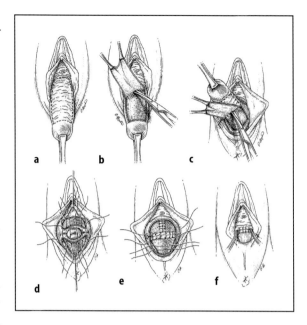

Figure 30.9 LeFort colpocleisis: **a** An incision is made in the anterior vaginal mucosa. **b** A rectangular segment of anterior vaginal mucosa is excised. **c** A rectangular flap of posterior vaginal mucosa is excised. **d** The anterior and posterior vaginal mucosal flaps are approximated over the cervix. **e** The denuded anterior and posterior vaginal walls are approximated. **f** Tunnels at the lateral edges of the re-approximated vaginal walls, indicated by Kelly clamps, allow for drainage of cervical secretions. [From Thompson JD, Rock JA, TeLinde's Operative Gynecology, 7th edition. JB Lippincott, Philadelphia, 1992.]

and uterine secretions by the creation of vaginal drainage canals (see Figure 30.9).

The most obvious disadvantage to colpocleisis or complete colpectomy is the loss of the vagina, but there are other potential disadvantages as well. The anatomical defects associated with complete uterovaginal prolapse are not really repaired by these operations, only covered over to alleviate the symptoms they produce. When the vagina is closed in this fashion, the continence mechanism may be altered with subsequent development of urinary incontinence. The potential development of this problem must be addressed in the preoperative evaluation of the patient, since additional bladder neck surgery may be required at the time of vaginal closure.[19,20] If a LeFort-type operation is performed, the uterus and cervix are not removed, but they then become inaccessible after surgery. The patient must have normal cervical cytology and a normal endometrial biopsy before undergoing a LeFort operation, since these organs will no longer be accessible for evaluation postoperatively.

30.3 Prevention of Prolapse

Prolapse is difficult to prevent because the aetiology is not completely understood and many different factors seem to influence its development. Since muscular support of the pelvic floor appears to be critical in maintaining normal function, it may be that regular pelvic muscle exercises will prevent the development of prolapse or ameliorate its early stages. Better obstetric care, including the judicious use of caesarean delivery in patients who appear to be at high risk for the future development of prolapse, is undoubtedly important. Avoiding things that lead to chronic increases in intra-abdominal pressure, such as heavy occupational lifting and chronic straining at stool, should be encouraged. Cessation of smoking and effective treatment of chronic pulmonary diseases are also important. Hormone replacement therapy in postmenopausal women is also likely to be helpful in many cases.

References

1. Wu V, Farrell SA, Baskett TF, Flowerdew G A (1997) Simplified protocol for pessary management. Obstet Gynecol 90: 990.
2. Richardson AC, Edmonds PB, Williams NL (1981) Treatment of stress urinary incontinence due to paravaginal fascial defect, Obstet Gynecol 57: 357.
3. Youngblood JP. Paravaginal repair for cystourethrocele (1993) Clin Obstet Gynecol 36: 960.
4. Paulina W, Harkin LH, Masterson BJ, Ross MH (1991) Subperitoneal layer of elastic fibers in the female pelvis. Clin Anat 4: 447.
5. Richardson AC (1993) The rectovaginal septum revisited: Its relationship to rectocele and its importance in rectocele repair. Clin Obstet Gynecol 36: 976.
6. Morley GW, DeLancey JOL (1988) Sacrospinous ligament fixation for eversion of the vagina. Am J Obstet Gynecol 158: 872
7. Chapin DS. Teaching sacrospinous colpopexy (1997) Am J Obstet Gynecol 177: 1330.
8. Richter K, Albrich W (1981) Longterm results following fixation on the vaginal sacrospinous ligament by the vaginal route: vaginaefixation sacrospinous vaginalis. Am J Obstet Gynecol 141: 811.
9. DeLancey JOL, Morley G (1997) Total colpocleisis for vaginal eversion. Am J Obstet Gynecol 176: 1228.
10. Benson JT, McClellan E (1989) The effect of vaginal dissection on the pudendal nerve. Obstet Gynecol 161: 97.
11. Holley RL, Varner RE, Gleason BP, et al. (1995) Recurrent pelvic support defects after sacrospinous ligament fixation for vaginal vault prolapse. J Am Coll Surg 180: 444.
12. Raz S, Nitti VW, Bregg KJ (1993) Transvaginal repair of enterocele. J Urol 149: 724.
13. Pasley WW (1995) Sacrospinous suspension: a local practitioner's experience. Am J Obstet Gynecol 173: 440.
14. Birnbaum SJ (1973) Rational therapy for the prolapsed vagina. Am J Obstet Gynecol 115: 411.
15. Cowan W, Morgan HR (1980) Abdominal sacrocolpopexy. Am J Obstet Gynecol 138: 348.
16. Menefee SA, Miller KF, Wall LL. Results of abdominal sacral colpopexy using polyester mesh for post-hysterectomy vaginal vault prolapse. Journal of Pelvic Surgery 1999; 5: 136–142.
17. Hardiman PJ, Drutz HP(1996) Sacrospinous vault suspension and abdominal colposacropexy: Success rates and complications. Am J Obstet Gynecol 175: 612.
18. Benson JT, Lucente V, McClellan E: Vaginal versus abdominal reconstructive surgery for the treatment of pelvic support defects: a prospective randomized study with longterm outcome evaluation. Am J Obstet Gynecol 175: 1418, 1996
19. Ridley JH (1972) Evaluation of the colpocleisis operation. A report of fifty-eight cases. Am J Obstet Gynecol 113: 1114.
20. Langmade CF, Oliver JA (1986) Partial colpocleisis. Am J Obstet Gynecol 154: 1200.

VI Complementary Therapies

31 Osteopathy

Y. Dereix

The osteopathic approach to incontinence is based mainly on the role of manipulative therapy in accordance with one of the basic principles of osteopathy – "structure governs function". Osteopathic techniques address "structural" issues such as:

- scarred and fibrosed tissue
- sliding surfaces of the peritoneum, subperitoneal pelvic space and perineum
- bladder and uterine positions, the related fascia and ligamentous tension and laxity
- structural involvement around the central and autonomic nervous systems.

The aim of treatment is to diagnose any loss of mobility within the body and bring about a correction.[1] However, more research is necessary to quantify and qualify the recommendations given in this chapter.

Manipulations of sacro-iliac (SI) joints or sacral pumping techniques can often be effective, especially for incontinence following chronic low back pain and lumbo-sacral dysfunction, and also in children and adults with nocturia and bowel dysfunction.

Manipulations of the thoracic spine and upper lumbar spine are also known to have possible effects on incontinence through L1 origins of the lumbar splanchnic nerve and the inferior mesenteric ganglia. Manipulation of the T10–L1 region can also influence the intermediolateral column which carries connections from the brain stem detrusor motor nuclei to detrusor motor neurons.

It is postulated that rib raising may pull on the fasciae shared between the rib head and adjacent sympathetic ganglia, thus activating reflex sympathetic response in related organs and also triggering slow sympathetic fibres as far as medullary centres, which in turn may have a long acting inhibitory response.

Manipulations to the occiput–atlas–axis group and craniosacral manoeuvres also have a major role to play on the parasympathetic nervous system as well as on the direct link through the dura mater between the occipital base (foramen magnum) and the sacrum. In craniosacral therapy, the balance of mobility between sphenoid and occiput are said to be in synergy with that of the sacrum and ilea.[2] Cranial manipulation is also a treatment of choice for patients with bowel disorders.

In addition, manipulation techniques of the different organs and soft tissues of the lower abdominal cavity and pelvis have been developed around their anatomical (structural) links, such as the position of the uterus and the tension on the uterosacral ligament, broad ligament, round ligament and their neurovascular content.

Furthermore, it is now accepted practice to treat and relieve certain chronic lumbar and sacroiliac problems through the treatment of certain muscles e.g. piriformis and ilio-psoas, as well as the manipulation and "re-orientation" of pelvic organs, especially the uterus.

Lymphatic drainage techniques may also reduce congestion and improve homeostasis in genital and bowel dysfunction.

31.1 Assessment

Most of the important symptoms arising from diseases of internal viscera are reflex in nature. In order to understand these symptoms, one must study the innervation of the various viscera and the interrelationship which exists between them, also the interrelationship which exists between the viscera and the skeletal structures.[3]

This sets the scene for the assessment procedure leading to the choice of osteopathic methods.

31.1.1 Vertebral column

Every patients' vertebral column should be examined in order to establish any possible derangement at any vertebral level, which could affect innervation, circulation and good function. The thoraco-lumbar and lumbo-sacral spine are certainly involved in many incontinence and pelvic pain disorders. To correct visceral dysfunction only at a local level would probably allow the condition to recur.

31.1.2 Trigger and Reflex Points

Different trigger points and Chapman's reflex points will provide useful information and means of treatment.[4]

31.1.3 Mobility

> Osteopathy is the art of diagnosing a loss of mobility within the body and bringing about a correction.[5]

For example, a bladder in a posterior position does not necessarily mean that the problem comes from this position; of greater importance is whether the pubovesical ligaments (anterior anchorage system) contract without restriction during a retention effort test. Likewise, a retroverted uterus can be acceptable if mobile but will definitely benefit from manipulative treatment if fixed, in order to restore functional mobility.

31.1.4 Motility

As opposed to mobility which can easily be tested by practitioners, motility is an intrinsic motion of a structure with a periodicity of approximately 7 Hz. The "listening" to slow and discreet oscillatory movements will be in "expire" and "inspire" ranges, where an organ is said to expire when it moves closer to the medial axis and inspire when it moves away. Medial organs are said to expire when moving posteriorly and vice versa.

31.1.5 Listening

Listening is used in craniosacral and visceral osteopathy to obtain information about the body as a whole (general listening) and about specific restrictions (local listening). It can be done by placing your hand very lightly on an area and passively concentrating on the motion of the tissues.

With practice, your hand will be drawn to the most restricted area.[6]

31.1.6 Tests

In addition to any standard physical tests carried out in allopathic practice, there are a few tests specific to osteopathic practice.

31.1.6.1 Completed Lasègue Test

Where a sciatica with genital involvement is suspected, reduction of symptoms may be obtained when performing an external inhibiting pressure on the pelvic zone in conflict.

31.1.6.2 Genitohumeral Test

Same as for the Lasègue test, but this time the pain produced by the abduction or external rotation of the shoulder (candlestick position) will be relieved with pelvic inhibition.

31.1.6.3 Hip Articulation Test

Improvement of hip mobility with ipsilateral pelvic inhibition.

31.1.6.4 Obturator Internus Stretching Test

The adduction and internal rotation of the thigh may cause an increase in pain or discomfort and an urge to urinate in restricted bladders as this test will pull on the obturator internus muscle (abductor/external rotator of the hip) and its origin from the obturator fascia, if there is some degree of fibrosis of the fascia. Similar symptoms can be obtained when testing the piriformis muscles in hip rotation or the acetabular ligaments which stretch from the hip joint to the internal obturator fascia and bladder.

31.1.6.5 Sacral Compression Test

A postero-anterior compression of the sacrum in prone lying will test the uterosacral ligament with its insertion from S2 to S4. Both bilateral and unilateral restrictions of the uterosacral ligaments should be confirmed by the lateral test of the cervix.

31.1.6.6 Uterosacral Ligaments Internal Test

This internal examination will indicate if there is pain or restricted mobility by pushing the posterior part of the cervix anterolaterally; any tension or tear of the uterosacral ligaments and the posterior portion of the broad ligaments can be detected.

31.1.6.7 Pubovesical and Uterovesical Ligaments Test

This internal examination will show if any of the ligaments restrict movement of the bladder or uterus. A retroflexion of the cervix indicates a hyperlaxity or damage of the uterovesical ligaments and an anteflexion occurs with fibrosed ligaments.

31.1.6.8 Bent Knee Test

This is used to test the sacrospinous and sacrotuberous ligaments by mobility test of the sacrococcygeal joint in unipodal standing.

31.1.6.9 Sacrococcygeal Rectal Test

This tests the anterior and posterior sacrococcygeal ligaments.

31.2 Treatments

Osteopathy incorporates a holistic approach to patients' health, and one condition is frequently linked with another. This chapter considers regional disorders rather than conditions.

Some conditions will respond more to treatment aimed at restoring good mobility of soft tissues, whereas others will be improved as a result of promoting good circulation. This increase in circulation can facilitate the healing and anti-inflammatory state of body tissues, which is dependent on the ability of the body to remove waste products from the tissues and to deliver oxygen and other nutrients to the area of tissue dysfunction.

Similarly, visceral irritation and disease, together with increased visceral afferent nerve activity, are often associated with hypersympathetic bombardment of the associated organs. Sympathetic nerve impulses may protect the body from external dangers but when they remain hyperactive, owing to spinal facilitation, they may inhibit rapid healing and restoration of good health.

31.2.1 Colon Disorders

In most disorders of the colon a treatment that enhances the homeostasis mechanisms of the patient and restores a harmony of sympathetic and parasympathetic impulses will be the optimum choice.

31.2.1.1 Constipation, Abdominal Pain, Flatulence and Distension

These conditions are usually related to hypersympathetic activity and the practitioner is encouraged to use the following techniques:

- Treatment by light circular pressure, kneading and stretching of trigger points and reflex points on the anterior part of the iliotibial band and a triangular area located on the lumbar spine between the two iliac crests and L2.
- Rib-raising techniques to T10–T12 together with paraspinal soft tissue techniques to T12–L2 and the lumbosacral region. The rib-raising manoeuvre is performed with the practitioner standing at the head of the patient who is in supine lying. The patient is asked to hold his hands together around the practitioner's waist or a belt. The practitioner then applies pressure with his hands on the rib angles and pulls upwards as the patient breathes in, then relaxes. The paraspinal soft tissue techniques will be a careful controlled and rhythmic inhibitory pressure to produce a palpable relaxation of the tissues.
- To facilitate lymphatic drainage from the colon, start at the thoracic inlet by restoring good mobility of the first and secnd ribs and manubrium of the sternum as well as T1–T4. Good mobility of the six lower ribs and the xiphoid process together with L1–L3 will free the abdominal diaphragm and provide the effective pressure gradients needed to pump lymph from abdomen to the thorax.
- Relaxation of the pelvic diaphragm through ischiorectal fossa techniques (or vaginal and anal digital inhibition techniques) should relieve congestion and perineural oedema of the pelvic parasympathetic and pudendal nerves (S2–S4). The ischiorectal fossa fascial release will be done with the patient in side lying, hips and knees flexed at 90º, with the side to be treated on top (away from the couch). The practitioner will then apply gentle and progressive pressure to compress the fat and fascia of the fossa with the fingertips while the other hand applies a counterbalance on the hip.

31.2.1.2 Diarrhoea, Cramps and Colon Pain

Usually related to an increase in the parasympathetic activity, treatment of these conditions is generally divided into right- and left-sided disorders. The right vagus nerve innervates the right colon, and examination and manipulation of the occipito-atlas and atlo-axoid joints together with the occipitomastoid cranial suture may be indicated. Condylar decompression and cranial techniques can promote occipitotemporal harmony. In addition, any symptomatic dysfunction of the cervical spine in C3–C5 should be corrected to ensure a good function of the phrenic nerve and abdominal diaphragm.

In left colon dysfunctions, manipulation of the lumbosacral region, sacrum and iliac bones should harmonise the pelvic splanchnic nerve (S2–S4). Sacral rocking is a technique of choice.

31.2.1.3 Irritable Bowel Syndrome

Irritable bowel syndrome (IBS) is considered to be a functional condition without a known cause, but characterised by certain identifiable and physiological reactions.[7] Harmonisation of the autonomic nervous system together with good lymphatic drainage and normal joint function may promote an improvement of the condition and increased comfort for the patient. Within weeks, the patient should be in a position to monitor the triggering factors and the relieving actions. Osteopathic manipulations, lymphatic drainage and self-care together with dietary modification and pharmacological help is the treatment of choice. Many IBS sufferers improve after treatment to the vertebral column.

Osteopathic treatment of IBS will include:

- rib raising
- thoracolumbar soft tissue techniques
- inhibitory ventral abdominal techniques on the midline between the xiphoid process and the umbilicus
- trigger points and Chapman's reflexes on the iliotibial bands and intercostal spaces 8, 9 and 10
- sacral rocking
- manipulation of the sacroiliac joints (S2–S4)
- harmonisation of occipito-atlas, atlo-axoid joints, C2, lambdoidal (or occipitoparietal) sutures near the jugular foramen together with the occipitomastoid cranial suture
- lymphatic drainage techniques as previously described.

31.2.2 Urological Disorders

This section addresses the osteopathic approach to the treatment of urge incontinence, stress incontinence and prostatitis.

31.2.2.1 Urge Incontinence

The detrusor muscle is activated by parasympathetic nerves and inhibited by sympathetic nerves. The internal urethral sphincter and ureteric orifices are activated by sympathetic and inhibited by parasympathetic nerves. The external urethral sphincter is innervated by the pudendal nerve.

The very nature of the pathophysiology of urge incontinence requires a treatment that will promote homeostasis and be complementary to bladder re-education (increase of volume) and pelvic floor exercises.

Osteopathic treatment will mainly be manipulative at the thoracolumbar level (lumbar splanchnic and inferior mesenteric ganglia), lumbosacral and sacroiliac region (S2–S4, pelvic and pudendal nerves). Treatment to the pelvic diaphragm by intravaginal fascial release may also help in controlling the urge. This is done by placing the fingers in the frontal plane of the vagina to open the orifice; on coughing at least three times, the fascia and muscular diaphragm are stretched and this should induce a functional relaxation.

31.2.2.2 Stress Incontinence

Stress incontinence can be divided into three bladder types:

- in type A (anterior) the bladder and urethral wall are pressed against the pubis by adhesion or sclerosis of the anterior system (pubovesical and pubourethral ligaments)
- in type P (posterior) the bladder collapses posteriorly due to dysfunction of the posterolateral system (uterosacral ligament and parametrium) and the bladder neck junction with the urethra moves outside the pressure zone of the abdomen
- the mixed type is a combination of both.

Depending on the functional mobility of the pelvic organs, the following manipulative techniques are recommended:

Median and Medial Umbilical Ligament Patient resting on her knees and elbows: the practitioner controls the stretching with one hand on the ligament and rotates the sacrum with the other hand.

Pubovesical Ligaments This technique can be done in different positions but the knee–elbow position presents the great advantage of disengaging the intestine from the pelvis and the abdominal muscles are relaxed. By placing your fingers on the lower abdominal wall, behind the pubis, it is possible to stretch the ligaments.

Anterior Part of the Perineum The fingers should be placed on both sides of the closed labia majora, a stretching manoeuvre of the superficial perineal aponeurosis and transverse perineal muscle should be performed in a posterolateral direction. This also affects the pudendal nerve.

Obturator Foramen Patient in supine with hip in flexion, abduction and external rotation; place your thumb under the pectineus and adductor magnus with your palm on the inner thigh, while adducting and internally rotating the hip turn your thumb gently to progress onto the foramen and stretch.

Bladder With one finger on the anterior wall of the vagina and the other hand on the abdomen with your fingers behind the pubis, move the bladder in all three dimensions. This will test and treat a lot of adhesions.

Bladder Neck Same position as above but this time you should aim to "scoop" the bladder with your fingers and lift up (in the patient's cephalic direction) to stretch any adhesions.

In posterior bladder necks, a repeated anterior manoeuvre of the neck with the intravaginal finger can restore a good mobility.

Urethra While keeping the bladder against the pubis, pull the uterus towards the bladder with your finger directly under the trigone. With the abdominal fingers, push up the bladder.

31.2.2.3 Prostatitis

Bacterial prostatitis may be treated pharmacologically and ischiorectal fossa release can also help homeostasis. Non-bacterial prostatitis may benefit from prostatic massage at regular intervals and pelvic floor exercises which will physiologically massage the prostate. Manipulation of T12–L2 and S2–S4 could be necessary to correct any somatic dysfunction.

Prostatodynia is the painful male urethral syndrome (PMUS) and can be accompanied by urgency, frequency, nocturia, dysuria, etc. The manual treatment includes pelvic floor exercises, treatment of the sympathetic system as well as possible vertebral manipulation.

31.2.3 Utero-vaginal Disorders

This section concentrates mainly on the treatment of some anomalies which may directly or indirectly cause incontinence or pelvic pain.

31.2.3.1 External Uterine Manipulation

Not to be performed if patient has an intrauterine device (IUD). Although this manipulation can be done in all positions, the knee–elbow position is preferred as it allows the disengagement of the intestines from the pelvis and the abdominal muscles to be relaxed. In addition the uterus will be anteverted and more palpable. By placing your hand on the abdomen lateral to the uterus, mobilise as required. If a uterovesical restriction is present, push the sacrum into flexion with your other hand.

31.2.3.2 Sacral and Sacrococcygeal Pumping

Both techniques are fairly similar and only vary in the level of application. Sacral pumping addresses the uterosacral ligament and sacrococcygeal pumping the anococcygeal ligament. It should be performed with the patient in prone, and the practitioner's hands on the sacrum should successively push anteroinferiorly, anteriorly and anterosuperiorly.

31.2.3.3 Sacrospinous and Sacrotuberous Ligaments Stretch

In supine, ask the patient to bring her knee towards the opposite shoulder while the other leg remains straight. This will cause a flexion, adduction and internal rotation of the hip and stretch these ligaments which share an aponeurosis with the pelvic organs.

31.2.3.4 Biceps Femoris Stretch

Patient sitting with both legs straight, bend trunk forward towards the non-treated side while moving her leg on the treated side into internal (medial) rotation.

31.2.3.5 Uterine Decongestion

Patient on her knees with her head and chest down (the pelvis is raised above the knees). Gravity will pull the abdominal viscera out of the pelvis and decongest the uterus.

31.2.3.6 Manipulation of Uterine Anteversion with Cervical Anteposition

Patient in supine, the practitioner places a hand on the abdomen over the uterus (fundus) and a finger of the opposite hand on the superoanterior part of the vaginal wall. Mobilisation will be in a postero-inferior direction then in a posterior one.

31.2.3.7 Manipulation of Uterine Retroversion with Cervical Anteposition

Patient in supine, the practitioner puts one hand on the uterus (fundus) and a finger on the supero-anterior part of the vaginal wall. Mobilisation will be in a posterior direction while the abdominal hand will attract the uterus forward.

31.2.3.8 Manipulation of Uterine Anteversion with Cervical Retroposition

Patient in lateral recumbent position, the practitioner puts one hand on the uterus (fundus) and a finger on the superoposterior part of the vaginal wall. Mobilisation will be in an anterior direction while the abdominal hand will push the uterus backward.

31.2.3.9 Manipulation of Uterine Retroversion with Cervical Retroposition

Patient in lateral recumbent position, the practitioner puts one hand on the uterus (fundus) and a finger on the superoposterior part of the vaginal wall. Mobilisation will be in an anterior direction while the abdominal hand will pull the uterus forward.

31.2.3.10 Prolapsed Uterus

The technique described here aims only to produce a temporary release of restriction and congestion of the uterosacral and broad ligaments. Optimum results are obtained by the uterine decongestion exercise in the knee–chest position described previously. The patient is in prone with a soft wedge or cushion under her anterosuperior iliac spines; the manipulation is carried out with two intravaginal fingers pushing on the lateral pouches or the cervical border while the abdominal hand pulls the uterus in a cephalic direction.

31.2.4 Sexual Disorders

31.2.4.1 Impotence or Erectile Dysfunction

The pudendal nerve and the parasympathetic system are both involved in the erectile mechanism; consequently, manipulation of sacroiliac joints and ischiorectal fossa release can sometimes be effective.

31.2.4.2 Premature Ejaculation

Ejaculation is activated through the lumbar splanchnic and the hypogastric nerves (L1 and L2) and so manual treatment of somatic dysfunction of the upper lumbar region may help. The sacroiliac joints may also be involved and should be addressed.

31.2.4.3 Dyspareunia or Painful Coitus

This may be due to a number of disorders including vaginal spasm, poor vaginal lubrication and pelvic floor spasm. Osteopathic treatment will concentrate on the dysfunction of the pelvic diaphragm and normalisation of the parasympathetic reflex. Relaxation of the pelvic diaphragm through ischio-rectal fossa technique (or vaginal and anal digital inhibition techniques) should relieve congestion and perineural oedema of the pelvic parasympathetic nerves and pudendal nerve (S2–S4).

31.3 Contraindications and Precautions

There are many situations in which structural manipulations or mobilisations of joints or soft tissues should be avoided or carried out only after careful consideration of possible side-effects. In all cases, informed consent to assessment and treatment should be obtained.

31.3.1 Contraindications Specific to Vertebral Manipulations

Any doubt on the precise nature of the lesion, suspicion of a tumour or a fracture, other soft tissue fragility, hip replacements, other surgical procedures and pregnancy may need special care in the chosen technique. Extra care should be taken when treating neurological conditions that may be exacerbated by manipulation, and with patients on anticoagulant therapy.

31.3.2 Contraindications Specific to Urogenital Manipulations

Virginity is an absolute contraindication to vaginal examination and manipulations. These procedures are also not advisable in the case of pregnancy and following radiotherapy to the pelvis. A woman with an abnormal mass or pain and menorrhagia should be referred for a complete gynaecological examination before any osteopathic manipulation. Hypersensitivity, infection, endometriosis, slight bleeding and IUD should encourage extra care in urogenital manipulations.

31.3.3 Contraindications Specific to Abdominal Visceral Manipulations

- open surgical wound
- aortic aneurysm
- friable and enlarged liver
- enlarged spleen
- inflammation of the appendix
- perineal, anal or rectal abscess
- rib and vertebral fractures.

31.4 Conclusion

Osteopathic techniques are not exclusive and should never exclude other forms of treatment. The aim of osteopathy is to restore and maintain good function with sound structures of the body promoting good homeostasis. It must not be thought of as a system-atic method of manipulating structures "back into place". Someone's deviation or asymmetry may be perfectly functional and to correct it for the sake of achieving textbook anatomy would upset the whole individual's equilibrium.

Although certain gentle techniques like general and local listening of tissue motion, motility perception, induction and craniosacral manipulation have been mentioned in this chapter, it has not been detailed. Techniques described herein need to be expanded, and practical experience is necessary for complete understanding. Furthermore, more research is needed to evaluate all the procedures listed.

The subject of incontinence, pelvic pain and dysfunction is a delicate one because of the many psychological and social factors involved. This makes it even more important to give these patients every chance of improving their condition.

References

1. Stoddard A (1969) Manual of Osteopathic Practice. Hutchinson Medical, London.
2. Upledger JE, Vredevoogd JD (1983) Craniosacral Therapy. Eastland Press, Seattle, Wa.
3. Pottenger FM (1953) Symptoms of Visceral Disease (7th ed). Mosby, St. Louis, Mo.
4. Travell JG, Simons DG (1983) Myofascial Pain and Dysfunction: a Trigger Point Manual. Williams & Wilkins, Baltimore, Md.
5. Barral J-P (1993) Urogenital Manipulation. Eastland Press, Seattle, Wa.
6. Barral J-P (1989) Visceral Manipulation. Eastland Press, Seattle, Wa.
7. Kutchera ML, Kutchera WA (1994) Osteopathic Considerations in Systemic Dysfunction. Original Works Books, Greyden Press, Columbus, Oh.

32 Acupuncture

N. Ellis

The existence of traditional Chinese medicine (TCM), of which acupuncture is a part, can be traced back through written manuscripts for more than 3000 years. It is founded on the holistic concept of treatment, and an acknowledgement of the body's ability to return to its balanced state of health, given the correct stimulus to do so. The two forces that need to be in balance are *yin* (negative) and *yang* (positive). Energy or *qi* circulates within a specified system of 12 channels and their collaterals that are controlled by the major organs of the body. Disruption of the smooth flow of *qi* results in imbalance and disease. It is important to remember that 3000 years ago there were no X-rays or laboratory tests that could be used to examine blood and other body substances. The doctor had to rely on the patient's own description of their problem and observation of the body surface, its temperature, colour of the tongue, pulses and the colour and nature of body secretions such as sputum, urine or faeces, to form a diagnosis.

The various syndromes described in TCM are based on the function of the organs rather than actual changes within these organs as understood in western medicine. For example, Lung *qi* deficiency indicates a lack of energy in the Lung organ and might be demonstrated as a problem in fluid metabolism or in the condition of the skin, both of these being part of Lung function according to TCM.

It is interesting to note that the circulation of blood pumped round the body by the heart was described in TCM 1700 years before western medicine came to that conclusion. However, in TCM the Heart also governs the mind, and could be the cause of some psychological problems.

The local heavy or numbing effect achieved when the needle is inserted into an acupoint is known as *deqi*. This sensation indicates that type II and III afferent nerves fibres in the area of the acupoint are stimulated to trigger the body's physiological response through the spinal cord, midbrain and pituitary, which release transmitter chemicals (endorphins and monoamines) that block noxious impulses.[1]

A great deal of work has been done in the west to evaluate the effect of acupuncture on pain.[2-4] However, the research evidence to support the effectiveness of acupuncture on urinary and faecal incontinence is sparse. Kubista et al. in 1976 showed in a controlled trial that acupuncture could increase the closing mechanism strength of the female urethra.[5]

This chapter includes the interpretation of TCM in relation to the signs and symptoms presented in incontinence problems. The clinician wishing to use acupuncture effectively and safely ideally needs to have a knowledge and practice of TCM in diagnosis and treatment. These traditional diagnostic techniques enable the practitioner to work out the most effective treatment based on established practice that has been recorded for many hundreds of years. However, it is possible to use acupuncture to augment physiotherapy treatment using some acupoints that can be effective in particular problems met in clinical practice.

32.1 Urinary Incontinence

The signs and symptoms of urinary incontinence are described as two major syndromes.[6]

32.1.1 Lung *Qi* Deficiency

The patient will present with frequent urge to urinate and inability to contain urine. There may be dribbling of urine, leaking when coughing or exercising. There may also be shortness of breath, weak voice and slight sweating. The latter three signs and symptoms, together with the urinary signs, indicate Lung *qi* deficiency in TCM. To confirm this impression the tongue will appear pale and the pulse weak.

The principle of treatment is to tonify Lung *qi*. The acupoints suggested are:

- BL13 (*Feishu*) and GV12 (*Shenzhu*) (Figure 32.1). These points are particularly effective to tonify Lung *qi* and can be heated with moxa. This is a dried herb (mugwort) that can be used in several ways. In the most convenient presentation it is compressed into the form of a cigar-shaped stick. This is then lit up to glow and is held 2 cm above the surface of the skin over the acupoint until the patient feels warmth in the area.

- GV20 (*Bahui*) positioned on the midline of the head at the transection of a line between the highest point of the ears, can be heated with moxa to help raise *qi* and support the pelvic floor.

- LU7 (*Lieque*) (Figure 32.2). This affects the water passages.

- CV6 (*Qihai*) (Figure 32.3). Tonifies *qi*, particularly in the lower abdomen.

- BL23 (*Shenshu*) (Figure 32.1). Heated with moxa to reduce urination and tonify kidneys.

- BL28 (*Pangguanshu*) and BL53 (*Baohuang*) (Figure 32.1). Strengthens the bladder function.

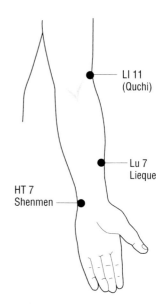

Figure 32.2   Acupuncture points: HT7 (*Shenmen*), LU7 (*Lieque*).

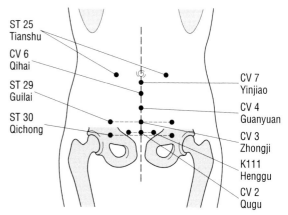

Figure 32.3   Acupuncture points: ST25 (*Tian Shu*), ST29 (*Guilai*), ST30 (*Qichong*), CV2 (*Qugu*), CV3 (*Zhongi*), CV4 (*Guanyuan*), CV6 (*Qihai*), CV7 (*Yinjiao*), KI11 (*Henggu*).

A selection of these points should be stimulated to achieve *deqi* and the needles left in place for 15–20 min.

32.1.2 Kidney *Yang* Deficiency

The patient with Kidney *yang* deficiency will present with frequency of urine, nocturia, slight dribbling, nocturnal enuresis in children, incontinence in the elderly. The urine will be pale, there may well be dizziness, exhaustion, tinnitus, weak and sore back

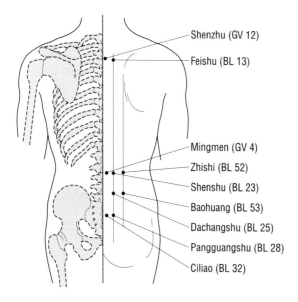

Figure 32.1   Acupuncture points: GV12 (*Shenzhu*), BL13 (*Feishu*) BL23 (*Shenshu*), BL28 (*Pangguanshu*), BL32 (*Ciliao*), BL52 (*Zhishi*), BL53 (*Baohuang*).

and a feeling of cold. The tongue will appear pale and wet and the pulse deep and weak.[6]

The treatment principle is to tonify and warm the Kidneys. Suggested sets of acupoints are:

- BL23 (*Shenshu*) (Figure 32.1); CV4 (*Guanyuan*) (Figure 32.3); SP6 (*Sanyinjiao*) (Figure 32.4) to strengthen Kidney *yang* and generally tonify the Kidneys.
- CV4 (*Guanyuan*), CV3 (*Zhongji*) (Figure 32.3), BL23 (*Shenshu*) (Figure 32.1), BL28 (*Pangguanshu*) (Figure 32.1) and KI3 (*Taixi*) (found posterior to medial malleolus above upper border of calcaneum) to strengthen the Bladder and tonify generally.

These two sets of points can be used alternately in treatment sessions. Treatment for both these syndromes should be twice weekly in the first 2–3 weeks and then weekly thereafter. Clinical experience suggests that a maximum of 12 treatments is usually sufficient if the acupuncture is going to be effective.

In many cases met in clinical practice there is an element of anxiety and stress. This is particularly so in childhood enuresis. In TCM the Heart plays an important role in stress-related conditions, and HT7 (*Shenmen*) (Figure 32.2) can be added to the other points to calm the Heart (*Shen*).

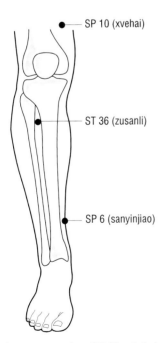

Figure 32.4 Acupuncture points: SP6 (*Sanyinjiao*), SP10 (*Xuehai*), K3 (*Taixi*). ST36 (*Zusanli*).

32.1.2.1 Treating Children

Treating a hyperactive child with needles can be a somewhat traumatic experience for practitioner and patient alike. Needles can be quickly inserted and withdrawn with good effect. This is because the *qi* or energy in children is much more accessible than in adults.

If the patient is under 16 years of age, consent from a parent or guardian is normally necessary before embarking on acupuncture treatment.

31.2 Faecal Incontinence

This can be described as a *qi* deficiency syndrome. The tongue will appear flabby and have a white coat and the pulse will be slow and weak. Points used to address this could include a selection of the following:

- GV1 (*Changqiang*) which lies between the anus and coccyx
- GV4 (*Mingmen*) (Figure 32.1) and GV20 (*Bahui*), ST25 (*Tian Shu*), CV6 (*Qihai*) (Figure 32.3) and ST36 (*Zusanli*) (Figure 32.4)

Acupuncture can be combined with electrical stimulation of the pelvic floor e.g. SP6 (*Sanyinjiao*) (Fig. 32.4) and GV20 (*Bahui*).

SP6 and GV20 are easily accessible for patients to give themselves acupressure at home. They are advised to press the points until a dull ache is felt and to hold the pressure for a minute. They can do this daily.

Lifestyle advice is of great importance as well. Regular exercise and a well-balanced diet should always be encouraged.

Many elderly patients suffering arthritic pain referred for physiotherapy have urinary problems, particularly at night. Inclusion of SP6 in the acupuncture treatment can be effective in reducing the number of times they have to empty their bladder at night.[7]

Combining acupuncture techniques with standard physiotherapy practice can be rewarding in treating these conditions. A programme of pelvic floor exercise should always be included in a treatment programme.

31.3 Pelvic Pain

The conditions addressed in this section are haemorrhoids, symphysis pubis pain and dysmenorrhoea

32.3.1 Haemorrhoids

This is a painful condition experienced by both men and women. In TCM terms the body *qi* or energy is weak and cannot properly support the structures of the pelvis. The most effective treatment is to use moxa on GV1 (*Changqiang*) and GV20. Needles can also be used, but can be very uncomfortable if there is inflammation local to the anus. The number of times of moxibustion is calculated by dividing a man's age by 8 and a woman's age by 7. Care should be taken to keep hair clear of GV20!

32.3.2 Symphysis Pubis Pain

This is a musculoskeletal problem. Needles are placed locally and distally to the pain and left in place for 15–20 minutes. Suggested points are:

- local: CV2 (*Qugu*), KI 11(*Henggu*), ST 29 (*Guilai*), ST 30 (*Qichong*) (Figure 32.3)
- distal point could be ST36 (*Zusanli*) (Figure 32.4). This gives both short- and long-term pain relief.[1]

Do not forget that the sacroiliac joints are often involved and acupoints local to these joints can also be used, e.g. BL28 or BL53 (Figure 32.1).

Electrical stimulation can enhance the effect of the needles. This is best achieved by a stimulator that gives a dense disperse current at both high and low frequency. The high frequency current (100– 150 Hz) gives an immediate effect and the low-frequency current (2–4 Hz) stimulates through the higher centres to raise the pain threshold and give a sustained effect after the stimulation is stopped.[4] The length of stimulation should be 10–20 min.

At most times it is safe to use needles to stimulate acupoints anywhere in the body, but it should be noted that traditionally, acupuncture should not be attempted in the first trimester of pregnancy, as there is anecdotal evidence of miscarriage. In the later stages of pregnancy, experienced practitioners do use acupuncture, but electrical stimulation is not to be used on these points.

TENS, acupressure or interferential therapy are all possible alternatives to needling. One should be aware, however, of the possible adverse effects of electrical stimulation even though needles are not inserted into the points.

Acute pain should be addressed in up to 6 treatments; however, chronic pain may need 6–8 treatments before there is improvement in symptoms.[1]

32.3.3 Dysmenorrhoea

The nature of pelvic pain experienced during the menses can vary a great deal. The blood flow, the type of pain and the duration relative to the monthly cycle are all significant factors. The most influential organs in the menstrual function are the Kidney, Liver and Spleen.

There are two main types of pain in dysmenorrhoea:

- Pain due to stagnation of *qi* and blood in the Uterus. Signs and symptoms are sharp pain and clots of blood in the discharge. Treatment should aim at moving the *qi* and Blood to restore normal flow.
- Dull aching pain indicative of deficiency and internal cold. The classic response is to press a hot-water bottle on the abdomen. The acupuncture treatment in this case would be directed to using points that have a warming effect and also support the Kidney and Liver.

32.3.3.1 Stagnant Liver Qi

May be associated with suppressed anger or stress in daily life. There may be resentment at the restricting aspect of the monthly cycle.

32.3.3.2 Stagnant Kidney Qi

This may be brought about mainly by an ongoing fear of loss of control in daily living. There is fear of letting go and possible fear of sexuality and pregnancy.

32.3.3.3 Deficiency of Qi and Blood

General fatigue and debility following overwork, illness or stress produces internal problems such as damp heat which inhibits the movement of *qi* and Blood.

Treatment is given once a week and can be undertaken between periods and immediately prior to them. Between the periods one is addressing the underlying deficiencies of the organ causing the problem. Treatment immediately prior to the menses is aimed at moving the *qi* and Blood. Improvement in symptoms should be measured over a three- month period in order to assess the efficacy of the treatment.

Points which can be effectively used for all the different causes of pain are:

- CV3, ST29 (Figure 32.3)
- LI4 (*Hegu*) located on the back of the hand between the first and second metacarpals
- SP6 (Figure 32.4).

This basic formula can be modified and used according to the changing needs of the patient.[8]

An important aspect of the treatment of dysmenorrhoea is exercise and this should be combined with the acupuncture treatment. Movement that uses the abdominal muscles assists the motivation of *qi* and enhances the effect of acupuncture treatment.

32.4 Prolapse

This is described as resulting from a spleen deficiency syndrome. Treatment should be focused on supporting the Spleen and raising the *qi*. The two major points to address this problem are:

- SP6 (*Sanyinjiao*) (Figure 32.4) for supporting the Spleen
- GV20 (*Bahui*) for raising *qi*.

These points can be augmented by ST36 (*Zusanli*) (Figure 32.4) which supports *qi* in the meridian system.

32.5 Conclusion

Acupuncture is a useful modality when addressing incontinence, pelvic pain and prolapse. Unfortunately there is as yet little acceptable research evidence to support these claims, and it is an area of investigation which urgently needs addressing.

References

1. Ellis N (1996) Acupuncture in Clinical Practice: A guide for health professionals, Chapter 8. Stanley Thornes, Cheltenham.
2. Andersson S, Lundberg T (1995) Acupuncture – from empiricism to science: functional background to acupuncture effects in pain and disease. Med Hypothesis 45: 271–81.
3. Han JS (1990) Differential release of enkephalin and dymorphin by low and high frequency electro-acupuncture in the central nervous system. Acupunct Sci Int J 1: 19–27.
4. Lewith G, Machin D (1983) An evaluation of the clinical effects of acupuncture. Pain 16: 111–27.
5. Kubista E, Altmann P, Kucera H, Rudelstorfer B (1976) Electro-acupuncture's influence on the closure mechanism of the female urethra in incontinence. Am J Chin Med 4(2): 177–81.
6. Maciocia G (1994) Enuresis and incontinence. In: Macioca G (ed) The Practice of Chinese Medicine: the treatment of diseases with acupuncture and Chinese herbs. Churchill Livingstone, Edinburgh, UK, pp. 526–8.
7. Ellis N (1993) A pilot study to evaluate the effect of acupuncture on nocturia in the elderly. Comp Th Med 1: 164–7.
8. Ross J (1995) Acupuncture Point Combinations: The key to clinical success. Churchill Livingstone, Edinburgh, UK, pp. 404–6.

33 Reflex Therapy

D. Isherwood

The term "reflex therapy", adopted in 1992 by the Association of Chartered Physiotherapists in Reflex Therapy (ACPIRT), is intended to encompass the practice of a variety of micro-pressure techniques on the premise that all body parts have corresponding reflex points on the feet (see Fig. 33.1) and other areas including hands (see Fig. 33.2), ears and spine.

The ancient practice of stimulating the healing energies of the body through pressure points belies the complexity of interactions taking place between the patient and practitioner. With practise and experience, sensitivity develops in the fingertips, which can detect very subtle changes in the reflex areas.

The Association of Reflexologists (a member of the Parliamentary Group for Alternative and Complementary Medicine) has produced a compilation of international research reports. A data collection network to simplify the collection of the large quantities of data necessary for analysis and research is currently being compiled. The Association of Chartered Physiotherapists in Bioenergy Therapies was formed in 1998 as a positive step towards gathering experienced researchers into the field of bioenergy therapies, including reflex therapy. Until there is research evidence of its effectiveness, any claims to the efficacy of the reflex therapy must be based on opinion.

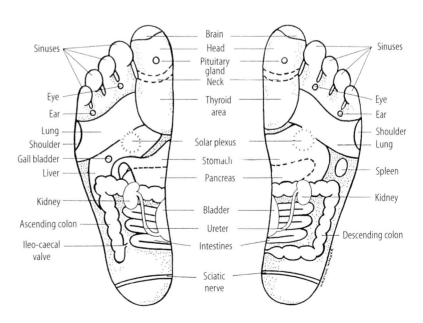

Figure 33.1 Reflex points on the soles of the feet. Reproduced by permission of the Association of Reflexologists.

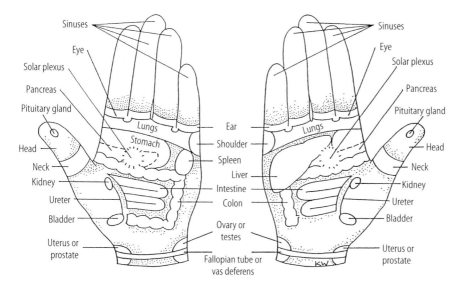

Figure 33.2 Reflex points on the palms of the hands.

33.1 Assessment

Before selecting reflex therapy as the preferred mode of treatment, a detailed assessment of the patient's medical history, current health and lifestyle must be made, followed by a detailed examination of the feet. The contraindications and special precautions relevant to reflex therapy[1] are shown in Table 33.1

Observation of the feet in standing and walking show weight-bearing pressures exerted on the reflex zones before a more detailed examination. The assessment continues with the patient covered and supported in a comfortable position, allowing access to the feet and a clear view of the patient's face. A visual followed by a palpatory assessment then takes place (see Table 33.2) and a diagram of the feet used to record initial findings for clarity and ease of reference.

Table 33.2. Visual and palpatory assessment of the feet

Visual assessment	Structure of the feet, including any arthritic changes, signs of hallux valgus and relative length and shape of the toes Presence, and particularly the position, of any corns, calluses, scars and fissures Pattern of skin colour Presence and distribution of oedema
Palpatory assessment	Reaction to initial handling of the feet Pattern of skin temperature Tissue tonus Mobility of structure Reaction to precise pressure on the reflex points of the feet

Table 33.1. Contraindications and special precautions for using reflex therapy

Contraindications	Deep vein thrombosis Pregnancies which are unstable or at risk
Special precautions	Infectious fevers and disease Acute inflammation of the venous and lymphatic systems Phlebitis Syncope Psychotic disturbance Implants, e.g. joint replacements, pacemakers and inter-uterine devices Medication, including chemotherapy

Table 33.3. Possible transient symptoms and post treatment reactions

Possible transient symptoms	Faintness Nausea Sweating Tearfulness
Possible post-treatment reactions	Changes in sleep pattern Variations in volume, colour and odour of urine and faeces Vaginal discharge, often acidic and irritating Change in menstrual flow Brief episode of fever Old, poorly healed scar tissue may become painful

Before patients are able to give informed consent, they must be aware of the possible reactions that may occur with reflex therapy.[1] These can be divided into possible transient symptoms and post-treatment reactions (see Table 33.3).

33.2 Treatment

Ideally, the patient should be treated in a comfortably warm and calm environment in order to relax, and have the opportunity to express any emotions which may surface. Reflex therapy complements other therapies such as pelvic floor exercises and bladder training, which may be used to alleviate the presenting problems.

The length of each treatment, the frequency and number of sessions required depend on the acute or chronic nature of the condition. Treatment may last from 10 min daily for 5 days, to 45 min weekly over 6 weeks. Acute conditions usually respond to short, frequent sessions over a limited period of time; chronic conditions need less intense input over a longer period with the possibility of adapting to an acute episode, which may be triggered during treatment.

The patient's general health and tolerance of any reactions that may arise are also taken into account, along with their ability to practise any self-help measures which may be advised, e.g. giving pressure on the reflex point of the uterus on the hands for dysmenorrhoea (see Fig. 33.2).

Both therapist and patient should be alert to any sweating, indicating general hypersensitivity, or chilliness, which can occur when the current limit of tolerance to the treatment has been exceeded. Care is taken at all times to assess and review any changes and to adapt the treatment accordingly. The patient remains warm and comfortable for at least 5 min at the close of treatment, to assimilate any changes that may have been experienced during the session.

For each condition the general routine is the same, consisting of relaxing massage techniques to familiarise the patient with the touch of the therapist, followed by an exploration of the current sensitivities of reflexes within the feet. Pressure is applied gradually and smoothly through the fingertips or thumbs with sufficient depth to elicit a response without inflicting unacceptable pain. Although the feet may be approached individually, a more comprehensive pattern emerges when the feet are treated together.

In treating specific conditions, reflex therapy deals with the underlying concerns that may surface as healing takes place. Anxieties and fears are common emotions that may be released during treatment. Practitioners specialising in treating conditions affecting the pelvic floor will be aware of possible underlying traumas, which may affect the patient's response to treatment. Women suffering traumatic deliveries may be victims of post-traumatic stress disorder over many years.[2] This can give rise to dyspareunia, bladder and bowel disturbances and weakness of the pelvic floor, among other physical and psychological disorders, which are unresponsive to conventional methods of treatment. Reflex therapy complements all other treatments including psychotherapy.

33.3 Changes that May Be Found During Treatment of Pelvic Conditions

The following information should be considered.

33.3.1 Menstrual Cycle

The size and sensitivity of the reproductive organs are affected by the menstrual cycle; the reflex point of the relevant ovary usually becomes swollen and sensitive just before ovulation, and the uterus point demonstrates similar responses premenstrually. The reflexes of the fallopian tubes can also become very sensitive around ovulation, particularly in cases of pelvic inflammatory disease. During menstruation, firm holds can be used over the uterine reflex to ease dysmenorrhoea. Fig. 33.3 illustrates the relevant areas.

Caution is necessary when an intrauterine device (IUD) is being used because of the possibility of rejection of the device during treatment.

33.3.2 Pregnancy

Reflexes of the endocrine system, particularly the pituitary gland, show changes in size and sensitivity, especially during the days leading up to delivery. The reflex area of the uterus enlarges during pregnancy, before gradually reducing postnatally, and a discernible rise in heat can be felt from the very early stages.

Reflex therapy is contraindicated in 'at risk' pregnancies. Due to the possibility of miscarriage in the first 12 weeks, treatment may be delayed until the second trimester. Some women respond well to treatment in the early stages, however, especially in alleviating fatigue and nausea.

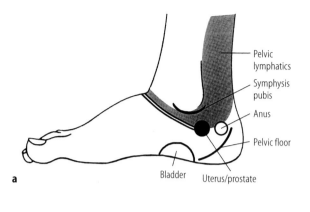

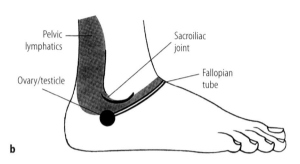

Figure 33.3 Reflex areas on the medial (**a**) and lateral (**b**) aspects of the ankle. Reproduced by permission of the Midland School of Reflextherapy.

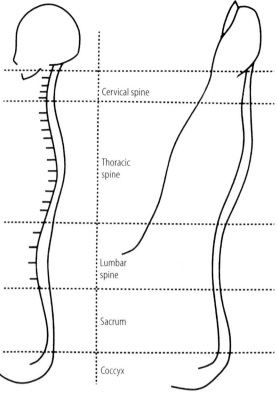

Figure 33.4 Relation of spinal levels to locations on the foot.

33.3.3 Spine

Palpation of the spinal reflexes (see Fig. 33. 4) can detect sensitivity over nerve roots, which may be involved in dysfunction in the pelvic organs. For instance, sensitivity may be found over the nerve roots of T11–L3 and S2–4. Any trauma to the coccyx can also be revealed during exploratory palpation.

33.3.4 Pelvic Joints

Palpation of the reflex points in standing, whilst observing the relative degree of pronation of the feet and structure of the arches, can provide a better understanding of pelvic imbalance. Increased sensitivity and heat over the reflex point of the symphysis pubis may be detected in the presence of inflammatory changes, and variation in sensitivity may be felt between the reflexes of the sacroiliac joints.

33.3.5 Lymphatic System

The reflexes of the pelvic lymphatics are found around the ankle joints (see Fig. 33.3); oedema in this area can indicate congestion within the pelvis, as well as inefficient circulation in the lower limbs. The initial assessment should identify the patients suffering from other conditions that could give rise to similar oedema and treatment adapted accordingly. Particular vigilance is necessary during pregnancy, when there may be a risk of pre-eclampsia.

33.3.6 Prostate and Testes

The reflex of the prostate gland may also show increased size and sensitivity if the prostate enlarges. The testes reflexes may be mobile and show sensitivity, even in a healthy state (see Fig. 33.3).

Table 33.4. Glossary of terms used in reflex therapy

Reflex points	Specific small points which reflect the body part, e.g. pituitary gland reflex found on the pad of the big toe
Reflex areas	Larger areas containing specific points, e.g. pelvic reflex area containing uterine, ovarian, anal and bladder points, found around the heel and the ankle
General relaxation	Massage of each foot and passive movement of all joints within pain-free range
Sedative holds	Holding the reflex with continuous gradual pressure of sufficient depth and length of time to elicit a calming response
Linking holds	Connecting the appropriate reflexes using two or more fingertips e.g. solar plexus with bladder reflexes to help calm an irritable bladder
Balancing of the systems	Reflex therapy encourages homeostasis by treating the reflexes of each system of the body e.g. excretory, digestive, musculoskeletal, endocrine, by either toning or sedating as necessary

33.4 Conditions Illustrated by Case Studies

The glossary of terms (see Table 33.4) will be helpful in gaining a fuller understanding of the reflex therapy treatment undertaken.

33.4.1 Bladder and Pelvic Floor

The amount of urine contained within the bladder and detrusor tone can affect the bladder reflex. When there is weakness of the pelvic floor muscles, the reflexes usually show decreased sensitivity and tone, although there may be areas of sensitivity over old scar tissue following surgery.

3.4.1.1 Case Study: Urge Incontinence

A 37-year-old primiparous woman presented 6 weeks postpartum complaining of urge incontinence, dragging pain in her perineum and a feeling of emotional upheaval.

Assessment revealed pale, cold feet with generally decreased tone. The arches were flat and the ankles showed resistance to passive ankle rotation. There was minimal oedema around the ankles and hard skin around the edge of both heels.

Palpation revealed sensitivity over the reflex points of the bladder, uterus, pelvic floor, lumbar spine, sacrum, coccyx, diaphragm, solar plexus and pelvic lymphatics. The reflex points of the pituitary, thyroid and adrenals were sunken.

Eight reflex therapy treatments over 2 months began with general relaxation techniques and balancing of the systems. The stimulation of the lymphatic system was followed by specific work on the pelvic lymphatics, helping to clear congestion. During the course of treatment, her feet became warm and more responsive, her energy levels rose and sensitivity of all affected reflexes normalised. She experienced considerable reduction in pain in her perineum and felt more able to concentrate on her exercise regimen. The urgency diminished, although she continued to have occasional episodes when confronting stressful situations. On review 2 months later, she had returned to work part-time, was pain free and reported no problem with urgency.

3.4.1.2 Case Study: Urinary Stress Incontinence

A 58-year-old female patient with three children and a husband in poor health presented with high stress levels. She was intermittently on hormone replacement therapy for night sweats and outbreaks of bad temper. She also suffered with insomnia and recurrent urinary stress incontinence over the past 2 years.

Her assessment revealed broad, flat, feet with inflexible joints and bilateral hallux valgus. The temperature graduated from hot toes to cool heels on both feet and the skin was dry. The right foot was initially intolerant to handling and the reflexes of the solar plexus (see Fig. 33.1) were depressed and hyposensitive on both feet. The bladder reflex point was hard and pale.

The first treatment consisted of relaxation techniques including comfort holds over the solar plexus reflex that was linked with the reflexes of the urinary system. Following the treatment she suffered pain in the right foot for 24 h, but the insomnia improved and she was having deep, short naps in the middle of the day.

During the course of six treatment sessions, she expressed her resentment and grief at allowing herself to be a "doormat"; she also revealed that her stress incontinence was most troublesome during housework, which she hated.

She sank into a deeply relaxed state during the treatment. Although she declined a vaginal assessment she followed a pelvic floor exercise programme. Improvement was made and she reported fewer incidents of urinary incontinence.

Progress became more erratic following a fall, but as she became more aware of her need to take time for herself, she began to enjoy a much improved sleeping pattern and felt that she could manage her own continence without further treatment.

33.4.2 Colon

Variations of tone and sensitivity along the reflexes of the colon, rectum and anus can be detected as areas of congestion or irritability are stimulated. The reflexes of the rectum and anus may be particularly sensitive in patients suffering from haemorrhoids.

3.4.2.1 Case Study: Faecal Incontinence

A 30-year-old female patient with normal deliveries of two children presented for treatment for faecal incontinence with little warning, usually after a meal.

Assessment revealed hot, swollen, difficult to palpate feet, with reflexes protected by oedema. The reflex areas of the pituitary and thyroid glands were particularly swollen; however, no sensitivities were elicited.

The first two treatments consisted of relaxation techniques and linking holds over the pelvic reflex area and the solar plexus. Although the heat began to diminish, the swelling and lack of sensitivity remained the same.

During the third treatment, she sobbed for much of the session. Her feet became cool and she was aware of sensitivity over the reflex area of the solar plexus.

The next two treatments revealed increased sensitivity over the reflexes of the small intestine, pituitary and thyroid. The reflexes of the anus, rectum and colon showed minimal sensitivity.

During the next session, there was a marked decrease in swelling and lymphatic drainage was begun. Stimulation of the reflexes of the anus and rectum, along with pelvic floor muscle exercises led to increased sensitivity and awareness of her pelvic floor and anus.

Treatment is on going, along with counselling, as the multifaceted nature of the problem is being addressed with the support of her doctor.

3.4.2.2 Case Study: Constipation

A 58-year-old female patient with adult children presented with chronic constipation.

Her assessment revealed warm mobile feet with patches of dry skin over the reflex area of the small intestine. Palpation elicited sensitivity over the pelvic lymphatic reflexes, particularly on the left foot, and over the reflexes of the cervical spine and lower thoracic area, with increased heat over the reflexes of the descending colon.

During the first treatment there was an immediate response in the digestive system. Extra stimulation was given to the pelvic lymphatic reflexes and holds were given over the affected spinal reflexes. Following the treatment, she had a normal bowel movement. By the third treatment, the whole of the digestive tract felt much improved and she was prepared to stop taking senna on a regular basis. Sensitivity over the pelvic lymphatics was minimal.

As she was about to go travelling for several months, she was shown how to stimulate the colon by giving a deep circular massage to the palm of each hand (see Fig. 33.2)

33.5 Summary

Reflex therapy, along with all other therapies, has its limitations, but there is great potential as the original concept expands to include working on the meridians and exploring the energy fields of the feet.

References

1. CSP (1997) Standards and Guidance for Good Practice in Reflex Therapy. Chartered Society of Physiotherapy, London.
2. Charles C (1997) When the dream goes wrong. . . Post-traumatic stress disorder. Midwives 110: 250–2.

Further Reading

Dougans I, Ellis S (1992) The Art of Reflexology. Element Books, Shaftesbury, Dorset.
Grinberg A (1993) Foot Analysis. Samuel Weisner Inc, York Beach, Maine.
Hall N (1994) Reflexology for Women. Thorsons, London.
Marquardt H (1983) Reflex Zone Therapy of the Feet. Thorsons, Wellingborough.
Reid E, Enzer S (1997) Maternity Reflexology – A Guide For Reflexologists, Born To Be Free, and Soul To Sole. Pymble, NSW, Australia.
Stormer C (1995) Reflexology–The Definitive Guide. Hodder & Stoughton, London.
Wagner F (1987) Reflex Zone Massage. Thorsons, Wellingborough.

34 Homeopathy

J. Worden

34.1 What Is Homeopathy and How Does It Work?

Homeopathy is a therapy based on the principle of "let like be treated by like". An amount of a substance usually toxic to the body is given in a very dilute and specially treated form to try to correct the symptoms that a large or material dose of the same substance would cause. Homeopathy considers the whole person, not just the particular symptoms of ill-health.

Nobody really knows how homeopathy works; although detailed studies of the atomic structure of liquids suggests evidence for molecules of water retaining a "memory" of substances mixed with them. This may be how the ultra-low dilutions of homeopathic remedies can be effective. There is a large body of research to support homeopathy[1-3] and five NHS-funded homeopathic hospitals. These hospitals contribute greatly to the growing volume of evidence for homeopathy, as does the Research Council for Complementary Medicine.[4,5]

Homeopathic medicine may be not only of plant origin but also mineral or animal origin, such as lachesis (snake venom) and apis (bee), in which no residue of the animal product remains, only its energy. The essential process in making a homeopathic remedy is succussing or shaking the remedy in between dilutions. It is this action that potentises or activates the remedy and makes it effective.

34.2 How Is a Remedy Chosen?

Extensive information is needed to make a homeopathic prescription, a new patient requiring 45 minutes minimum. A full medical history, including drugs and family and social history, is taken and then a homeopathic history. This includes questions about the patient's personality ("mentals"), factors affecting their symptoms such as temperature and weather ("physicals") and information about their general preferences, e.g. whether they like certain foods or not ("generals"). Seven or eight significant facts from the history covering the mental, physical and general symptoms are used to find the remedy that best encompasses the assessment.

The easiest approach for somebody inexperienced in homeopathy is the "three-legged stool" approach, where one mental, one physical and one general symptom is chosen; this method is quick and easy to apply. When discussing individual remedies for use in incontinence, the information given is with the latter method in mind.

34.3 How Can Homeopathy Help Continence?

The four main areas that are usually helped by homeopathy are stress incontinence, interstitial cystitis, enuresis and nocturia. The important thing to remember is that homeopathy can help not only on a superficial, or physical level, but also on a deeper, or mental, level. The first change in symptoms that patients normally notice is a feeling of well-being. This is an important symptom and one to ask a patient when seeing them for the first time after homeopathic treatment. When treating a chronic condition, it is normal to allow 4 weeks in between consultations as it can take some time for the gentle effect of homeopathy to become apparent. Conversely, when treating an acute urinary tract infection (UTI), the patient can feel effects within 24 h.

Unlike conventional drugs, homeopathic remedies can safely be taken by patients of all ages, from birth through to old age, and throughout pregnancy. There are no contraindications to its use by breast-feeding mothers and recent research[5] has shown an excellent safety profile. Homeopathy can be used alone or as an adjunct to conventional therapy.

A course of treatment may vary from a single tablet to continuous therapy. With a long-standing problem, it can take several consultations to see the symptom picture clearly and it always helps to be realistic with patients rather than overly optimistic.

34.4 Homeopathic Remedies for the Urinary Tract

34.4.1 Stress Incontinence

Causticum is probably the leading remedy for stress incontinence. Mentally, this remedy is suited to someone who is inclined to be weepy and pessimistic but with sympathy for others, and who can be proud. Physically, tenesmus and then incontinence of urine is common, or post-operatively urine retention. Generally, they are very sensitive to the cold, particularly dry and frosty weather.

Sepia is a key remedy where stress incontinence is due to a cystocele. Mentally, the women are depressed with a lack of libido. They often seem to be little affected by their loved ones and weep easily. Physically, they complain of the feeling of a dragging feeling, even in the absence of a prolapse. Generally, they are chilly, but when feeling well, love to dance. They enjoy spicy food but can become nauseated when hungry.

Pulsatilla helps many urinary symptoms. Incontinence from coughing or changing position is typical. Mentally, patients are mild mannered and weep easily, enjoying consolation or sympathy, unlike sepia patients who become irritable when offered sympathy. They are typically changeable, with changing mood and changing symptoms. Physically, they can experience a severe urge to pass urine but can only pass it drop by drop. Generally, they dislike stuffy rooms but can become chilled. They feel better for gentle exercise in the fresh air; they have a sweet tooth and enjoy ice-cream and cream cakes, although they find that the latter can upset them.

34.4.2 Interstitial Cystitis

Staphisagria is one of the most used remedies for this syndrome of dysuria, urgency and frequency but with negative bacteriology tests on urine culture. Incontinence is a not uncommon side effect although patients often complain that if delaying urination they then cannot pass urine and their discomfort increases. Mentally, staphisagria patients are very sensitive emotionally, especially to criticism, and tend to bottle up their anger or indignation although they are seething inside. Although not demonstrating a high libido, they nevertheless think about sex quite often. If their temper flares, they are liable to throw things. Physically, their urinary symptoms are often worse after emotional upheaval. The peculiar symptom of feeling that urine is trickling down the urethra is common and also burning pains around the bladder and urethra when not passing urine. Staphisagria is also indicated when urinary symptoms seem related to first sexual intercourse or "honeymoon cystitis", or a history of physical or mental abuse. Generally, patients are chilly and enjoy eating bread and sweet things.

Apis is also a useful remedy. Mentally, apis patients feel that they must keep busy, rather like the bee from which the remedy is made. Physically, they complain of a stinging or burning sensation around the urethra, which can persist for some time after passing urine. They may have localised swelling of the genital area with extreme sensitivity to touch. Generally, they are hot and are intolerant of heat.

Petroselinum is almost specific for interstitial cystitis. There are no particular mental or general symptoms for this remedy but physically there is burning and stinging throughout the whole perineum to the urethra, with a sudden urgency; if delayed, they are incontinent. The pain on passing urine is extreme, leading to the patient dancing around the room in agony.

Cantharis is similar in its physical attributes to petroselinum in that patients needing this remedy have an irresistible desire to pass urine, but cantharis patients are more restless and excited. Cantharis is made from Spanish fly and the vision of somebody infuriated by the burning pains of these biting insects should help when deciding whether to prescribe cantharis or another remedy. Haematuria is common, with a relief from pain if lying down. Generally, patients feel better for warmth and rest and worse for drinking coffee, which can exacerbate their urinary symptoms severely.

34.4.3 Enuresis

The involuntary passage of urine at night may occur because of an acute UTI or simple inability to get to the toilet quickly enough. When referring to enuresis in this section, I will be suggesting remedies that can be used where the control of urination is lost while sleeping.

Terebinthina is a remedy particularly suited to the elderly. Mentally, there is tiredness and difficulty with concentration of thoughts. There may be confusion or depression. Physically, strangury may precede incontinence, with pain on micturition. Generally, patients feel worse in damp, cold weather, tend to get a bloated stomach after eating and feel better when warm and taking some exercise.

Tuberculinum is extremely safe to use in all age groups and works well for enuresis. If using it in a child, look for sensitivity but with underlying irritability with a tendency to throw temper tantrums. They tend to have a poor resistance to infections and suffer from lots of coughs, colds or tonsillitis. Generally, they are hungry and love to drink cold milk but can remain surprisingly thin. They do not sleep well and may suffer from nightmares. Adults requiring tub.bov., as it is abbreviated, will often complain of chronic tiredness and appear somewhat dissatisfied with life. They love to travel and want to do different things all the time but can become weary of life if thwarted in this. Generally, they sleep badly, feeling tired in the day, but are unable to rest at night. They particularly desire smoked meat, and also salty and refreshing foods. They dislike changes in weather, especially if it is damp and cold and feel better for fresh air. There may, or may not be, a family history of TB.

34.4.4 Nocturia

Lycopodium is a remedy that not only encompasses acute and chronic UTIs but is very useful for the treatment of nocturia, particularly where the cause of the symptom is prostatism. Mentally, patients often feel weak and inadequate and incapable of fulfilling their responsibilities. They can overcompensate for these feelings and present a picture of extrovert friendliness and courage. Bullying behaviour is the extreme manifestation of this aspect of their personality. They can be sensitive and weep when emotional. Physically, impotence is a common associated problem despite a strong sexual drive. Indigestion and the ability to feel full after small meals with abdominal bloating immediately after eating is also a common complaint of patients requiring this remedy. Generally, lycopodium patients are chilly with cold hands and feet. They like warm drinks as opposed to cold ones and have a marked sweet tooth.

Sabal serrulata is another common nocturia remedy that is also available in a herbal form. It is also useful for enuresis and has been termed the "homeopathic catheter" for urinary retention due to enlarged prostate. Although usually prescribed on its physical attributes, sabal serrulata's mental attributes include a dislike of sympathy and tendency to brood on perceived sufferings or wrongdoings. They fear to fall asleep in case something should happen in the night. Physically, there is a constant desire to pass urine in the night with strangury and a feeling of bladder coldness that can extend to the genitals. Generally, patients are better after sleep and dislike cold, damp, cloudy weather; they like milk.

Nux vomica is another remedy that can be used for both enuresis and nocturia. It is commonly seen as a male remedy but can in fact be used for either sex. Mentally, patients are angry and impatient with a poor pain threshold. There is a tendency to eat, drink and work too much, which is why it is often referred to as the "executive" remedy. Physically, the bladder is irritable with frequent visits to the toilet but with only small amounts of urine passed each time. Renal colic may have been a problem in the past or urethral stricture. Generally, patients are worse for cold and in the early morning. Stress also affects them to a severe degree as does coffee, alcohol and drugs. Resting is the one thing guaranteed to make them feel better.

34.5 Doses of Homeopathic Remedies

The doses of homeopathic remedies are much more variable than those of conventional drugs. Most of the over-the-counter remedies are a 6C strength, which should be taken as described on the packet. Professional homeopaths would normally suggest a 30C strength taken daily for a limited period of time of 7–10 days. For a long-standing problem, a daily dosage of a 6X remedy might be suggested. Generally the higher the number, the more potent the remedy. X remedies are the weakest, then C and finally M. The more potent the remedy, the more the chance of an aggravation of symptoms. There is no particular need to take age into consideration, except when treating the very young, when a weaker remedy is usually suggested. Homeopathic tablets are safe in overdose.

34.6 Finding and Choosing a Homeopath

The training of homeopaths is variable, without statutory guidelines, although the Faculty of Homeopathy in London oversees the training of medically qualified homeopaths and will be conducting ongoing training and re-accreditation for its members. Associate membership of the Faculty is open to doctors, nurses, veterinary surgeons, dentists, podiatrists, midwives and pharmacists. Doctors and veterinary surgeons may become members by taking a rigorous exam after a prescribed period of training. The Society of Homeopaths is one of the largest organisations promoting homeopathy through its non-medically qualified members, and being on its Register indicates a certain level of experience. Both organisations are actively campaigning to increase the availability of homeopathy within the NHS.

Homeopathy is part of NHS services via the homeopathic hospitals and trained general practitioners. The remedies are available on NHS FP10 GP prescriptions, although not all of the combination types are allowed. Some high-street chemists are training their pharmacists in homeopathic prescribing and now stock homeopathic remedies, which may be bought over the counter without prescription.

References

1. Kleijnen J, Knipschild P, Ter Rief G (1991) Clinical trials of homeopathy. BMJ 302: 316–23.
2. Linde K, Clausius N, Ramiraz G et al. (1997) Are the clinical effects of homeopathy placebo effects? A meta-analysis of placebo-controlled trials. Lancet 350: 834–43.
3. Anonymous (1997) Complementary medicine. What works for you ? Health Which (June): 84–7.
4. Reilly D (1998) The Evidence for Homeopathy (3rd ed). Academic Departments of Homeopathy, Glasgow.
5. Royal London Homeopathic Hospitals NHS Trust (1999) The Evidence Base for Complementary Medicine (2nd ed). Royal London Homeopathic Hospitals NHS Trust, London.

VII Professional Issues

35 Research Trials in Incontinence

P. Assassa and F. Mensah

Current health care has often evolved by trial and error over many years, any intervention seemingly causing improvement becoming incorporated into practice. However, many of these interventions are not able to stand up to close scrutiny. To determine current best practice more investigations need to be undertaken in evaluating current treatments and also before new treatments are incorporated into practice.

35.1 Randomised Controlled Trials

The most powerful methodology for investigating the effectiveness of treatments is the randomised controlled trial (RCT). This is a true prospective experiment in which investigators randomly assign an eligible sample of patients to one or more treatment groups and follow patients' outcomes. The fundamental feature of a RCT is that the response of the patients receiving the intervention under investigation is compared to the response of a control group receiving a standard intervention or placebo. To make this comparison unbiased the two groups must be similar in every respect other than the intervention. Obvious confounding variables that are likely to influence the results of the trial such as age, sex, marital status, or social class will be randomly distributed between the groups. Less easily definable and obvious variables (for example patients' willingness to comply with treatment), which might influence treatment response, will also be randomly distributed.

Uncontrolled trials are not advisable in incontinence as the condition is prone to spontaneous variation over time. It has been shown that incontinent people may spontaneously remit at a rate of about 10% per year.[1,2]

RCTs provide valuable evidence in the evaluation of treatments and services for incontinence. They must, however, be well organised and conducted to proper ethical and scientific standards. A good RCT has a clear hypothesis stating the study population, the condition to be treated, the intervention under investigation, and the outcome or response to treatment.

35.2 Study Population

It is important to use a suitable case definition when selecting patients to take part in a trial; this should be clearly decided in terms of the source of cases and any criteria such as age, gender or diagnosis used for selection. For example, in a drug treatment for patients with detrusor instability, we would need to make a diagnosis based on accepted guidelines such as those put forward by the International Continence Society.[3] However, in a primary care continence service, we would want to include all patients within the community with significant urinary leakage. This may be defined by reported symptoms, e.g. leakage several times per month[4] or clinical assessment, e.g. a urine pad loss of more than 10 g.[5] In the second example, case definition might be expanded beyond incontinence to include storage abnormality symptoms such as urgency, urinary frequency and nocturia.

The definition of a case should include patients in whom the intervention is likely to produce benefit and should preferably include all groups who may receive the intervention in the future. It is advisable to exclude as few patients from a trial as possible. Some exclusions are unavoidable, such as patients with medical contraindications to receiving the active treatment, e.g. patients with glaucoma in anticholinergic drug trials. However, some trials have excluded elderly and frail patients. Within these groups there is a high prevalence of incontinence and a great need for effective treatment. Extrapolation of the results of trials that have excluded such groups may be misleading if applied to them. In general, if a group is likely to receive treatment in the future on the basis of the trial results, they should be included as cases within the trial. A good trial will, as far as possible, be generalisable to future practice and inclusion and exclusion criteria will be explicitly specified and reasonable.

The source of cases needs to be considered carefully. Patients are probably best recruited from the place where the treatment under investigation is likely to be offered in the future. The prevalence of the condition to be treated should be known. If a relatively rare condition is to be investigated there is likely to be a need for multi-centre collaboration to recruit enough patients.

35.3 Size of Trial

The sample size must be large enough to be able to give reliable estimates of the response to treatment of each of the treatment groups, and thus powerful enough to detect a difference between the treatments, if there is one. A sample size calculation should be carried out during the planning phase of the trial to ensure that it is feasible to recruit an adequately sized sample. This statistical calculation will be based on the expected response to the standard or control treatment, the minimum difference between the treatments you wish to be able to detect and the ability of the trial (power) to detect this difference.

35.4 Randomisation and Blinding

As described above, randomisation of eligible participants within the trial is essential. To do this practically a list of allocations is drawn up before recruitment starts, using a simple method such as random tables or a computerised statistical package. When a patient consents to enter the trial, allocation to a treatment can then be achieved by referring to this list. Such methods include opening a sealed envelope containing the treatment to be allocated, or

a hospital pharmacy dispensing pre-randomised numbered packages of drug treatments. If feasible, the trial should be double blind; this is achieved by ensuring that both the patient and anyone involved in assessment or treatment are unaware of which treatment group the patient has been allocated to. The purpose of this is to remove any influences which may be present due to knowledge about which treatment a patient is receiving.

35.5 Interventions and Controls

A wide ranges of interventions is available for continence care. These may be very specific such as drug or surgical therapies, or may be more general such as service packages or health promotion. The intervention should have a good scientific basis and warrant further investigation. A literature search should be performed to describe this and the key elements of the intervention. The intervention should be formally described and follow pre-defined protocols. It is important that the intervention follows accepted best practice, e.g. using the right dose of drug, so that it is not open to criticism later. An accurate description will help others repeat the trial or transfer it into general clinical practice. The length of the intervention should be long enough for any treatment effects to be apparent, but an over-long intervention period may result in excessive withdrawals from the trial.

Selection of the control is important. In comparative studies an accepted treatment may be compared to a new treatment. The result of such a study will show if the new treatment is better, worse or comparable to accepted treatment. However, the implications of this will depend on the efficacy of the accepted treatment. If the accepted treatment is poor then a comparable treatment will be just as poor. To truly measure efficacy, a placebo must be used. Most studies in incontinence have found a large degree of improvement in people receiving placebo.[6] It is the ability of an intervention to show improvement above this placebo effect that is the true efficacy of that treatment. As far as possible, apart from the experimental intervention, the treatment and care the groups receive should be identical.

35.6 Assessment

It is important to perform a thorough assessment of each patient at the beginning of the trial. This will measure the baseline condition of each patient, a repeat assessment at the study end will show any change.

Questioning the patient using a structured questionnaire is usually easy. However, it is important that the questions have been validated, and suitable questionnaires are available.[7,8] Incontinence is a socially disabling and hygienic problem to patients and so the outcome of an intervention should be measured from a patients' perspective. The questions should ask about the severity of the condition but should also explore the effect of the condition on the patient's quality of life in terms of psycho-social morbidity.[9] Questionnaires are, however, open to influence by the person administering them. As far as possible, an independent observer who is unaware of which intervention the patient has received should perform questionnaires used as outcome measures, e.g. surgeons should not question patients about the outcome of their own surgery.

Many clinicians believe that objective assessment of bladder function is the best form of outcome assessment. The use of a well-structured, easily completed voiding diary can be achieved in the majority of patients, provided detailed verbal and written instructions are given. This should give information on frequency of micturition (by both day and night), frequency of incontinence, and an estimation of types and volumes of fluid ingestion. Measurement of the volume of each void will allow calculation of mean voided volume and functional bladder capacity (maximum void). Diaries are only as good as the patients' ability to fill them in accurately. They should therefore not be over-complex or performed over too long a period of time.

Another objective measurement often used in incontinence is the pad test. Pre-weighed pads can be worn by a patient and then re-weighed to calculate the amount of urine lost. The pad can be worn while a standard set of exercises are performed, such as during the ICS 1h pad test,[3] or can be worn and collected over a period of time in the patient's normal environment.

Objective measurements used as outcome measurements should be performed under as similar conditions as possible and be performed on the same day of the week, in the same place, etc. Other outcomes that may be important are compliance and side-effects of the interventions used, as well as the patient's satisfaction with the intervention. These help to show how easily the intervention might be used outside the study. In modern health care it is also important to perform some economic evaluation. This should take into account both the cost of the intervention and any improvement in the financial burden of the condition on the patient or the health service.

35.7 Ethical Considerations

Before commencing a study a complete protocol should be assembled. As part of this, patient information material should be produced which ensures informed consent to participate in the study is obtained. All protocols, information material and consent forms must be submitted to the relevant medical ethical committee for approval before commencing recruitment.

35.8 Analysis

The aim of analysis of an RCT is to compare the response of each of the treatment groups, to try to estimate whether there are differences between the treatments, and the size of any difference. Various analysis techniques are available to do this ranging from a simple t-test to more complicated modelling and survival analysis.[10,11] The involvement of a medical statistician early in planning the trial is to be encouraged as the type of analytical techniques that can be used will depend on the trial design, the hypothesis to be tested and the outcome measures used. Specific issues which need to be thought about carefully include how to analyse patients who change from the intervention they were originally allocated to (for some reason such as intolerable side effects), and how to cope when the data collected is incomplete.

35.9 Conclusion

Properly conducted clinical trials require careful planning and are often difficult to perform. However, it is the results of such trials that will determine future organisation and delivery of healthcare provision. They are therefore important and rewarding in terms of ensuring that patients receive the best possible standard of health care in the future.

References

1. Herzog AR, Diokno AC, Brown MB, Normolle DP, Brock BM (1990) Two-year incidence, remission, and change patterns of urinary incontinence in non institutionalized older adults. J Gerontol 45(2): 67–74.

2. Nygaard IE, Lemke JH (1996) Urinary incontinence in rural older women: prevalence, incidence and remission. J Am Geriatr Soc 44(9): 1049–54.
3. Abrams P, Blaivas JG, Stanton SL, Andersen JT (1998) The standardisation of terminology of lower urinary tract function. Scand J Urol Nephrol Suppl 114: 5–19.
4. O'Brien J, Austin M, Sethi P, O'Boyle P (1991) Urinary incontinence: prevalence, need for treatment, and effectiveness of intervention by nurse. BMJ 303: 1308–12.
5. Jeyaseelan SM, Oldham JA, Roe BH (1997) The use of perineal pad testing to assess urinary incontinence. Rev Clin Gerontol 7: 83–92.
6. Tapp A, Fall M, Norgaard J et al. (1989) Terodiline: a dose titrated, multicenter study of the treatment of idiopathic detrusor instability in women. J Urol 142(4): 1027–31.
7. Jackson S, Donovan J, Brookes S et al. (1996) The Bristol Female Lower Urinary Tract Symptoms questionnaire: development and psychometric testing. Br J Urol 77(6): 805–12.
8. Donovan JL, Abrams P, Peters TJ et al. (1996) The ICS-'BPH' Study: the psychometric validity and reliability of the ICSmale questionnaire. Br J Urol 77(4): 554–62.
9. Kelleher CJ, Cardozo LD, Khullar V, Salvatore S (1997) A new questionnaire to assess the quality of life of urinary incontinent women. Br J Obstet Gynaecol 104(12): 1374–9.
10. Pocock SJ (1983) Clinical Trials: A practical approach. John Wiley & Sons, Chichester, UK.
11. Armitage P, Berry G (1994) Statistical Methods in Medical Research (3rd ed). Blackwell Scientific Publications, Oxford.

36 Audit

J. Clayton

Three of the most important elements underpinning the provision of healthcare at the beginning of the twenty-first century, and supporting the central theme of health policy in the United Kingdom, are clinical governance, evidence-based practice and clinical effectiveness. Audit contributes in some way to measuring achievement in all three.

- Clinical governance involves the recognition of corporate responsibility and individual accountability to improve and maintain the quality of services,[1] and audit is one of the key components of the infrastructure required to support it.[2]
- Evidence-based healthcare involves "doing the right thing right".[3] One of the criteria identified for its introduction is to evaluate any changes that have resulted from applying the "evidence" to practice.
- Clinical effectiveness involves doing more good than harm,[4] and uses audit to confirm what is actually happening in practice.

36.1 Audit and the NHS Reforms

Audit came to the fore in healthcare in the UK with the introduction of the NHS reforms in 1990, as part of the drive to provide value for money. Initially the focus was on medical audit that used quantitative measures as indicators of the quality of care, for example, morbidity, mortality and cure rates. By 1992 the initiatives to introduce audit to all aspects of healthcare was widened to include nurses and the professions allied to medicine, and these groups tended to use more qualitative measures, for example, standards of care or criteria such as acceptability, appropriateness or timeliness as mea-

sures of their performance or as outcome measures of care.

By the middle of the decade these initiatives had been superseded by multidisciplinary or clinical audit in order to provide a more accurate evaluation of services and their impact on patients. This has since progressed to multi-agency audit involving non-clinical groups such as social services.

36.2 What Is Audit?

Audit is a systematic process that checks and reviews. It describes what has been done, how it was done and why, it explains different kinds of activity and their impact, using objective measures alongside subjective judgement to identify success or failure. It identifies and acknowledges good practice, provides a measure of the quality of patient care and examines the structures used to deliver services.[5]

Audit will examine and evaluate:

- the available resources to provide care: the quality of the service
- the treatments and interventions: the quality of care
- the outcomes of service provision and care provided in terms of quality of life
- the inputs of care to include costs, skills and workload and the outputs of care that include productivity (caseloads, throughput, cure rates, value for money, etc.) and patient outcomes (clinical response and satisfaction).

Methods similar to those used in research are often used in the measurement phase of audit, but it is clearly different from research. Several kinds of activities are used to collect audit data. They include checking records, equipment and computer files, asking questions as part of an interview or by using a questionnaire, and observation to see what is actually happening. The data is then analysed to provide a snapshot of activity in a certain place or at a particular time or used for comparison, e.g. over time, of different environments or of outcomes of different interventions used to treat similar problems.

The three key aspects of audit activity involve:

- being sure that audit is the appropriate activity to answer your questions
- designing and carrying out the audit
- maintaining or changing practice in response to your audit findings or results

In 1996 the Continence Foundation issued a purchasing guide for continence services[6] aimed at general practitioners, which included a framework for the evaluation of service provision. This framework suggested nine indicators of effectiveness, which could be applied to any element of a service. They include:

- access to the service
- full needs assessment
- evidence-based
- treatment outcomes
- patient satisfaction
- capacity and appropriate use
- availability of information
- cost and value for money.

These guidelines were complemented by a clinical audit scheme prepared and published by the Royal College of Physicians[7] which provides audit proforma for the management of incontinence in individual patients, multiple patient audit tools and facility audits to support the review of policies and procedures.

Some validated, standard instruments are also available which have been developed specifically for use with incontinent people and can be used to audit the impact and effectiveness of their treatment and management programmes. They include the Incontinence Impact Questionnaire,[8] described as a health-related quality of life tool, and the Male and Female ICS Questionnaire,[9] which measures clinical status alongside quality of life using the concept of "bothersomeness".

A government review of continence service was completed in 1999 and published in 2000[10] in which audit is recognised as one of the key elements of service provision linking local provision directly to

Health Improvement Programmes, National Service Frameworks, the National Institute for Clinical Excellence, the National Framework for Assessing Performance and the National Survey of Patient Experience as set out in the white paper, *A First Class Service*.[1]

36.3 Conclusion

Whatever interventions or regimes are used in the assessment and conservative treatment of incontinence and pelvic floor disorders, it is essential to monitor and review their impact and in some way measure their effectiveness. It is important to use audit to take account of clinical standards, costs and patients' views and to encompass all aspects of service provision, for example health education, health promotion and product use as well as direct clinical interventions or complementary therapies. Audit has become a routine part of healthcare provision and although its findings are not generalisable or directly transferable, as research findings should be, by sharing the experience of audit, practitioners help to improve the overall quality of patient care.

References

1. National Health Service Executive (1998) A First Class Service: Quality in the New NHS. Department of Health, London.
2. McSherry R, Haddock J (1999) Evidence-based health care: its place within clinical governance. Br J Nurs 8(2): 113–17.
3. Muir Gray JA (1996) Evidence-based Healthcare: How to make health policy and management decisions. Churchill Livingstone, Edinburgh, UK.
4. NHS Centre for Reviews and Dissemination (1999) Effective Healthcare; Getting evidence into practice. NHS Centre for Reviews and Dissemination, University of York.
5. Malby B (1995) Clinical Audit for Nurses and Therapists. Scutari Press, London.
6. Continence Foundation (1996) Purchasing Continence Services; A brief guide for general practitioners. Continence Foundation, London.
7. RCP (1998) Promoting Continence; Clinical audit scheme for the management of urinary and faecal incontinence. Royal College of Physicians, London.
8. Schumaker S, Wyman J, Hebersax J, McClish D, Fantl J (1994) Health related quality of life measures for women with urinary incontinence: the Incontinence Impact Questionnaire and the Urogenital Distress Inventory. Qual Life Res 3: 291–306.
9. Donovan J, Abrams P, Peters T et al. (1996) The ICS-BPH Study: the psychometric validity and reliability of the ICS male questionnaire. Br J Urol 177(4): 554–62.
10. DoH (2000) Good Practice in Continence Services. Department of Health, London.

37 Infection Control Issues

L. Barkess-Jones and J. Haslam

The following chapter refers to the UK, but the principles should be transferable to other countries.

The need to raise the profile of infection control has never been higher, owing to the development of clinical governance within the NHS,[1] which is at the heart of the Government's recent white papers (see Chapter 36).[2,3] The principal aim is to ensure that care is consistent and that quality is afforded the same focus as financial management.

Within the clinical governance framework, all professional staff are required to ensure that the guidance is implemented fully. They must be conversant with their equipment and be fully competent, knowledgeable and experienced to implement the associated operating processes. Furthermore, clinical governance seeks to build on existing good practices, utilising evidence-based practice and research and thus engendering a culture of continuous professional development.

The introduction of a controls assurance function seeks to assure that existing guidance is implemented in order to standardise and endorse good practice within the NHS. This includes clinical risk assessment, clinical audit, the development of a learning culture, patient feedback, accreditation schemes and the use of evidence based clinical practice. Clinical Governance and its controls assurances apply to all clinical practitioners in both primary and secondary care organisations.

The first controls assurance is in infection control,[4] and this should be considered in conjunction with the Department of Health Safety Action Bulletin 108 on the decontamination of vaginal instrumentation[5] and decontamination of medical devices.[6] The issue of infection control encompasses not only the decontamination of equipment before and after use, but also includes consideration of the environment and risk assessment of the patient and staff, and incorporates any product or company guidance as appropriate. This information should form the basis of any infection control policy to be agreed between the professional user-groups and the infection control department and then approved by the local infection control committee. Each policy should include the names of the authors, the names of those who have agreed it, the date it was agreed and the date it should be reviewed, so that any clinician who reads or implements the policy can clarify any points or changes in practice required.

37.1 Background

The following background information should be considered when formulating infection control policies.

37.1.1 The Environment

The environment must be free from dust to ensure that micro-organisms are kept to a minimum. The majority of dust is made up of skin scales, and within it some micro-organisms can survive for long periods of time.[7] Working in a dusty environment helps to facilitate contamination of equipment and hands, so an acceptable standard of cleanliness for the working environment should be agreed with the domestic manager.[8]

The patient should be examined on a couch covered with either disposable paper sheeting or a clean sheet that is changed between patients. Any surfaces that have been contaminated must be cleaned adequately using detergents and water, and disinfected if required.[9,10] Each NHS Trust infection control department should have a decontamination policy and a list of recommended disinfectants. Tubes of lubricants can become contaminated, so it

243

is recommended that the first 2.5 cm of lubricant from the tube is discarded at the beginning of each day and the tube discarded after 1 week's usage. Otherwise an individual lubricant sachet should be used for each patient.

Within the room there should be appropriately allocated separate waste bins for domestic waste (black bin liner), and for clinical waste products (yellow bin liner). Clinical waste includes anything that has come into contact with the patient, or could be contaminated with the patient's body secretions or fluids. Domestic waste is any other waste that can be disposed of in a land-fill site.[9] There should also be a wash-basin for general cleaning, and a clinical hand-hygiene basin to prevent cross-contamination from the dirty aerosols caused by water splashing back on to the hands during the washing process along with air back-draft from the overflow recess.[11] Storage space (cupboards or drawers) should be used to prevent environmental contamination of gloves, aprons and other equipment.[7]

37.1.2 Risk Assessment

Risk assessments should be an integral part of patient care in order to help staff prioritise and manage any professional risks, and should be undertaken on each patient in order to identify any infections. An appropriate decision[7] can then be made either to postpone a required procedure and make an appropriate medical referral, or to adopt suitable protective clothing and ensure the decontamination of equipment, etc.

The management of risk assessment is the responsibility of the individual carrying out the procedure and is undertaken to protect both the clinician and the patient from the possibility of acquiring infection from one another.

37.2 Universal Precautions

"Universal precautions" (sometimes known as "standard body fluid precautions" or "blood and body fluid precautions") should be observed when there is an anticipated contact with blood or body fluids.[12] These precautions, in addition to appropriate protective clothing, are normally adequate to protect the clinician. The use of pressure probes, vaginal or anal electrodes, or cone therapy should not proceed if there is any cause for concern regarding possible communicable disease; guidance from the local infection control team should be sought.

37.2.1 Protective Clothing

Protective clothing is a two-way barrier to protect the patient as well as the clinician and should be worn if the risk assessment deems it appropriate. Gloves and apron should be worn to prevent clothing and hands from becoming contaminated with bacteria or body fluids if there is a possibility of contact with body fluids.[7] If there is a high risk of splashing, or aerosol spray, goggles should also be worn.[7] For routine vaginal assessment examination gloves (bulk boxed) should be worn. For any catheterisation procedure or examination of broken vaginal or vulval membranes, then appropriate sterile gloves and an apron must be worn.

All gloves must be checked before the examination of a patient to ensure that they are not damaged. When gloves are removed, care must be taken to ensure that there is no possibility of self-contamination with the patient's body fluids and the gloves must be discarded into a yellow clinical waste bag. The clinician must always wash their hands using an appropriate product before putting on and removing gloves.

37.2.2 Probe Sheaths and Condoms

The condom or probe sheath may be of latex or some other material, and is applied to cover the full length of the pressure device extending along any extension tube, or other equipment as appropriate. Condoms are deemed to be adequate protection for perineometers as perineometry does not use as vigorous a force as sexual activity (for which condoms have been shown to be impermeable to viruses with a 90–95% success rate).[13,14]

Hands must always be washed using an appropriate technique before placing a new sheath or condom on equipment; after use, the condom must be discarded into a clinical yellow bag. NB. Condoms that have a spermicide applied to them should not be used on patients having fertility investigations or problems.

37.2.3 Cautionary Note on Latex

Universal precautions still require the use of latex products as research shows that it provides proven protection against blood-borne viruses,[13,15] but research is ongoing into polyurethane and nitrile products as future alternatives. However, during the risk assessment, it should be ascertained whether the patient has any known latex problem. If a suspected latex irritation, sensitivity or allergy is reported, then no procedure using latex gloves or condoms should take place without prior medical consultation. Latex-free gloves (e.g. Dermaprene and Allegard), and latex-free condoms or sheaths (e.g. Femidom, Avanti, Trojan Supra) can readily be purchased. Also, there may be a need to provide a latex-free environment; NHS Trusts should therefore have latex allergy policies and action plans.

37.3 Hand Hygiene

Thorough hand-washing technique should be practised at all times to reduce the number of surface skin micro-organisms on the clinician's hands, along with any transient environmental or patient micro-organisms which may have been picked up inadvertently. Thorough hand washing is normally sufficient to remove surface and transient bacteria.[9]

The hand hygiene technique is more important in removing bacteria than the time spent washing hands. Clinicians can augment hand washing by using an antimicrobial soap, which will remove and destroy transient micro-organisms, but there is a risk that some users may develop skin disorders. Where rapid skin disinfection on the same patient is required, a 70% alcohol hand-rub solution can be used.[7,9] This use of alcohol solution is supplementary to the hand washing, not a substitute for it; requiring the same hand hygiene technique to distribute the alcohol across the surface of the skin.

An appropriate cover that is waterproof, bacteria-proof and virus-proof must be applied to cuts, abrasions, or eczema to protect from environmental micro-organisms and blood-borne pathogens.[7,9,12]

37.4 Inoculation Injuries

There should be a hospital NHS Trust reporting system for any accidents or incidents that place either patient or staff at risk. Any incidence of innoculation injuries should be reported in accordance with local policy to include the patient's risk assessment especially if there is any history of blood-borne or any sexually transmitted diseases. This will help to formulate the inoculation injury risk assessment, and enable the clinician to receive appropriate prophylactic treatment as required.[12] Incidents should be evaluated and audited to modify clinical procedures as appropriate.

37.5 Equipment

It is imperative under the controls assurance for infection control[4] and the Medical Device Agency guidance[16] that equipment is used in line with the manufacturers' stipulation with respect to its being:

- single use (used once then discarded)
- single patient use (used for one patient's treatment programme and decontaminated between appointments)
- multiple use (used on any patient provided that it is sterilised between each patient using appropriate infection control measures).

In view of the presence of normal skin and genital bacterial flora and other potential micro-organisms in the genital area, equipment must be protected and decontaminated after use.[5] Each individual piece of equipment requires risk assessment for the level of decontamination required.

Items that have contact with mucous membranes are considered medium risk and should be sterilised by an autoclave or appropriate chemical sterilant solution between patients. Where this is impossible, the equipment must be cleansed, disinfected and covered with a sterile sheath (agreement with the local infection control team should be sought). Items considered of lower risk are those in contact only with intact skin. In this case cleansing is sufficient.

When choosing any decontamination process, the issue of Consumer protection[17] and medical devices regulations[18] must be borne in mind at all times. An individual clinician must comply with a manufacturer's guidance or instructions on decontamination and reprocessing, otherwise any product liability will transfer to the clinician or NHS Trust.

Collaboration between the users and companies can lead to a greater harmonisation between healthcare decontamination facilities, product design to enable vaginal equipment to be sterilised in accordance with the requirements of Safety Action Bulletin 108[5] and the controls assurance for infection control.[4,10]

37.6 Decontamination

A decontamination process may include cleansing, disinfection and sterilisation, as described in Table 37.1. Equipment for disinfection or sterilisation must always be cleansed beforehand to decrease bacteria and organic debris present.

Table 37.1. Possible decontamination processes

Decontamination	Process	Method
Cleansing	The physical removal of contamination and many micro-organisms	Detergent and water at 50-55°C. Rinse
Disinfection	The physical reduction of the number of micro-organisms to a level at which they are not harmful. The process removes the majority of bacteria but spores will not usually be destroyed	Cleanse first as above. Temperatures of 90°C or chemical disinfectants
Sterilisation	The removal or destruction of all micro-organisms including spores	Cleanse first as above. Steam sterilisation at 121°C or chemical sterilisation

It is preferable that any decontamination process is undertaken by the hospital sterilisation and disinfection units (HSDU), as they are required to provide the required validation and documentation to enable batch tracing of sterilised items in the event of manufacturing problems. If a central sterilisation services department (CSSD) is responsible for decontamination and sterilisation of equipment they are required to comply with the controls assurance in infection control and implement the guidance on washer disinfectors (HTM2030)[19] and autoclaves (HTM2010)[20].

37.6.1 Benchtop Washer-Disinfectors and Steam Sterilisers

If decontamination is performed in a benchtop steam steriliser, it is necessary that the equipment be first cleansed in a washer-disinfector. Under the controls assurance, it is required that decontamination is undertaken by automated procedures which are documented and can be validated in accordance with HTM2030.[19] This document is guidance, endorsed under controls assurance, on the validation and testing that is required to be undertaken daily, weekly, monthly, quarterly and annually as shared functions between the clinician and the sterilising engineer to ensure that the washer-disinfector performs consistently. Hand washing of equipment does not meet this expectation as it introduces the potential for human error e.g. inappropriate water temperature and detergent and washing technique. In many NHS Trusts, decontamination of equipment is moving away from hand washing to automated processes under the control of HSDU/CSSD.

Where benchtop steam sterilisers are being used for the sterilisation of vaginal equipment, it is now expected that there is full compliance with sterilisation guidance:[20] benchtop steam sterilisers

guidance[21] for equipment for immediate use and benchtop vacuum steam sterilisers[22] for equipment placed into an autoclaving bag before sterilisation. This will protect equipment from environmental contamination for up to six months if stored in dry, non-humid conditions.

It is imperative that anyone using these washer-disinfectors and sterilisers reads the MDA documentation in order to evaluate whether local or centralised sterilisation is the most effective in terms of overall service provision. A transitionary period of 5 years (from 1999) has been allowed under the controls assurance for infection control[4] for Trusts to achieve compliance.

37.6.2 Use of Chemical Disinfectants and Sterilants

During the transition period allowed under the controls assurance for infection control[4] to comply with automated decontamination and sterilisation, chemical disinfectants or sterilants may continue to be used.

It is imperative that any clinicians engaged in the hand washing of equipment must be suitably protected to guard against the splashing of the eyes, and the contamination of hands and clothing, ensuring that the clinician is protected from both microbiological contamination and chemical exposure. When choosing chemical disinfectants and sterilants, the local health and safety officer should be consulted to ensure that the environment is suitably ventilated or recommend appropriate extraction equipment.

Equipment washing should only be performed in sinks dedicated to that purpose; separate washing and rinsing facilities are required.[4] The purpose of washing equipment before decontamination or sterilisation is to remove body fluid secretions and to reduce the level of micro-organisms present. When making up a solution of detergent it is imperative to

Table 37.2. Types of chemical disinfectants and sterilants

	Chemical	Trade names
Disinfectants	Hypochlorite solution	Milton
	Sodium dichloroisocyanurate	Sanichlor, Haztab
	Chlorine dioxides	Tristel
	Hydrogen peroxide	Virkon
Sterilants	Paracetic acid	Nu-Cidex Steris, Peraclean, Perasafe

follow the dilution instructions recommended. Insufficient detergent will not break down grease and proteinaceous material; excessive detergent may not be rinsed off, which could result in the neutralisation of some disinfectants and sterilants.[11] Most detergents are activated at 40–55°C; as this is at the upper limit of being "hand-hot" it reinforces the need for hand protection, i.e. the wearing of gloves.

The difference between disinfection and sterilisation is that the latter eradicates all microbial contamination including spores, whereas the former may not necessarily remove or inactivate all microorganisms from the surface of the equipment.[9] The types of chemical disinfectants and sterilants that may be used are shown in Table 37.2.

The concentration of disinfectant or sterilant normally used should be of sufficient strength to kill off viruses (refer to manufacturer's guidance). It should be noted that in the UK there is a move away from using aldehyde products because of the Control of Substances Hazardous to Health (COSHH) regulations on potential exposure to fumes.[23] Compatibility with the equipment manufacturer's specifications must be ensured before choosing any disinfectant or sterilant.

After use the disinfectant must be rinsed off, using either sterile or distilled water, to avoid environmental contamination and to remove chemical residue. It is recommended that a condom or sheath be used on the equipment prior to clinical procedure, ensuring compliance with Safety Action Bulletin 108.[5] However, after the use of a sterilant, this must be rinsed off with sterile water only in order to avoid desterilising the equipment, and to avoid exposing the patient to the risk of chemical irritation of the mucous membranes. Providing this is done effectively, then a condom or sheath should not be required before the clinical procedure.

However, where these manual processes cannot be validated, it is recommended that a condom or sheath should be used for each clinical intervention.

This inability to validate hand decontamination processes is the main reason for the introduction of validated and verified automated processes in the NHS. The added benefit of this automation is that condoms or sheaths will not be required, which will also reduce the risk of latex sensitisation in future.

37.6.3 Decontamination of Specific Equipment

Wherever possible all equipment not designated for single-use should be cleansed and disinfected or sterilised in accordance with Table 37.1. There may be instances where equipment cannot be disassembled for automated immersion decontamination, e.g. an ultrasound bladder scanner head. In such cases, the scan head should be cleansed using 5 ml (1 teaspoon) of detergent to 5 L of hand-hot water, rinsed, dried and wiped over with a 60–80% ethanol or isopropanol alcohol wipe between patient examinations.[7]

37.6.4 Decontamination of Equipment for Home Use

Each patient should be given full written instructions regarding the use and decontamination of equipment for home usage. This includes vaginal cones or any electrodes used for home stimulation or biofeedback. For example, in the case of vaginal cones these instructions should include information that the vaginal cones are intended for personal use only. Instructions should state that the hands must be washed thoroughly before using the cones and before first usage the cones must be disassembled, washed in warm, soapy water, rinsed and dried thoroughly (this requires 5 ml of detergent to 5 L of hand-hot water). After use the cones should again be disassembled, the same procedure followed and then stored in a dry container. It should also be stated that it is not recommended to use cones during menstruation or if there is thought to be any vaginal infection present and finally, that the use of the cones should be discontinued if there is any discharge or discomfort. A contact telephone number should be provided.

37.7 Summary

Infection control procedures will alter in light of future research and legislation. It is imperative for the clinician to receive current updates by liaison with their infection control specialist.

References

1. NHS Executive (1999) Health Service Circular: Governance in the new NHS: Controls Assurance Statements 1999/2000. Risk Management and Organisational Control. HSC 1999/123. NHS Executive, London.
2. Department of Health (1997) The New NHS: Modern, Dependable. HMSO, London.
3. Department of Health (1998) A First Class Service: Quality in the New NHS. HMSO, London.
4. NHS Executive (1999) Health Service Circular: Controls Assurance in Infection Control: Decontamination of Medical Devices. HSC 1999/179. NHS Executive, London.
5. DoH (1994) Safety Action Bulletin No 108: Instruments and Appliances Used in the Vagina and Cervix: Recommended Methods for Decontamination. SAB(94)22. Department of Health, London.
6. NHS Estates (2000) Decontamination of Medical Devices. HSC 2000/032. NHS Estates, Leeds.
7. Ayliffe GAJ, Babb JR, Taylor LJ (1999) Hospital-Acquired Infection: Principles and Prevention, 3rd Edition. Butterworth-Heinemann, Oxford.
8. ICNA/ADM (1999) Standards for Environmental Cleanliness in Hospitals. Infection Control Nurses Association and Association of Domestic Management, London.
9. Ayliffe GAJ, Fraise AP, Geddes AM, Mitchell K (2000) Control of Hospital Infection: A Practical Handbook (4th ed). Arnold, London.
10. MDA (1999) Sterilization, Disinfection and Cleaning of Medical Equipment: Guidance on Decontamination from the Microbiology Advisory Committee to Department of Health. Medical Devices Agency, London.
11. Maurer IM (1984) Hospital Hygiene (3rd ed). Arnold, London.
12. UK Health Departments (1998) Guidance for Clinical Health Care Workers: Protection against Infection with Blood-borne Viruses. Department of Health, London.
13. Judson FN, Ehret JM, Bodin GF, Levin MJ, Rietmeijer CAM (1989) In vitro evaluations of condoms with and without nonoxynol-9 as physical and chemical barriers against Chlamydia trachomatis, herpes simplex virus type 2, and humanimmunodeficiency virus. Sex Transmitted Dis 16(2): 51–6.
14. de Vincenzi I (1994) A longitudinal study of HIV transmission by heterosexual partners. N Engl J Med 331(6): 341–6.
15. MDA (1996) Device Bulletin: Latex Sensitisation in the Health Care Setting (Use of Latex Gloves). MDA DB9607. Medical Devices Agency, London.
16. MDA (2000) Single Use Medical Devices: Implications and Consequences of Reuse. MDA Device Bulletin DB2000(04). Medical Devices Agency, London.
17. Consumer Protection Act 1987. HMSO, London.
18. Consumer Protection: The Medical Devices Regulations 1994, Statutory Instrument No 3017. HMSO, London.
19. NHS Estates (1997) Washer-Disinfectors: Operational Management. Health Technical Memorandum 2030. NHS Estates, Leeds.
20. NHS Estates (1997) Sterilization. Health Technical Memorandum 2010. HMSO, London.
21. MDA (1996) Device Bulletin: The Purchase, Operation and Maintenance of Benchtop Steam Sterilisers. MDA DB 9605. Medical Devices Agency, London.
22. MDA (1998) The Validation and Periodic Testing of Benchtop Steam Sterilizers. MDA Device Bulletin 9804. Medical Devices Agency, London.
23. Control of Substances Hazardous to Health Regulations 1988. HMSO, London.

Appendix 1
Bladder Record Chart

BLADDER RECORD CHART (FREQUENCY AND VOLUME)

Name .... Date................................ *Please complete this chart and bring it with you*

	Day 1				Day 2				Day 3				Day 4			Instructions		
	In	Out	Wet		In	Out	Wet		In	Out	Wet		In	Out	Wet			
6 am																**In**	When you have a drink, place a tick in this column opposite the appropriate time.	
7 am																		
8 am																		
9 am																		
10 am																		
11 am																		
12 noon																		
1 pm																		
2 pm																		
3 pm																**Out**	Measure the amount of urine passed in a jug, and record the amount in this column opposite the appropriate time. If you are unable to measure, place a tick in the column.	
4 pm																		
5 pm																		
6 pm																		
7 pm																		
8 pm																		
9 pm																		
10 pm																		
11 pm																		
12 mn																**Wet**	Place a W in this column each time you wet yourself. This includes one drop or enough to wet your clothes.	
1 am																		
2 am																		
3 am																		
4 am																		
5 am																		
Total																		

Appendix 2
Urinary Continence Assessment Form

URINARY CONTINENCE ASSESSMENT FORM

Name: .... DOB .... Age ....

Address: ....

Tel. No: Home .... Work ....

Occupation/Hobbies .... Referral ....

Problem ....

Duration .... GP ....

Symptoms	Initial	Disch	Severity	Initial	Disch
Stress			Daily		
Urgency			>1/week		
Urge Incontinence			<1/week		
Frequency			>1/month		
Nocturia			<1/month		
Nocturnal Enuresis					
Incomplete Emptying			Few drops		
Pain			Wets underwear		
Hesitancy			Wets outerwear		
Family History			Runs down legs		
Childhood Problems					
Other: e.g. Dyspareunia			No. of pads per day		
Coital Incontinence			Size of pads		
Frequency Volume Chart					
Freq. Of void/24 hrs.					
Freq. Of incont/24 hrs.					
Max. voided volume					
Min. voided volume					
No. of drinks/24 hrs.					
Caffeine/24 hrs.			Stop test – not permitted		

History

Parity..

Wt. Heaviest Baby ....

Types of Delivery.....................................

Menopausal State ....

Pregnant   Yes/No/Planning

HRT   Yes/No

When commenced HRT ....

Smear test ....

Surgical History

....

....

....

Bowels: B/O ....week

Faecal incontinence ....

Faecal urgency ....

Constipation ....

Stool consistency ....

250

Medical History

Cystitis ....   Height ....

Smoking...   Weight ....

Respiratory Problems ....

Allergies ....   **Investigations:**

Cardiac ....   MSU ....

Diabetes ....   Urodynamics ....

Back/Neck Problems ....   Other ....

Other ....

Current Medication ....

....

Previous treatment (including medication) ....

....

On Examination   Informed consent

Dermatomes ....

Myotomes ....

Reflexes ....

Abdominal Examination ....

Pelvic Floor – Digital

	Initial	Discharge
012345 Oxford Grading		
Endurance		
Repetitions		
Fast contractions		
Perineometer (type) reading		
Hold with cough		

If you were to spend the rest of your life with your urinary condition just the way it is now, how would you feel about that?

Quality of life due to urinary symptoms	Delighted	Pleased	Mostly Satisfied	Mixed equally satisfied and dissatisfied	Mostly Dissatisfied	Unhappy	Terrible
Initial							
Discharge							

Signature ....   Date: ....

Comments

Appendix 3
Exercise Diary

Practise . . . contractions, each lasting . . . seconds
Also practise . . .. fast contractions at each exercise session
Please indicate on the chart below each time that you exercise.
Remember to brace your pelvic floor each time that you cough, laugh, sneeze, lift or shout.

Monday	Tuesday	Wednesday	Thursday	Friday	Saturday	Sunday

Any further special instructions:

Appendix 4
Fluid Intake and Bladder Diary

Start your diary on ...   ID Number ...

Time	Record drinks taken type and amount	Record volume of urine passed (in ml)	Tick when you changed a pad/panty liner	Each time you leak urine, circle whether you were
6am				Almost dry Damp Wet Soaked
7 am				Almost dry Damp Wet Soaked
8am				Almost dry Damp Wet Soaked
9am				Almost dry Damp Wet Soaked
10am				Almost dry Damp Wet Soaked
11am				Almost dry Damp Wet Soaked
Midday				Almost dry Damp Wet Soaked
1pm				Almost dry Damp Wet Soaked
2pm				Almost dry Damp Wet Soaked
3pm				Almost dry Damp Wet Soaked
4pm				Almost dry Damp Wet Soaked
5pm				Almost dry Damp Wet Soaked
6pm				Almost dry Damp Wet Soaked
7pm				Almost dry Damp Wet Soaked
8pm				Almost dry Damp Wet Soaked
9pm				Almost dry Damp Wet Soaked
10pm				Almost dry Damp Wet Soaked
11pm				Almost dry Damp Wet Soaked
Midnight				Almost dry Damp Wet Soaked
1am				Almost dry Damp Wet Soaked
2am				Almost dry Damp Wet Soaked
3am				Almost dry Damp Wet Soaked
4am				Almost dry Damp Wet Soaked
5am				Almost dry Damp Wet Soaked

One day of 3 days' charts provided to patients. (Courtesy of Leicestershire MRC Incontinence Study).

Reminders for Completing the Charts for the Leicestershire MRC Incontinence Study

- Don't forget to record the time you woke up in the morning and the time you went to sleep.
- Don't forget to record what happened overnight when you get up in the morning.
- Try and make a record of things just after they happen in case you forget them later on.
- Record things to the nearest hour.
- Record type and amount of drinks taken (e.g. 2 cups of tea, 1 mug of coffee, 1 can of coke, 1 glass of water/wine/juice, 2 pints of beer).
- Start a new sheet for each new day.

Appendix 5
Useful Addresses and Websites

International

- International Continence Society (ICS) *www.icsoffice.org* Full details of organisations in many countries can be found by following links on the website.

United Kingdom

Organisations

- Association for Continence Advice (ACA) *www.aca.uk.com* Email: *info@aca.uk.com*
- Association of Chartered Physiotherapists in Women's Health (ACPWH) *www.womensphysio.com*
- Association of Reflexologists, 27 Old Gloucester Street, London WC1N 3XX.
- British School – Reflex Zone Therapy, 23 Marsh Hall, Talisman Way, Wembley Park, Middlesex HA9 8JJ.
- The Continence Foundation *www.continence-foundation.org.uk*
  Email: *continence.foundation@dial. pipex.com*
- Enuresis Resource and Information Centre (ERIC) *www.eric.org.uk* Email: *enuresis@compuserve.com*
- Faculty of Homeopathy, 15 Clerkenwell Close, London.EC1R 0AA.
- ICS (UK) *www.icsuk.org.uk*
- InconTact *www.incontact.org* Email: *edu@incontact.demon.co.uk*
- Midland School of Reflextherapy, 5 Church Street, Warwick CV34 4AB.
- Society of Homeopaths, 2 Artizan Road, Northampton, NN1 4HU.

Useful UK Companies

- Aquaflex *www.aquaflexcones.com*
- Educational and Scientific Products Ltd *www.espmodels.co.uk* Email: *sales@espmodels.co.uk*
- Genesis Medical Ltd *www.genmedhealth.com* Email: *info@genmedhealth.com*
- Isis Medical Ltd *www.isis-medical.com*
- NEEN Healthcare *www.neenhealth.com* Email: *info@neenhealth.com*
- Physio Med Services Ltd *www.physio-med.com* Email: *webmail@physio-med.com*
- Sissel UK Ltd, 10 Moderna Business Park, Mytholmroyd, West Yorkshire HX7 5RH Tel: 01422 885433 Fax: 01422 882143 *www.sisseluk.com*
- Verity Medical Ltd *www.veritymedical.co.uk* Email: *sales@veritymedical.co.uk*

Index